The Metabolic Typing Diet

The Metabolic Typing Diet

*Customize Your Diet for: Permanent Weight Loss,
Optimum Health, Preventing and Reversing Disease,
Staying Young at Any Age*

William L. Wolcott
and Trish Fahey

BROADWAY BOOKS
New York

BROADWAY

A hardcover edition of this book was originally published in 2000
by Doubleday, a division of Random House, Inc. It is here reprinted
by arrangement with Doubleday.

THE METABOLIC TYPING DIET. Copyright © 2000
by William L. Wolcott and Trish Fahey.
For information, address: Broadway Books,
a division of Random House, Inc.,
1540 Broadway, New York, NY 10036.

Broadway Books titles may be purchased for business or promotional use or for special sales.
For information, please write to:
Special Markets Department, Random House, Inc.
1540 Broadway, New York, New York 10036.

PRINTED IN THE UNITED STATES OF AMERICA

BROADWAY BOOKS and its logo, a letter B bisected on the diagonal, are
trademarks of Broadway Books, a division of Random House, Inc.

Visit our website at www.broadwaybooks.com

First Broadway Books trade paperback edition published 2002

Designed by Tina Thompson
Illustrated by Einat Peled and Yina Zhang

Library of Congress Cataloging-in-Publication Data
Wolcott, William L. (William Linz)
The metabolic typing diet : customize your diet for permanent weight loss, optimum
health, preventing and reversing disease, staying young at any age / William L. Wolcott
and Trish Fahey.
p. cm.
Originally published: New York : Doubleday, 2000 (without a subtitle).
Includes bibliographical references and index.
1. Reducing diets. 2. Metabolism. I. Fahey, Trish. II. Title.

RM222.2 .W583   2002
613.2'5—dc21
2001043831

ISBN 0-7679-0564-4

9   10   8

*To RKS, to whom I owe any good qualities I may possess,
and to my wife, Suzi, for her love and her generous heart.*

W.L.W.

For Bob and Sherri Maver

T.F.

CONTENTS

ACKNOWLEDGMENTS

It's impossible to adequately acknowledge and thank the scores of people who contributed to the development of this book.

Like many people involved in nutritional research, I'm very grateful for the scientific legacy of great innovators such as Weston Price, D.D.S.; Francis Pottenger, M.D.; Royal Lee, D.D.S.; Roger Williams, Ph.D.; George Watson, Ph.D.; Henry Harrower, M.D.; Henry Bieler, M.D.; Melvin Page, D.D.S.; Elliott Abravanel, M.D.; James D'Adamo, N.D.; Peter D'Adamo, N.D.; Dietrich Klinghardt, M.D.; and the remarkable Emanuel Revici, M.D.

I'm especially indebted to William Donald Kelley, D.D.S., for his brilliant contributions in the field of clinical nutrition and for his central role in launching the exciting and evolving field of metabolic typing. We are also very grateful to Guy Schenker, D.C., whose pioneering work in metabolic individuality is an ongoing inspiration.

Very special thanks go to Ron Hoffman, M.D.; Don Davis, Ph.D.; Leo Roy, M.D.; Ron Hunninghake, M.D.; Sherry Rogers, M.D.; Daniel Fahey, M.D.; Anne Louise Gittleman, M.S.; Milo Siewert, M.D.; Gabriel Cousens, M.D.; Harold Grams, D.C.; Doris Rapp, M.D.; Peter Konigs, N.D.; Etienne Callebout, M.D.; David Vaughan, N.C.; Andreanna Vaughan, R.N.; Karen Gorney, R.N.; and the extraordinary Paul Chek.

My heartfelt appreciation goes to Harold and Adele Smith and to Scott Baker for their many years of exceptional work and collaboration. I'm also deeply indebted to June Hutchins, Leni Felton, Sam Biser, William Fioretti, and Sam Caster.

A very special thank you goes to Judy Kern and Michael Palgon at Random House, and to the fine editorial team at Broadway Books, including Ann Campbell and Amanda Gross. Thanks also to our agent, Katherine Cowles; to our talented illustrators, Einat Peled and Yina Zhang; and to Tina Thompson and Chris Fortunato, who did such an excellent job designing and producing the book.

We're very grateful for the support and keen insights of Anita Shapiro, Dennis Gronek, Michael Calvey, Jodie Garay, Laura Hinthorn, Mark Worthington, Joan Fahey, Henry Lin, Lery Lin, Elaine Schweitzer, Jo Schweitzer, Ruth Moss, Diana De Lucia, Adrian Van Caneghem, Debra Lesser, Michaelyn Harris, Penny Lucas, Steve Pollack, and Laurie Cowan.

Pat Connolly and the entire team at the Price-Pottenger Nutrition Foundation are treasures, and we're all deeply indebted to them for their many years of invaluable work. We're also very grateful to the brilliant Audrey Kramer, whose efforts dating back many years were so instrumental in putting this process in motion. Thanks also to Kenny Kramer, Allyson Kramer, and Kathleen McCann.

A special acknowledgment goes to Sherri Maver and to the late Robert W. Maver, F.S.A., whose life and legacy as a pioneer in alternative medicine continue to inspire us all. In addition, this project would not have been possible without the talent, support, and generosity of Mary Jo Fahey, Bruce Anderson, Peter King, Barbara Tanis, David Schmuller, Penny Lucas, and Kathleen Mulcahy.

Dodie Hayes Anderson deserves very special thanks for vital contributions to the practical portions of the text, and for extraordinary leadership, insights, and expertise as a health educator.

Above all, I'd like to thank my family, especially my wife, Suzi, whose remarkable talents, wisdom, and dedication have made so much possible for so many.

Finally, I don't know how to begin to thank Trish Fahey, whom I am so fortunate to have as my coauthor. The book could not have been written without her unique talents, vision, and depth of knowledge. I owe her a debt of gratitude I'll never find words to express.

—William L. Wolcott

FOREWORD

I first began to investigate metabolic typing almost fifteen years ago, after hearing reports of the exceptional clinical results that people were achieving with it. I was intrigued when I learned of this novel nutritional technology, one that somehow enabled clinicians to identify the highly specific dietary needs of individuals. At the same time, I was skeptical. It sounded a little too good to be true and was based on concepts that seemed highly unconventional, even within the context of alternative medicine. Nonetheless, I decided to follow up on the subject, in case there was something of value I might discover.

Back in the 1980s I was, like many other clinicians, a true believer in the value of diet and nutrition. But like everyone else, I was continually frustrated by the contradictions and complexity inherent in nutritional science. Nutritional therapy clearly held a great deal of potential as a primary therapeutic approach, yet there were many practical challenges involved in applying it in clinical settings. Health professionals simply had no reliable means of evaluating people's dietary deficiencies and recommending predictably effective nutritional protocols. Time and again I had encountered the same frustrating dilemma: A dietary program that worked very well for one person would produce little or no beneficial results for someone else. There seemed to be no readily available solutions on the horizon.

Then in the mid-1980s I heard about a group of scientists and clinicians in the United States who had, over a period of years, evolved a unique way of addressing this problem, with a system they called metabolic typing. Researchers such as William Kelley, George

Watson, and Roger Williams had built upon the work of scientists and clinicians of an earlier era: men like Weston Price, Frances Pottenger, and Royal Lee. What they all shared was a profound interest in a concept that Williams described as "biochemical individuality," or the idea that no two individuals are alike on a biochemical or physiological level.

As far back as the 1930s, Weston Price embarked on extraordinary anthropological expeditions to remote corners of the globe and uncovered the link between modern eating habits and the incidence of chronic degenerative illness. He also discovered that there is no such thing as a standard "healthy diet." Due to tremendous variations in climate, indigenous food supplies, environmental conditions, and the principles of evolution, adaptation, and heredity, different cultural and ethnic groups, over a period of many centuries, developed distinctly different kinds of dietary requirements.

In later years, Watson, Kelley, and others did remarkable work in examining what these variations in genetically based nutritional needs were all about from a metabolic or biochemical perspective. They knew that a given diet upon which some people might thrive could easily cause other people to be sick. But why? What was the underlying scientific explanation for this phenomenon?

One of the factors they discovered early on was the pivotal role that the involuntary or autonomic nervous system (ANS) plays in determining metabolic individuality and in influencing health and disease. There are two separate branches of the autonomic nervous system. One of these branches, the sympathetic system, controls bodily processes that have to do with energy utilization; it is sometimes referred to as the "fight or flight" branch. The other branch, the parasympathetic system, controls bodily activities that pertain to energy conservation; it is often thought of as the "rest and digest" branch.

In most people, one branch tends to be stronger or more dominant than the other, which creates a certain amount of biochemical or metabolic imbalance. If this imbalance becomes too pronounced, disease processes can develop. Interestingly, specific foods and nutrients have the natural capacity to strengthen whichever side of the autonomic system is weaker. As a result, metabolic typing enables people to establish balance within the ANS. This is important, since the ANS is the master regulator of metabolism.

Another primary determinant of what kind of food a person needs in order to be healthy pertains to the *rate* at which their cells convert food into energy, or the rate of cellular oxidation. The oxidative rate, which is also largely determined by heredity, needs to be kept in balance if the body is to function properly. Some people are fast oxidizers, which means that their cells rapidly convert food into energy. To sustain metabolic balance, these people need foods that burn slowly, such as heavier proteins and fats. On the other hand, slow oxidizers are able to maintain metabolic balance with lighter food (carbohydrates) that burns faster than protein and fat.

In the late 1970s and early '80s, the nascent science of metabolic typing got a tremendous push forward when Bill Wolcott entered the picture and made a breakthrough discovery pertaining to the interrelationship between the Autonomic Nervous System and the Oxidative System. This discovery, which he termed "the Dominance Factor," enabled him to predict, with far greater levels of accuracy and precision than ever before, exactly what kinds of foods and nutrients a person would need to establish metabolic balance. In the years since then, he has single-handedly expanded and refined the foundational principles of metabolic typing to an extraordinary degree. The practical results have proven to be nothing short of spectacular.

By providing dietary solutions that are effectively tailored to people's highly individualized biochemical needs, Bill has shown us the true potential of diet and nutrition, and demonstrated the body's superior capacity to regulate and heal itself, once it's given the right raw materials to work with. His methodology resolves a great many of the bewildering contradictions and limitations of modern nutritional science. He really has taken the guesswork out of dietary therapy.

One of the many unique aspects of metabolic typing is that it's not something clinicians use to "treat" specific diseases or symptoms. Rather, it's a "non-specific" approach that allows us to look beyond symptoms, and to analyze the physiological imbalances and biochemical disturbances that underlie chronic health disorders. That's why people who use metabolic typing have the ability to build health and wellness from the ground up, rather than simply trying to address disparate symptoms in a piecemeal fashion. This foundational approach to diet and nutrition produces a health-inducing "domino effect" on all the body's systems and leads to the elimination of multiple symptoms at the same time.

I have used metabolic typing in my clinical practice for a long time, and I'm convinced that it is an unrivaled method for conducting dietary evaluations and developing dietary recommendations. I have found it to be very successful in resolving and/or alleviating the severity of all manner of health problems: allergies, digestive disturbances, chronic fatigue, anemia, obesity, hormonal imbalances, mood swings, poor concentration, depression, high blood pressure, diabetes, low blood sugar, arthritis, and so on. Yet it's important to realize that metabolic typing does a lot more than eliminate symptoms. Because when you balance body chemistry, you then have the capacity to be vibrantly, glowingly healthy, not merely free of nagging aches and pains and ailments.

Unlike other methods of determining dietary individuality, such as blood typing and body typing, metabolic typing is a dynamic, comprehensive system that encompasses all of the body's known adaptation or homeostatic mechanisms. In other words, it doesn't just measure a single fixed variable such as your blood type or body type. Instead, it takes into account many different types of biochemical or metabolic variables, which are subject to continual change and flux over the course of your lifetime.

That's why metabolic typing is a very accurate dietary discipline, not subject to the laws of chance. This is also why it is a very advanced academic discipline, even though it's also a practical, easy-to-use nutritional technology.

There are so many levels to metabolic typing that I am sure it will go on being a wonderfully advanced clinical technology for health professionals. But what is exciting is that this book now provides health consumers with what they have desperately needed for so long: a simple, rapid, and dependable way to identify their metabolic type and eat accordingly, and to adjust their dietary regimes as the need arises.

The term "revolutionary" is too frequently overused in our modern era. But in the case of metabolic typing, it's a very apt description. I think you will agree with me when you read Bill Wolcott's marvelous book.

—Etienne Callebout, M.D.
Harley Street, London
1999

PREFACE

Over the last quarter century we've witnessed a profound cultural shift in our perspectives toward health and wellness. We've awakened to the realization that modern medical science has no "magic bullet" solutions for the majority of human ailments, and that good health and longevity are somehow inextricably linked to diet and lifestyle management. Thus, it's axiomatic these days that, in order to remain free of pain, illness, and excess weight, or to enjoy high levels of health and well-being, one needs to pursue the right dietary and nutritional regimen. On some levels, this seems like it ought to be a simple enough task. And yet, identifying a truly effective diet has long been, for most of us, an elusive goal, an objective that somehow remains just beyond our reach.

One of the problems is that we're continually bombarded with complex and often sharply contradictory information about what constitutes a healthy diet. There's widespread disagreement among dietary experts about what we should be eating, and it's virtually impossible to make sense of the cacophony of conflicting opinions. On top of that, most of us are paralyzed by the sheer volume of miscellaneous dietary tips, nutritional advice, and product information that comes our way through the media. How or where would we even begin to sort through it all?

Yet there's another, even more fundamental obstacle that has long prevented us from achieving the kind of dietary success we yearn for. Here's the problem: For many years nutritional science has been based on a generic or standardized or mass market approach to health and nutrition. That's why virtually all of the world's leading dietary experts have established single, one-size-fits-all dietary solutions, which they believe can be universally applied to everyone. But this is a false assumption, and one that has proved to have very limited clinical success.

Standardized diets and nutritional approaches fail to recognize that, for genetic reasons, people are all very different from one another on a biochemical or metabolic level. In other words, we're all different in the way that our bodies process foods and utilize nutrients. Thus we all have highly individualized nutritional requirements. In the same way that certain car engines are designed to run on gasoline and others can't run without diesel fuel, your body has its own unique "engines of metabolism," and requires specific kinds of "body fuel" in order to function efficiently.

We all take it for granted that human beings are very different on an external level, with respect to hair texture and color, skin color, facial features, height, weight, skeletal structure, and so on. Yet we're largely unaware of, or inattentive to, the biological diversity that exists internally. Just as no two individuals share the same fingerprints, and no two snowflakes are alike, there is infinite variety among people from a metabolic and physiological perspective.

As a result, human beings have endlessly variable needs for foods and nutrients. For example, with respect to proteins, carbohydrates, and fats (the "macronutrients"), those essential dietary building blocks, people's needs fall along a broad continuum. At one end of the spectrum are people who thrive on diets high in protein and fat (heavy foods such as meat and cheese). At the other end of the spectrum are people who function best on high carbohydrate, low-fat diets (lighter foods such as grains, vegetables, and fruit). You may fall into one of these two distinctly opposite categories, or your nutritional needs may fall anywhere in between.

Your dietary needs are largely determined by your ancestral heritage, and your ancestors' dietary needs were the result of evolution and adaptation to many unique aspects of their natural habitat, including geographical location, climate, naturally occurring vegetation, and available food sources. As you can imagine, a diet that could effectively support the health of people living in one part of the world, say, equatorial Africa, would be very different from a diet that could support the health of people in Nordic countries.

Unfortunately, we've all been misled by the diet and nutrition industry, which has promulgated the fallacy of the "healthy diet" for many years. There is no such thing as a healthy diet, and there never has been. There's nothing intrinsically healthy or unhealthy about any given food. All that matters is how well a particular food or dietary regimen can fulfill your unique, genetically inherited metabolic requirements.

Nutrition's best-kept secret is this: A diet or nutrient that works well for one person may have no effect on a second person, and may make a third person worse. Here's a more precise or technical way of describing the same principle: Any food or nutrient can have virtually opposite biochemical influences in different people. This is the concept that lies at the heart of metabolic typing.

What is metabolic typing? It's actually many things to many people. For instance, for almost fifteen years, my company has provided health professionals with an advanced, computer-based form of metabolic typing. Clinicians use this technology to evaluate people's nutritional requirements, and to design individualized nutritional protocols. Metabolic typing is also the culmination of seventy years of pioneering efforts and interrelated discoveries by a whole series of remarkable medical researchers, including physicians, biochemists, dentists, physiologists, clinical nutritionists, and psychologists. It's also an exciting and continually evolving academic discipline that many contemporary researchers regard as the "missing link" in modern nutritional science.

And now, for the first time ever, thanks to the introduction of this book, metabolic typing is also a very simple, user-friendly methodology that anyone can use to customize a diet to his or her own unique body chemistry. Just by using the written self-test (questionnaire) contained in Chapter 6, you'll be able to identify your "metabolic type" rapidly and easily. You can then use this information to select the specific foods and combinations of foods that will enable your body to function at peak efficiency.

Unlike existing dietary approaches, metabolic typing is a dynamic process that does far more than simply assign you to a broad, fixed category that roughly approximates your nutritional needs. It's much more precise and flexible than that. Included in this book, for example, you'll find a whole series of additional self tests and "fine-tuning" techniques that you can use to tailor your diet with a very high degree of accuracy and precision.

Since metabolic typing is not a static system, the tools contained here allow you to adjust your diet if your metabolism shifts. It's important to realize that your metabolic type is not carved in stone. Although you were born with a specific set of dietary requirements dictated by your genetic heritage, your needs can shift for any number of reasons, such as illness, stress, aging, or nutrient deficiencies or excesses. Where metabolism is concerned, everything is highly individualized and continually in flux. That's why testing your metabolic type and fine-tuning your diet are techniques you'll want to employ from time to time on an ongoing basis.

Once you discover your metabolic type and begin to eat accordingly, it will be a very liberating experience on many levels. Even if you're currently consuming only the highest-quality and most healthful foods and food supplements available, it's entirely possible that you're malnourished, i.e., very deficient in the specific foods and nutrients that your particular metabolism requires to function properly.

In the short-term, a metabolically appropriate diet will put an end to food cravings, hunger, blood sugar imbalances, many forms of digestive problems, headaches, depression, irritability, and other nagging ailments. You'll have plenty of physical and mental energy, and your food will be efficiently converted to energy rather than stored as fat.

If you stick to a diet that's tailored to your metabolic type, there are plenty of long-term benefits you can expect as well, including permanent weight loss without struggle, deprivation, or calorie restriction; strengthened immunity; ongoing energy and endurance; a slowing of the aging process; and the ability to prevent and reverse many types of chronic illness.

How do I know this is what you can achieve? Because metabolic typing is far from a new dietary fad, theory, or experiment. It's been around for a long time, and tens of thousands of people have used it with unprecedented success. The empirical evidence is overwhelming. Of course, your personal experience is the only litmus test that ultimately counts. I encourage you to discover for yourself the benefits to be derived from pursuing a diet that's customized just for you.

Chapter 1

ONE MAN'S FOOD IS
ANOTHER'S POISON

The Wisdom of Ancestral Diets

Would you believe that in certain remote regions of the world there are old and indigenous cultures in which our modern epidemics—obesity, heart disease, cancer, diabetes, colitis, hypertension, arthritis, and the like—are virtually unknown?

For many years scientists have observed isolated cultures in which people maintain levels of health and fitness that are vastly superior to the health status of those of us who live in modern societies.

Yet these remarkably strong people live in primitive environments very far removed from the industrial mainstream, where there are none of the vast resources so widely available in "advanced" civilizations—no high-tech medicine, no scientists or clinicians or academic institutions, no multibillion-dollar research programs, no health officials or government advisory boards, no vitamin industry, fitness clubs, health spas, weight loss clinics, or health-oriented media.

Oddly enough, the native diets of these old and indigenous cultures are far from what you and I might consider healthful.

Imagine: Traditional Alaskan Eskimos with excellent immunity and cardiovascular health thriving on large quantities of fat and several pounds of meat a day. Daily diets centered around caribou, kelp, salmon, moose, seal, and whale blubber.

Today there are Aboriginal people in remote regions of the Australian Outback with the strength and fitness levels of Olympic athletes. They still live as their ancestors did, on diets comprised of insects, beetles, grubs, berries, and meat from the kangaroo and wallaby.

Consider this: Swiss people with superior constitutions and longevity living in isloated mountain villages, eating primitive diets of whole rye bread and large quantities of high-fat cheese and cream and raw goat's milk, supplemented by wine and small amounts of meat. Villagers of all ages enjoying robust health despite rustic living conditions and the challenges of glacial winters.

Similarly: African Masai tribes, renowned for extraordinary physical and mental development, still living as they have for centuries, primarily on meat and milk and blood that is carefully extracted in small doses from live cattle at regular intervals.

And in other isolated places—high in the Andes Mountains, deep in the Amazon rain forest, in remote villages of the South Pacific islands—native people who consume the primitive diets of their ancestors consistently demonstrate the same kind of remarkable strength, stamina, and resistance to disease, often living well past one hundred.

Researchers have discovered that people who live in primitive cultures consistently display an astonishing range of physical attributes rarely seen in modern cultures: virtually no birth defects or physical deformities or weight problems. Exceptionally well-shaped bones and skeletal frames. Wide and symmetrical faces with expansive, highly functional nasal and respiratory passages. Strong jaws with perfect dental alignment and flawless teeth and gums that rarely if ever succumb to decay and disease.

But when these same people are exposed to the foods and dietary customs of modern civilization, their health rapidly deteriorates and they fall victim to the very same diseases that have long permeated industrialized societies.

The most noteworthy observer of the declining health of primitive cultures was Dr. Weston Price, a remarkable medical researcher who began his career as a dentist in Ohio in the early part of the twentieth century. Price first became interested in malnutrition in an attempt to understand why so many Americans suffered with extensive tooth decay and gum disease, along with severe structural deficiencies such as small dental palates crowded with poorly developed and crooked teeth.

Dr. Price knew that people in undeveloped regions of the world had no such problems—no need of orthodontia, metal fillings, gum surgeries, root canals, or elaborate restorative work. He wanted to find out why.

So in 1934 he began a series of investigative expeditions to remote corners of the world. He visited indigenous cultures and closely examined the diets and health status of native populations in Africa, northern Europe, Canada, Alaska, Australia, and the South Pacific.

Time and again Price found indigenous cultures to be free of the chronic disease and physical disabilities that were very much the norm in the United States and other "advanced" societies. He also observed that whenever primitive cultures abandoned their native diets and adopted modern eating habits, they would rapidly develop the kinds of health problems prevalent in the advanced cultures to which they'd been exposed.

In 1938 Dr. Price documented his findings in the classic *Nutrition and Physical Degeneration.* This book includes a wealth of dramatic photographs that clearly illustrate the rapid physical deterioration of many indigenous cultures throughout the world.

The Myth of the Universal Diet

Over thousands of years of evolutionary history, people in different parts of the world developed very distinct nutritional needs in response to a whole range of variables, including climate and geography and whatever plant and animal life their environments had to offer.

As a result, people today have widely varying nutrient requirements, especially with regard to *macronutrients*—the *proteins*, *carbohydrates,* and *fats* that are the fundamental dietary "building blocks,"

INDIGENOUS PEOPLE ON NATIVE DIETS

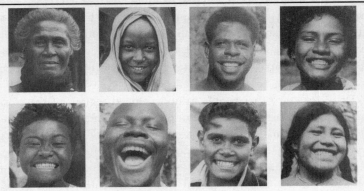

In the 1930s, Dr. Weston Price conducted anthropological investigations of isolated, pre-industrialized cultures all over the world. He consistently found that people who adhered to their native diets were free of physical degeneration, structural deformities, and disease. These people are typical of indigenous cultures everywhere who avoid modern eating habits. They all have well-developed skeletal structures, including well-developed, perfectly proportioned facial bones. This facilitates broad dental arches and nasal passages and perfectly aligned jaws and teeth, and helps optimize respiration, digestion, and other metabolic functions.

INDIGENOUS PEOPLE ON MODERN DIETS

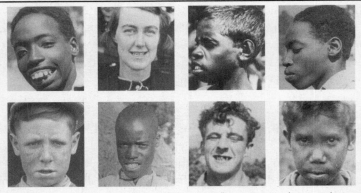

Physical deformities and chronic illness become rapidly apparent (within a single generation) when isolated cultures adopt modern eating habits and depart from their genetically-based nutritional requirements. Remarkably, people of every race and color develop the very same kinds of physical deformities and diseases. These young people were born with multiple problems. The most visible of these are: poorly developed skeletal structures, compressed facial bones, inadequately developed jaws and nasal passages, and small dental palates crowded with severely misaligned and cavity-filled teeth.

that is, the compounds most essential to sustaining life. Most foods from either animal or plant sources contain at least some amount of each of the macronutrients.

For example, many people who currently inhabit tropical or equatorial regions have a strong hereditary need for diets high in carbohydrates such as vegetables and fruits and grains and legumes. These foods provide the kind of body fuel that is most compatible with the unique body chemistry of people who are genetically programmed to lead active lifestyles in warm and humid regions of the world. Their systems are simply not designed to process or utilize large quantities of animal protein and fat.

Conversely, people from cold, harsh northern climates are not genetically equipped to survive on light vegetarian food. They tend to burn body fuel quickly, so they need heavier foods to sustain themselves. Eskimos, for example, can easily digest and assimilate large

MACRONUTRIENT CHART			
	PROTEIN	**CARBOHYDRATE**	**FAT**
Food source	Meat, poultry, dairy	Fruits, vegetables, grains	Oil, nuts, meat, cheese
Molecular structure	Breaks down into peptides and amino acids	Breaks down into sugar and starch	Breaks down into triglycerides and fatty acids
Metabolic role	The main structural ingredient of human cells, and the enzymes that keep them running	A primary source of energy for all living things, and a structural component of cell walls and plasma membranes	A structural component of cell membranes, a source of insulation, and a means of energy storage

quantities of heavy protein and fat—the very types of foods that would overwhelm the digestive tracts of people from, say, the Mediterranean basin.

The bottom line is that a diet considered healthful in one part of the world is frequently disastrous for people elsewhere in the world.

For instance, well-known dietary expert Nathan Pritikin pointed out that Bantu tribes in Africa eat a very low-fat diet, one that is widely regarded as very healthful in the United States and other industrialized societies. Not surprisingly, coronary artery disease among the Bantu is almost nonexistent.

Pritikin's successors and other leading health professionals have long advocated low-fat diets for everyone. Yet this "one-size-fits-all" approach has clearly failed to reduce obesity and cardiovascular disease in large segments of our population. Like all other *universal* dietary recommendations, it overlooks the enormous amount of *biochemical* and *physiological diversity* among individuals.

As an example, Scottish, Welsh, Celtic, and Irish people have certain nutritional requirements that are just the opposite of the Bantu. The ancestral diets of the Scots and Irish and related cultures have always been very high in fatty fish. For this and other reasons they have a hereditary need for more fat than other populations. Remarkably, the low-fat diets that *prevent* heart disease in the Bantu can actually *cause* heart disease in many people of Anglo-Saxon descent.

This principle of diet being linked to genetic requirements is seen throughout nature. Every animal species is genetically programmed to feed on specific sources of food. They're not guided in their food selection by their taste buds or manipulated by high-concept advertising strategies about what's "good to eat."

Unlike man, who applies free will to his dietary choices, animals eat according to their natural instincts and genetic dictates. Consequently, insects, reptiles, fish, birds, and mammals (except man) are not plagued with degenerative health disorders like cancer, heart disease, diabetes, arthritis, allergies, and multiple sclerosis—to name but a few.

In his book *Happiness Is a Healthy Life*, Lendon Smith, M.D., writes: "The trick of eating is to figure out your racial/ethnic background and try to imitate it." It's a great idea, but there's just one problem: Few of us today have a clear-cut ethnic or genetic heritage, particularly in the United States, where we've become a true genetic "melting pot."

People from different ethnic and cultural backgrounds have moved from continent to continent and country to country and mixed and mingled like crazy. So most of us have lots of different blood running through our veins. A little of this and a little of that.

Maybe you're part Irish and part German with traces of Mexican blood. Your best friend might be half Italian and half Japanese. Perhaps your neighbor has a Swedish mother and a Lebanese father and a maternal grandmother who was part Jamaican. The permutations are endless. There have been so many cultural shifts and so much inter-marriage in the modern world that it's just not possible for most of us to identify with any degree of precision exactly what our ancestral diets might be.

And even if you could, it might be pretty tricky to try to imitate it. If you're of pure Native American descent, you could have a hard time obtaining cactus or buffalo meat on a regular basis. Or if you're of full-blooded Austrian descent, it could get challenging (if not monotonous) to base most of your meals on large quantities of raw goat's milk and stone-ground grains.

Of course, it's entirely possible that your native dietary needs are both clearly defined and none too hard to fulfill. For instance, maybe both your parents come from a purebred Greek lineage, in which case you'd have little trouble accessing fish, pasta, garlic, olive oil, salads, beans, and wine—roughly the kinds of foods that kept your ancestors healthy and fit. Similarly, if you're of Asian extraction, you'd likely do well with rice and sea vegetables and soy.

But here's a major caveat: While your ancestral diet is of critical importance in figuring out what foods might be ideal for you, it's not the only factor. Our nutrient requirements are also heavily influenced by our environments and the kinds of lifestyles we lead. And both those factors have shifted dramatically over the course of the last century.

It took all of us thousands of years to adapt to our earthly sur-roundings, yet in the last hundred years (the evolutionary blink of an eye) many of the essential qualities of our air and water and soil have been altered, suddenly and profoundly. The delicate symbiosis that our ancestors developed with their natural habitats has been seriously disrupted. In many ways the environment can't sustain human health as it once could.

The same applies to our lifestyles. We've all been genetically bred over the millennia for a great deal of physical activity—to run and walk and plant and hunt and fish and ride and herd. But in a very short span of time that all changed. Now we spend huge blocks of time indoors under artificial light, exposed to all kinds of foreign chemicals, leading sedentary lives in front of TVs or computers or riding around in planes, trains, and automobiles.

So, identifying the diet that will best support your health is considerably more complicated than simply trying to determine your ethnic and cultural heritage. There are just too many factors besides heredity that influence your nutritional needs.

Not to mention the fact that your nutritional needs are not static. Your body is a dynamic homeostatic system, meaning it's always in flux, always attempting to regulate itself, achieve a healthy balance, and adjust to shifting environmental conditions.

Your dietary needs can change from year to year, season to season, day to day, even hour by hour, due to cyclical (circadian) rhythms that cause predictable shifts in your body chemistry every twenty-four hours.

Fortunately, there is a breakthrough technology you can use to quickly and easily identify which foods are right for you, a technology you'll be reading about very shortly. In the meantime, here's a quick recap of important points so far:

1. *Lots of people worldwide have no chronic illness.*
For many years scientists have observed isolated or primitive cultures that are completely free of all the major degenerative diseases of modern civilizations.

2. *Modern diets cause serious illness in healthy indigenous cultures.*
When isolated or primitive cultures abandon their native diets and take up modern diets, they develop all the same chronic diseases now epidemic in modern societies.

3. *Different indigenous cultures require different diets.*
There is no such thing as a healthful diet. A diet that promotes health
and vigor in one culture can cause serious illness in another.

4. *Heredity plays a major role in your dietary requirements.*
You are genetically programmed to require the same kinds of foods and
nutrients your ancestors depended upon for survival. But other factors
play a role—such as environmental conditions, specific nutrient deficiencies, and your level of stress or physical activity, for example.

5. *Your nutritional needs are highly unique.*
Just as we all differ tremendously with regard to outward physical
characteristics, we are all unique on an internal (biochemical and
physiological) level as well. Thus we all process foods and utilize
nutrients differently.

6. *You'll need technological assistance to identify your unique dietary needs.*
Most of us have no clear-cut ancestral lineage. For this and other
important reasons, identifying your individual dietary needs is difficult, if not impossible. Fortunately, metabolic typing can provide you
with a simple solution to this complex problem.

Beyond Mass-Market Nutrition

Contemporary dietary wisdom is analogous to modern pharmaceutical science. The drug industry is entirely focused on the "magic bullet" medical concept, i.e., it seeks to develop single therapeutic
solutions that can be universally applied to anyone and everyone who
displays a particular health problem or set of symptoms. Modern
nutritional science also operates almost exclusively on this type of
"mass-market" approach.

Our government provides an excellent case in point. Health officials here in the United States dispense generic dietary recommendations based on a "one-size-fits-all" approach to nutrition, despite
the fact that America is one of the most heterogeneous societies on
earth—a true genetic melting pot.

The government's one-dimensional approach to healthful eating is represented by the omnipresent "food pyramid," a slightly more modern derivative of the old "4-food-group" approach to daily meal planning.

The mass-market approach to nutrition also dominates the private sector. Virtually every leading nutritional expert today has a single dietary formula or regimen that they believe will effectively optimize the health of anyone who adheres to it.

FOOD GUIDE PYRAMID
A GUIDE TO DAILY FOOD CHOICES

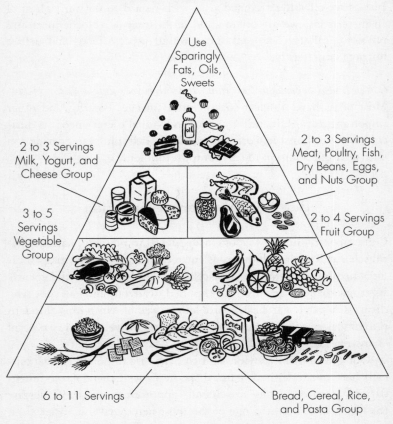

Use Sparingly
Fats, Oils, Sweets

2 to 3 Servings
Milk, Yogurt, and
Cheese Group

2 to 3 Servings
Meat, Poultry, Fish,
Dry Beans, Eggs,
and Nuts Group

3 to 5
Servings
Vegetable
Group

2 to 4 Servings
Fruit Group

6 to 11 Servings

Bread, Cereal, Rice,
and Pasta Group

Source: U.S. Department of Agriculture, U.S. Department of Health and Human Services

Yet today's best-seller diets are striking in their dissimilarity, especially with regard to the all-important issues of macronutrient consumption and macronutrient ratios—in other words, how much protein, carbohydrate, and fat people should be consuming, and in what combinations.

For example, some nutrition experts are big proponents of low-fat, low-protein, high-carbohydrate diets. They contend that diets that include meat, cheese, and vegetable oil will expand our waistlines, clog our arteries, and put us all on the fast track to senility and premature death. Many of these experts advise us to cut fat intake to a bare minimum and to stick to light vegetarian fare based on grains, fruits, and vegetables.

Other leading nutritional gurus advocate just the opposite: diets high in protein and fat and low in carbohydrates. They believe that the only way people can combat serious health disorders like obesity and heart disease is to heavily restrict their consumption of carbohydrates (like fruits, grains, breads, and pasta), while making proteins (meat and fish and poultry) the mainstay of every meal.

Still other experts are firm believers in "40-30-30" diets. In other words, they believe that all meals and snacks should be comprised of carbohydrate, protein and fat in a precise 40-30-30 ratio. In some people, this approach prevents certain kinds of unwanted hormonal shifts which, if left unchecked over time, contribute to serious chronic health problems, including obesity, atherosclerosis, cancer, diabetes, and chronic fatigue.

Countless other diets also compete for our attention, all promising similar kinds of long-lasting health benefits—energy and fitness and disease-free lives—despite the fact that they too offer sharply contradictory advice.

A quick stroll down the health and fitness aisle of your local bookstore reveals a dizzying array of choices: macrobiotic diets, raw-food diets, celebrity diets, organic-food diets, rotation diets, dairy-free diets, sugar-free diets, cardiovascular diets, cancer-prevention diets, diets for athletes, diets for women, diets to slow the aging process, diets to strengthen immunity, diets to combat depression or fatigue, cholesterol-free diets, hypoglycemic diets, and on and on.

The primary problem for health consumers is this: Since the market is flooded with so many dietary options, and so much conflicting advice and opinion, people are left feeling confused, not knowing how to make sense of it all.

Since people have no way to make rational dietary choices, they're forced into a process of endless experimentation, forced to play a never-ending game of "dietary roulette."

Although there are some people who do manage, on occasion, to win the gamble, or to hit upon a dietary solution that happens to be right for them, most of us are left in a state of perpetual empty-handedness.

In other words, mass-market diets do produce success, but only for some people—those for whom a given diet happens to be physiologically appropriate.

That's why many of today's dietary experts have significant numbers of followers who swear by their methods, and why all the best-selling authors can cite plenty of examples of clinical success.

But what the experts consistently fail to mention is the "silent

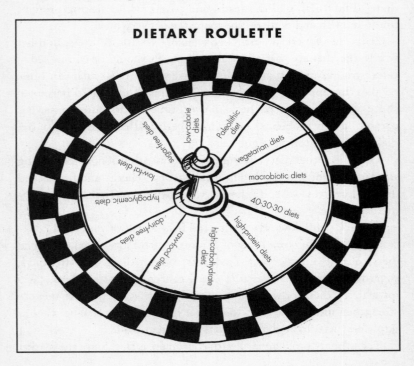

DIETARY ROULETTE

majority," those of us who don't do well on their diets and who are continually shuffling from one stop to the next on the long, well-beaten path of trial and error.

The sad truth is that the only real success modern nutritional science has been able to achieve is hit-or-miss success. Nutrition experts are simply unable to achieve consistent, predictable results with patients.

In fact, the inability to duplicate favorable outcomes in a consistent fashion is the secret frustration and primary professional challenge of virtually all health professionals currently engaged in clinical nutrition. It's the problem clinicians don't like to talk about, even among themselves.

Yet virtually everyone involved in the nutrition industry continues to overlook the most obvious solution, which is simply this:

Dietary solutions need to be tailored to individuals because what works for one person may have no effect on another person, and may make a third person worse.

The idea that foods and nutrients affect different people differently makes a lot of sense, doesn't it? Many of our ancestors thought so.

All the great classic medical traditions (from India, Egypt, Greece, Rome, and China) understood the importance of physiological individuality. As Lucretius, the oft-quoted Roman healer/philosopher, succinctly observed some two thousand years ago, "One man's food is another man's poison."

Ironically, modern nutritional science is very sophisticated in certain ways. After all, many of today's experts are extremely intelligent people who've spent years conducting state-of-the-art laboratory and clinical research. They've analyzed foods and nutrients and their mechanisms of action in exhaustive detail. The resulting body of information available to us is staggering in its scope, precision, and complexity.

But without individuality as the guiding principle of nutritional science, all our advanced research and impressive data and scientific expertise don't really translate into effective clinical solutions, at least not on a meaningful scale. If they did, Americans wouldn't be the fattest and unhealthiest people in the world.

Over the last two decades, we've witnessed an extraordinary nutrition revolution here in the United States. Yet this is the very same time frame during which the health of Americans has declined significantly.

Up until the late 1970s, few Americans paid much attention to the topic of nutrition. But in 1977 a landmark event occurred in Congress. The Senate Select Committee on Nutrition and Human Needs, cochaired by Senators George McGovern and Bob Dole, published a set of nutritional guidelines designed to help curb the nation's growing epidemic of chronic disease. Shortly thereafter, the National Institutes of Health began to allocate increased funding for nutrition-based research.

These events fueled public interest, which in turn stimulated investment activity in the private sector. Before long, a whole new nutrition industry was taking shape, one that gained enormous momentum throughout the 1980s and '90s.

For example, health food stores, once a rarity on the retail landscape, are now an integral part of every shopping mall in America. Annual sales of vitamins and natural food products have grown exponentially, from under $1 billion in 1980 to over $10 billion in 1996. And since 1980 the major food manufacturers have introduced scores of new health-oriented products, which have come to dominate supermarket shelves: low-fat foods, fat-free foods, cholesterol-free foods, fiber-rich foods, low-calorie foods, preservative-free foods, unprocessed foods, sugar-free foods.

The popularity of health- and nutrition-oriented media has also skyrocketed in the last fifteen years. Dozens of major university-based medical research centers have introduced nutrition newsletters for consumer and professional audiences. The lifestyle sections of newspapers and magazines have come to be dominated by articles and columns devoted to health and nutrition. Book sales on these topics have soared by more than thirty percent in the last decade alone.

But despite all the frantic consumption of diet and nutrition-based information and food products, we've not managed to slim down one iota, nor have we managed to put a dent in the incidence of any chronic illness. Consider that:

• The incidence of obesity in the United States increased by thirty-two percent in the last fifteen years.

• The National Institutes of Health recently reported that over ninety-seven million Americans are now either obese or significantly overweight.

• Obesity is a major contributor to heart disease, which now claims the lives of one out of every two Americans.

• Cancer, like heart disease, was largely unknown prior to the twentieth century. But today one out of every four Americans dies prematurely of cancer.

• The epidemic status of cancer, heart disease, obesity, diabetes, and many other chronic illnesses has resulted in significantly reduced longevity for Americans, who now live an average of five years less than people in other industrialized nations.

• Obesity among children in the United States has risen by 40 percent over the last sixteen years. Over 25 percent of children are now obese or significantly overweight.

• Chronic illnesses of all kinds are increasingly common among children and young adults. Today over 40 percent of young people who attempt to enter the Armed Services are rejected due to poor health.

There is only one logical explanation for why our health continues to decline despite all our herculean efforts to achieve some improvement. And that is this:

> *Our poor health is a direct result of serious dietary deficiencies or imbalances. But these problems persist simply because we have lacked the clinical technology to enable us to evaluate and correct nutritional problems on an individual or case-by-case basis.*

Fortunately, the technology to analyze individual nutritional differences now exists, and it's known as *metabolic typing*.

Metabolic typing is a groundbreaking technology that takes the guesswork out of nutritional science. It's a system you or anyone can use to cut rapidly through the information glut of confusing fact and opinion in order to identify your own unique nutritional requirements.

It's an extremely logical methodology that provides what has long been desperately needed: a systematic, testable, repeatable, verifiable means for each of us to find an answer to the question "What's right for me?"

Medicine's Missing Link

For the past twenty years, I've been involved in the research, development, and innovation of a unique field within the health care industry, a clinical technology that I believe may prove to be one of the most important nutritional breakthroughs of the twentieth century. It's called Metabolic Typing—the science of building health.

Since the late 1970s, I've provided technical consulting services to scores of health professionals involved in various forms of clinical nutrition—doctors, dentists, chiropractors, nutritionists, and other kinds of practitioners throughout the United States. In the process, I've personally developed many thousands of individualized metabolic typing profiles or analyses for their patients. I've also provided technical consulting services to vast numbers of clients who sought out my services directly.

Metabolic typing is really two separate and distinct disciplines. One is a simple, clinically oriented dietary technology that can be used by anyone, either health consumers or health professionals. It's an advanced but user-friendly technology that enables people to identify easily their individualized nutritional requirements.

But metabolic typing is also a complex and multidimensional *academic discipline*, one that integrates essential components of many scientific disciplines, including biochemistry, anatomy, physiology, and endocrinology.

In this book I'll be focusing almost exclusively on the clinically oriented dietary technology for health consumers. My goal is to provide you with lots of new, easy-to-use, practical insights about how you can greatly improve your health by managing your diet in a way that's compatible with your genetically determined metabolic needs.

When you eat according to your own unique hereditary requirements, as opposed to following some universal dos and don'ts or randomly prescribed dietary advice, it's entirely possible that you can achieve the same kind of robust good health and fitness your ancestors undoubtedly enjoyed. You can:

- prevent and reverse degenerative disease
- strengthen your immune system
- achieve and maintain your ideal weight
- optimize physical energy and mental clarity
- overcome mood swings and depression
- enhance athletic performance and endurance

As you may already know, *metabolism* is simply the sum total of all the chemical and biological activities that are necessary to sustain life. Although these life functions, or metabolic activities, are many and diverse, they can be summarized as follows: nutrition, transport, respiration, synthesis, regulation, growth, and reproduction.

But in order to sustain life, all these metabolic activities require energy. The air, water, sunlight, and food (nutrients) we acquire from our environment are used by our bodies to produce this vital, life-sustaining energy.

The raw materials in the foods we eat (vitamins, minerals, enzymes, etc.) are particularly important since they're used by our bodies to repair, rebuild, and heal tissue.

But foods and nutrients are also essential because they provide the fuel that is oxidized (or burned or combusted) in our cells to provide the energy for all our metabolic activities.

In fact every biochemical process in your body is entirely dependent on the rate, quality, and amount of energy available to you.

When optimum energy is available to your body on all levels—to all your cells, organs, glands, and systems—then optimum (balanced and efficient) functioning, or good health, is possible.

It is on the cellular level that all metabolic activity takes place and efficiency or inefficiency is determined. Each cell in your body is like a biochemical factory built to fulfill a specific metabolic function.

As food passes through the digestive tract, it is absorbed into the bloodstream, where it is transported to the cells. Once nutrients arrive at the cells, they are assimilated into the cells, and then utilized by the cells for the production of energy and for the fulfillment of each cell's "programmed" function.

We all need a full spectrum of nutrients. But different people have genetically programmed requirements for different amounts of various nutrients. It is these differing genetically based requirements that explain why a certain nutrient can cause one person to feel good, have no effect on another, and cause a third person to feel worse.

Each cell in the body "knows" how to be a perfect cell—it's designed to be healthy and to efficiently perform the functions for which it was created.

But unless the genetically required raw materials are available at the right place, at the right time, and in a form that can be utilized, inefficiency at a cellular level will result.

The bottom line is this: Unless you acquire all the nutrients for which you have a genetically programmed need, your cells' ability to perform their functions will be impaired.

As your cells lose the ability to produce adequate energy (because they lack sufficient nutrients), they also lose their ability to repair and rebuild tissue. Strong, healthy cells become replaced by weak, defective ones. This then exerts a domino effect on your whole system.

For example, as the cells of an organ become weakened and less able to fulfill their roles, the function of the organ itself becomes weak and inefficient. When this happens, stress is put on your entire system—with disease as the inevitable result.

On the other hand, when cells do get all the nutrients for which there is a genetically required need, they're capable of producing optimum amounts of energy. With adequate available energy, they can readily fulfill their genetic roles. And with the proper raw materials (nutrients), the cells can also repair and rebuild and reproduce efficiently and effectively.

When the cells are strong, healthy, and efficient, so, too, are the organs, glands, and systems they comprise, with good health as the natural result.

But in order to acquire the nutrients for which your body has a

CELLULAR METABOLISM

FUEL → **OXIDATION** → **ENERGY** = **METABOLISM**

CELL

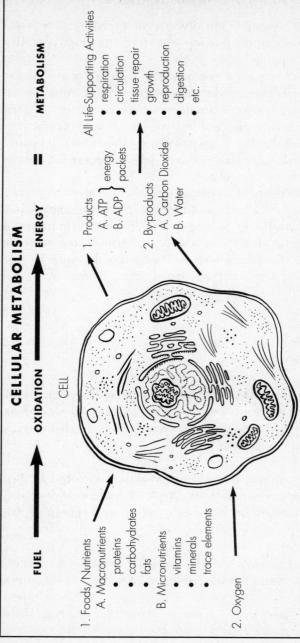

1. Foods/Nutrients
   A. Macronutrients
      • proteins
      • carbohydrates
      • fats
   B. Micronutrients
      • vitamins
      • minerals
      • trace elements

2. Oxygen

1. Products
   A. ATP
   B. ADP } energy packets

2. By-products
   A. Carbon Dioxide
   B. Water

All Life-Supporting Activities
   • respiration
   • circulation
   • tissue repair
   • growth
   • reproduction
   • digestion
   • etc.

All metabolic activity takes place at the cellular level. Each cell in your body is like a biochemical factory whose primary task is to oxidize (burn or combust) foods and nutrients to provide energy for all of the life-supporting (metabolic) activities your body carries out.

The quality of your health is largely dependent on the rate, quality, and amount of energy available to your metabolic processes. To optimize your energy production, you need a full spectrum of nutrients. But different people have genetically programmed requirements for different amounts of various nutrients.

genetic need, you must first identify what your needs are. That's why I develop metabolic typing profiles—they represent a kind of personalized dietary shopping list.

I should point out that a metabolic typing profile or analysis can take various forms, ranging from very simple to very complex.

But for most purposes, a simple metabolic typing analysis, one you can do in the convenience of your own home, without computer assistance, is sufficient. It will reveal plenty of essential information about how you can tailor your diet to effectively support and enhance your own unique body chemistry.

You can quickly and easily obtain a metabolic analysis on yourself simply by taking the self-test in Chapter 6. Once you tabulate your score, you'll immediately be able to identify your basic metabolic type. One important factor that is used to determine your metabolic type is your rate of cellular oxidation. Thus, one of the things we need to do is find out which of the following three characteristics may apply to you:

1. slow oxidizer
2. fast oxidizer
3. mixed oxidizer

Once you've identified your metabolic type, you can then use this essential information to choose the specific foods and food combinations that are best for you, especially with regard to the all-important macronutrients. For example:

1. Slow oxidizers require low-protein, low-fat, high-carbohydrate diets.
2. Fast oxidizers require high-protein, high-fat, low-carbohydrate diets.
3. Mixed oxidizers require relatively equal amounts of proteins, fats, and carbs.

Just how and why metabolic typing works is the key focus of this book, and something I'll be describing in great detail in subsequent chapters.

But for now, you may be interested to know that your body is continually offering up a very large and never-ending volume of information—through a distinct kind of "body language" that defines your unique chemical makeup and nutritional needs.

This information takes many forms, including all your physical, structural, emotional, psychological, and behavioral characteristics, even your dietary preferences and reactions to specific foods. Each bit of information is a critical "clue" in the overall biochemical "puzzle" that is you.

Taken together, all these external clues speak volumes about the way your body functions on an internal level, and the way your system processes food and utilizes nutrients.

Metabolic typing is the culmination of seventy years of pioneering efforts and interrelated discoveries by a whole series of remarkable medical researchers, including physicians, biochemists, physiologists, clinical nutritionists, dentists, and psychologists.

Although their names are not quite household words—Dr. George Watson, Dr. William Donald Kelley, Dr. Royal Lee, Dr. Weston Price, Dr. Francis Pottenger, Dr. Melvin Page, Dr. Roger Williams, Dr. Emanuel Revici, Dr. Henry Bieler—many are giants in their fields and world renowned in their respective scientific and clinical disciplines.

These and other individuals played vitally important roles in the evolution of metabolic typing. Of course, it would be impossible even to begin to adequately address each of their contributions. However, the achievements of some of these scientists, especially Williams, Kelley, Lee, Pottenger, and Watson, are central to understanding the science of metabolic typing. So I'll highlight the work of these men very briefly in the following chapter, and in greater detail later on.

In the meantime, what I can tell you with absolute certainty is this: When correctly applied at the clinical level, therapeutic regimens based on metabolic typing are extremely effective in *building or optimizing health*, and, in turn, *preventing or reversing chronic health disorders*. In fact, they're consistently more effective than other nutritional approaches.

To understand fully why metabolic typing is superior to other dietary or clinical methodologies, you'll want to read the entire book.

But for the moment, here are a few "big picture" criteria to help you quickly understand what distinguishes metabolic typing from other disciplines:

1. *Metabolic typing is applicable to chronic health disorders.*
Orthodox medicine excels in the treatment of acute medical emergencies such as traumatic injuries, childbirth, heart attacks, seizures, and other problems that necessitate rapid drug or surgical intervention. In contrast, metabolic typing is a clinical approach that is useful in the treatment and prevention of chronic health disorders—an enormous category of illness that accounts for eighty percent of all human health problems.

2. *Metabolic typing moves beyond symptom-oriented medicine.*
One of the primary limitations of orthodox medicine and modern nutritional science with respect to chronic health disorders is that they focus on treating conditions at the symptom level. Metabolic typing addresses health disorders at a much deeper level. It's geared toward building health by correcting the patterns of biochemical imbalance that underlie, or are at the root of, chronic health problems.

3. *Metabolic typing produces reliable, predictable clinical results.*
Modern nutritional science, like orthodox medicine, is primarily focused on the diagnosis and treatment of specific diseases. But when nutrition is used to treat specific symptoms or diseases, the results are unreliable and unpredictable. Sometimes it works and sometimes it doesn't. The reason is that two people with radically different physiological or metabolic problems may actually exhibit the same kinds of symptoms. Since metabolic typing focuses on the needs of the person with a given disease rather than on the disease itself, it offers a far more reliable methodology for evaluating and correcting real systemic problems.

4. *Metabolic typing offers a highly integrated approach to building health.*
Metabolic typing is based on the concept of optimizing health by building the strength of all the systems, organs, and glands simultaneously, in much the same way as a "rising tide lifts all boats." If you

try to treat just one part of the body at a time, it's the therapeutic equivalent of sweeping dirt under a carpet. You may get an initial positive effect, but after a while the health problem will just show up in another part of the body. In subsequent chapters, I'll tell you much more about this concept and the reason metabolic typing focuses on "balancing total body chemistry."

5. *Metabolic typing relies on the body's innate intelligence.*

As all scientists know, nothing we can invent in the laboratory can actually "cure" a degenerative illness or induce a true "healing response." It's the body itself that is the true healer, the ultimate source of wisdom that controls every authentic healing response. Although metabolic typing makes use of advanced computer technology, its ultimate effectiveness is owed not so much to science or technology, but to its ability to utilize simple, subtle, natural methods that support the body's own innate ability to regulate and heal itself.

6. *Metabolic typing represents a logical new paradigm shift.*

Although it's a discipline based on traditional scientific knowledge, metabolic typing actually represents a profound new paradigm shift within the realm of modern medical science. In other words, metabolic typing relies on the very same information that supports current, mainstream belief systems in medicine and nutrition. But it provides an entirely new way of interpreting that information, and in turn applying it, in a practical way, to people's everyday lives.

Chapter 2

A Brief History
of Metabolic Typing

Origins of a Breakthrough Technology

The evolution of metabolic typing has not been a linear progression. It happened gradually, with one advance slowly giving rise to another in an often serendipitous fashion, on and off over the course of the twentieth century. As is so often the case in science, the key discoveries didn't come from prestigious and well-funded research centers, but arose instead from unexpected sources, typically from maverick researchers or clinicians working apart from the medical/scientific mainstream.

The discovery of vitamins in the very early 1900s, and other early forays into nutritional science, paved the way for important breakthroughs related to metabolic typing in the decades that followed.

Yet nutrition was far from fashionable in the 1930s and 1940s when many scientists and physicians swarmed around the lucrative, rapidly growing, and seemingly miraculous realm of pharmaceutical science.

Dr. Roger Williams, however, was not particularly interested in conventional scientific pursuits.

In the 1930s the young biochemist had an odd experience while undergoing a surgical procedure, one that led him down a unique professional path.

Williams's physician attempted to get him to fall asleep by giving him a shot of morphine. But the morphine had just the opposite effect from what the doctor intended. Instead of going to sleep, Williams was jolted wide awake by the morphine, and his mind raced uncontrollably. The doctor tried larger doses of morphine, but Roger's torturous speeding episode only intensified.

Physicians insisted that the incident was a rare "idiosyncrasy," but Williams was skeptical. He wondered if there might be some logical explanation as to why he reacted so differently from most people to morphine.

Though Williams put the question aside for a number of years, the morphine incident lingered in the back of his mind and eventually triggered his interest in a new area of scientific inquiry, one he would take up in earnest by the late 1940s.

One day he happened to be reviewing the book *The Atlas of Human Anatomy* and was stunned to come across illustrations of "normal" human stomachs (carefully copied from autopsy specimens) depicting the organs in radically different shapes and sizes. Williams suddenly realized that the *internal* anatomical characteristics of human beings were every bit as variable as their external characteristics.

Even more surprising than the anatomical differences was the enormous degree of variation in the chemical composition of stomach digestive juices. For example, Williams found that the pepsin content of gastric juice among normal adults varied at least a thousandfold.

In 1956 Dr. Williams wrote a classic book called *Biochemical Individuality*. In it he asserted that:

- Individuality pervades every part of the human body.
- Human beings are highly distinctive on a microscopic as well as a gross anatomical level, in the functioning of their organs, and in the composition of their body fluids.
- Inherited differences extend to the structure and metabolism of

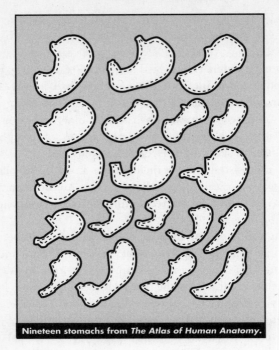

Nineteen stomachs from *The Atlas of Human Anatomy*.

every cell, and determine the speed and efficiency with which cells perform their essential functions.

• Unbalanced or inadequate nutrition at the cellular level is a major cause of human disease.

• People have genetically determined and highly individualized nutritional requirements.

Williams believed that medicine lacked the clinical tools necessary to diagnose and treat chronic health problems effectively. He called for the development of "metabolic profiles," which could be used to evaluate and treat patients with nutrition on a highly individualized basis.

Although Williams was a prestigious researcher who achieved fame for the discovery of pantothenic acid (vitamin B5) and other important accomplishments, his theories on biochemical individuality were largely ignored by mainstream medicine. But these theories did have a strong impact on a variety of independent, nutrition-oriented researchers and clinicians outside the mainstream.

One maverick clinician in particular, an orthodontist from a small town in Grapevine, Texas, was heavily influenced by Roger Williams's book on biochemical individuality.

William Donald Kelley, armed with degrees in biology, chemistry, and biochemistry, graduated from the dental college at Baylor University in Houston in 1957. When he moved into clinical practice with a specialty in orthodontics, his business and reputation flourished.

And like the distinguished Weston Price, a fellow dentist of an earlier generation, Dr. Kelley began to question what was causing so many crooked teeth and distorted, inadequately developed jaws and dental palates among Americans.

Kelley knew of Price's work with primitive cultures, and he had some familiarity with the connection between diet and degenerative disease. That understanding, along with his exceptional gifts as a researcher, clinician, and highly innovative thinker, would serve him well when a personal health crisis turned his life upside down.

In the mid-1960s Kelley broke the news to his family that he had developed pancreatic cancer, the most aggressive and untreatable form of the disease. His condition was inoperable and there were no chemotherapeutic agents that had ever been shown to extend the life of pancreatic cancer patients. His doctor told him he had only a few months to live, and suggested he go home and get his affairs in order.

Initially, Kelley was resigned to the grim prognosis. It was a very bleak prospect, since he had a wife and several children and was not yet forty years old. One member of his family, however, was not about to take the news lying down. Kelley's mother was a feisty, self-sufficient woman who'd grown up on a Kansas farm and spent most of her life struggling in tough, impoverished circumstances. She had little use for doctors, and though she had no formal education, she was a strong believer in the power of native intelligence and commonsense dietary traditions.

Velma Kelley lost no time demanding that her son abandon his modern eating habits and restrict his diet to fruits and vegetables and whole grains. Despite Dr. Kelley's strong academic interest in nutrition, he'd followed an extremely poor diet for years and consumed lots of candy and other junk foods on a daily basis.

But Kelley followed his mother's dietary advice and, to his surprise, within a few weeks his condition improved. His energy picked up dramatically, and the tumors in his abdomen, always readily apparent to the touch, diminished somewhat. Feeling encouraged, Kelley decided to visit the library to see if he could find any useful information about natural remedies in the treatment of pancreatic cancer.

He found much more than he anticipated. It turned out that scores of credible researchers around the world had been experimenting with many different kinds of natural, nontoxic methods to treat cancer for many years. Few if any of these approaches were sanctioned by the medical establishment. Nonetheless, many of the alternative methods that Kelley read about appeared to be just as promising, if not more so, as orthodox cancer treatments, which were limited to chemotherapy, radiation, and surgery.

Dr. Kelley decided to add some of these other therapeutic measures to the whole-foods, vegetarian diet recommended by his mother. He patched together a fairly crude yet comprehensive regimen for himself, which now included vitamins, minerals, enzymes, and detoxification techniques.

Kelley's approach was uniquely eclectic. He integrated whatever remedial measures made sense to him regardless of their source. As an example, he utilized a number of detoxification procedures, ranging from simple herbal tea formulas, which originated in medical folklore, to more elaborate procedures developed at mainstream medical institutions.

Months went by and Kelley had lots of ups and downs. At times the enzymes and other elements of the regimen overwhelmed his system, leaving him nauseated, weak, and unable to function. But Kelley soldiered on. He tinkered endlessly with the protocol, adjusting dosages of nutrients, trying out new foods and dietary supplements, all the while voraciously reading everything he could find that was relevant to his newly improvised therapy.

After a while he found himself having more good days than bad, with abdominal tumors that were becoming barely detectable. A year passed, then two, and Kelley's health was slowly and steadily improving. Most important, he had managed to survive well past the point at which his doctors were certain he would die.

Word of Kelley's highly unusual recovery spread quickly through his small Texas hometown and the surrounding area. Before long he was confronted by hordes of patients with cancer and other kinds of degenerative illnesses, all seeking his advice on diet-centered therapies. Suddenly nobody was interested in his orthodontic services.

Over the next few years Kelley began to produce impressive results working with all kinds of seriously ill people. By the early 1970s his reputation had spread far beyond Texas and he was emerging as a well-known and highly regarded figure within the nationwide alternative, or "holistic," medical community. He was encouraged by his ability to resolve the serious and often life-threatening conditions of many people. But at the same time, he was deeply troubled by the large number of patients for whom his methods just weren't working.

Then, in 1973, Kelley was faced with yet another personal crisis, one that would, once again, lead to a major turning point in his clinical education. His wife became inexplicably ill after being exposed to toxic paint fumes. She became very weak and was unable to function or get out of bed. Kelley attempted to treat her with the same nutrients and vegetarian diet that had worked so well for him. But instead of helping her, the protocol actually made her condition significantly worse.

Kelley scrambled to find a solution and repeatedly modified various aspects of his wife's regimen. But try as he might, nothing worked. Her condition deteriorated so badly that she was verging on becoming comatose. At this point Kelley began groping desperately for any stopgap measure that might bring her around.

He realized there was one last thing left to try—meat. It seemed like an absurd choice, but he'd run out of options. Kelley began by feeding his wife beef broth. She reacted well and gathered a bit of strength, so Kelley continued by feeding her small pieces of meat.

To his amazement, her recovery was swift and dramatic. Within twenty-four hours she was suddenly strong enough to sit up in bed, and in a short while she began to resume many of her normal activities. It was quite a "eureka moment" for Dr. Kelley. Suddenly it became clear to him that what constituted a healthy diet for some people—eating little or no meat—was a formula for disaster for others. Soon the dynamic Kelley was off and running once again. It was not long before he had created exactly what Williams, the distinguished biochemist, always hoped for: a clinical tool for assessing people's metabolic individuality.

He also invented novel methods for making his radical new approach to nutrition-based healing available to thousands of people worldwide. For these and other reasons, Kelley would become one of the most respected alternative medicine pioneers of the twentieth century, widely regarded as the "father of metabolic typing."

The Science of Customized Nutrition

I first heard the name William Donald Kelley in 1977, in the same way everybody did, by word of mouth. He had kept an unusually low profile for a clinician, and rarely appeared at public or professional gatherings. And he certainly didn't advertise or promote himself. But somehow the world really did seem to beat a path to his door.

By the mid-1970s it was no longer feasible for Kelley to treat patients directly. There were just too many people to handle, and it was clear he needed to free up his time for research. His primary interest was in developing and refining his metabolic protocol, and he knew there were endless possibilities in that regard.

Kelley's solution was to set up an educational institute that would provide services to other clinicians around the country who wanted to use his protocols in their own practices. This alleviated the strain on Kelley, while providing many more patients with access to his expertise. So in 1975 he packed up his home and office in the remote little Texas town of Grapevine and headed for an even more remote location—Winthrop, Washington, a rural area high in the Cascade Mountains, northeast of Seattle. He loved the pristine mountain air and uncontaminated physical surroundings. But he also wanted to remove himself, as much as possible, from the competitive scrutiny and inevitable hostility and political pressure on the part of the drug and surgically oriented medical establishment.

In those days he left his mountain sanctuary only rarely, mainly to attend weekend educational seminars sponsored by his institute. The seminars were designed to assist patients and clinicians utilizing Kelley's protocols. It was at one of these sessions that I first met Kelley, in the spring of 1978, after spending a year on a comprehensive nutritional program that had been tailored for me by his organization.

I'd struggled with serious allergies all my life and had tried every conceivable therapeutic approach under the sun. Nothing had worked. By age twenty-nine I'd just about given up all hope of ever getting off the antihistamines I was forced to take every day, all year round. They made me drowsy and their effectiveness was limited and quick to wear off. Nonetheless, I needed them badly in order to function.

Then, in 1977, a friend suggested I check out the Kelley program. I was intrigued from the start upon hearing of Kelley's "nonspecific" approach to dealing with chronic ailments. Word had it that he didn't treat diseases per se, but focused instead on balancing a patient's overall body chemistry, a method he called metabolic typing. Other aspects of Kelley's approach appealed to me as well, so I quickly followed up on my friend's suggestion to try it out. Actually, part of my motivation was to prove to myself that I already knew all I needed to know about nutrition. I'd spent a number of years studying nutrition, and considered myself quite an expert on the subject, despite my inability to resolve my own allergy problems.

But I was in for a very rude awakening. I was about to learn that I was dead wrong about my level of expertise. And over time I would come to realize that Kelley not only knew far more about nutrition than I did, but that he also knew much more than anyone else I had ever encountered.

So I began Kelley's regimen. It was not a quick fix, but over the course of a year my allergy symptoms gradually subsided to the point where I no longer needed the drugs I'd depended on for most of my life.

Shortly after starting, I also noticed an improvement in my energy level and mental outlook, along with an unusual resistance to colds and flu infections. Over a period of months my strength and energy and overall sense of well-being rose to a level I had never before experienced.

To be honest, I had no idea I could feel as good as I started to feel. I was living proof of Kelley's belief that most people in industrialized societies have no idea what really good health is, simply because they've never experienced it.

At that point I was convinced he was onto something, and I wanted to learn as much as I could about the science behind his program. So I flew to Chicago to attend one of his weekend seminars.

I was fascinated by the range and depth of the material that was presented. One of the primary topics Kelley addressed was the way in which the autonomic nervous system (ANS) could be used to pinpoint people's individual nutritional requirements.

Through his experiences with his wife and other patients, Kelley had stumbled across the realization that different people require different foods and nutrients. Later, he went on to learn about biochemical individuality from Roger Williams and other researchers.

But these insights alone were not enough. He still needed to find some systematic way of determining people's unique food and nutrient requirements. For example, he needed a reliable methodology that would allow him to predict which patients would do well on vegetarian diets versus meat-centered diets, and vice versa. Or which patients might require calcium or potassium or other specific nutrients.

That's when Kelley turned to the work of two of the century's leading pioneers in nutritional science: Francis Pottenger, M.D., and Royal Lee, D.D.S. Pottenger was a physician who practiced nutritional therapy and Lee was a dentist and the founder of Standard Process, one of the world's best-known vitamin companies.

In the 1930s and '40s both men conducted groundbreaking research with the ANS. They recognized that people have unique dietary requirements, and they discovered that the ANS holds very important clues that can be used to predict what types of foods and nutrients people need.

As you may know, the nervous system is divided into two parts: the *cerebrospinal* division and the *autonomic* division.

The *autonomic nervous system* is widely referred to as the "master regulator of metabolism" because it controls all the *involuntary activities* of the body—all those functions that are *not under your conscious control*. These include your heart rate, digestion, respiration, tissue repair and rebuilding, cellular activity, regulation of your body temperature, immune activity, and countless other functions.

It's also divided into two distinct branches: the *sympathetic branch* and the *parasympathetic branch*. Each of these two branches of the autonomic nervous system regulates a different set of metabolic activities. As the diagram on pages 34 and 35 indicates, some organs, glands, and systems are controlled by the *sympathetic system,* while others are controlled by the *parasympathetic system.*

Each system is in charge of "turning on," or "innervating," various functions of the body, while the opposite system has the task of "turning off," or inhibiting, those same functions. This dualistic, "push-pull" phenomenon is what enables the two branches of the autonomic nervous system to work together, in a synchronized fashion, to regulate all involuntary metabolic processes in the human body.

For example, the sympathetic system speeds up the heart rate, while the parasympathetic system slows it down. In the case of other involuntary functions, the roles can be reversed. For instance, the parasympathetic system turns on the activity of digestion—the secretion of hydrochloric acid, contractions of the stomach, and related functions.

But should a tiger appear while you're taking a lunch break, your sympathetic system would kick in, causing a "fight or flight" response. This would immediately shut off your digestion, send blood from your digestive organs to your muscular system, speed up your heart rate, and make all the other necessary metabolic preparations for your fight or flight.

Most people are neurologically influenced more strongly by either the sympathetic or the parasympathetic system. They also vary in the degree to which they are influenced by each of these two systems.

As a result of these inherited differences, people have many different physical, behavioral, and psychological characteristics, which

The Two Branches of the

Sympathetic Branch

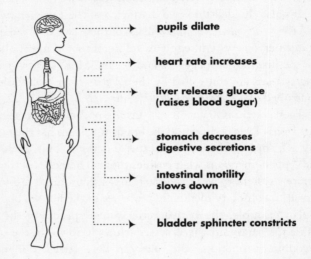

→ **pupils dilate**

→ **heart rate increases**

→ **liver releases glucose (raises blood sugar)**

→ **stomach decreases digestive secretions**

→ **intestinal motility slows down**

→ **bladder sphincter constricts**

Throughout the universe, on every level, we find evidence of cycles and the interplay of two opposing yet complementary forces, for example: night/day, dark/light, acid/alkaline, high tide/low tide, protons/electrons, and so on. This dualistic or "yin-yang" phenomenon is evidenced in the Autonomic Nervous System (ANS) as well.

The ANS is known as the "master regulator of metabolism," because it controls all bodily processes that are outside your conscious control, such as breathing, heart rate and digestion. It can be thought of as your body's automatic pilot, which keeps you alive without your being aware of it or participating in its activities.

The Autonomic Nervous System functions through the opposing yet complementary interaction of the sympathetic and parasympathetic branches. Most people are

Autonomic Nervous System

Parasympathetic Branch

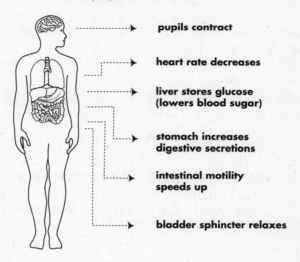

- **pupils contract**
- **heart rate decreases**
- **liver stores glucose (lowers blood sugar)**
- **stomach increases digestive secretions**
- **intestinal motility speeds up**
- **bladder sphincter relaxes**

neurologically influenced more strongly by one of these two branches, but everyone is different in the degree to which their bodies are influenced.

In general, the sympathetic system switches on organs and glands involved in energy utilization, such as the adrenals, thyroid, and pituitary. It is often referred to as the "fight or flight" branch. Conversely, the parasympathetic system is responsible for energy-conserving processes, and switches on organs and glands pertaining to digestion, elimination, repairing, and rebuilding. It is sometimes called the "rest and digest" branch.

Since different foods and nutrients exert different effects on the two branches of the ANS, metabolic balance can be strongly affected by the diet.

correlate with either "sympathetic dominance" or "parasympathetic dominance."

Both Pottenger and Lee realized that good health demands a balance between the two branches of the autonomic nervous system. They also recognized that nutrients play a crucial role in keeping the ANS in balance.

Some nutrients stimulate or strengthen the sympathetic system, while having just the opposite effect on the parasympathetic system. Other nutrients stimulate the parasympathetic system while having just the opposite effect on the sympathetic system.

Pottenger was the first to discover the value of addressing ANS imbalances in treating certain health problems. He began using calcium and potassium in an early attempt to bring the autonomic sys-

CHARACTERISTICS ASSOCIATED WITH

SYMPATHETIC DOMINANCE	VERSUS	PARASYMPATHETIC DOMINANCE
Physical Tendencies • indigestion • heartburn • insomnia • hypertension • high blood pressure • predisposed to infection • low appetite • angular facial structure • tendency to be tall, thin		*Physical Tendencies* • diarrhea • allergies • low blood sugar • irregular heartbeat • chronic fatigue • cold sores • excessive appetite • round face and skull • shorter, wider build
Psychological/Behavioral Tendencies • excellent concentration • highly motivated • cool emotionally • irritable • hyperactive • socially withdrawn		*Psychological/Behavioral Tendencies* • lethargy • procrastination • slow to anger • deliberate, cautious • warm emotionally • socially outgoing

tem into balance. Lee took things a step further by defining a broader range of health problems associated with autonomic imbalance, and expanding Pottenger's technique of using nutrients to establish autonomic balance.

But it was Kelley who took a giant leap forward in using the autonomic nervous system as a basis of determining metabolic individuality. In the process, he created a profound new paradigm shift, away from the conventional, specialty-driven approach to medicine and toward a new variety of integrated or "holistic" healing.

For instance, even though Pottenger and Lee were pioneers in nutritional science, they used nutrients the same way doctors use drugs and the same way most contemporary nutritionists still use nutrients—to treat specific diseases or to address ailments on a symptom-by-symptom basis.

Kelley's idea was different. He believed that trying to isolate health problems and treat them one at a time would only offer, at best, a temporary "fix." Since all the systems of the body have a complete and continual dependence on one another, Kelley believed that nutritional regimes should be used to build health rather than to treat disease.

In other words, he didn't believe in prescribing a nutrient here and a nutrient there for any given ache or pain. He was much more interested in feeding the body whatever raw materials it needed to create balance and efficiency at all levels within the body at the same time—at the cellular, tissue, organ, glandular, and systemic levels.

Kelley felt that if the body could just be given everything it needed—the right foods and the right combinations of nutrients—it could then heal itself far more effectively than any piecemeal regimen designed by a clinician. He called this approach nonspecific metabolic therapy.

By the late '70s Kelley had become the first researcher ever to use the autonomic nervous system as the foundation for classifying people into metabolic categories, or metabolic types, each with its own comprehensive nutritional protocol. These protocols ranged from vegetarian to meat-centered diets, and everything in between. They also included different vitamin and mineral combinations, all designed to address varying degrees of metabolic imbalance.

The real complexity of Kelley's approach to metabolic typing,

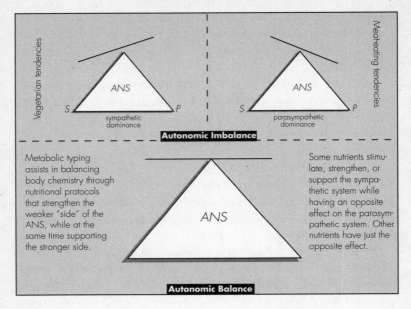

Vegetarian tendencies

ANS

S — sympathetic dominance — P

Meat-eating tendencies

ANS

S — parasympathetic dominance — P

Autonomic Imbalance

Metabolic typing assists in balancing body chemistry through nutritional protocols that strengthen the weaker "side" of the ANS, while at the same time supporting the stronger side.

ANS

Some nutrients stimulate, strengthen, or support the sympathetic system while having an opposite effect on the parasympathetic system. Other nutrients have just the opposite effect.

Autonomic Balance

even this early approach, is impossible to communicate in the space of these introductory passages, just as it was impossible to fully absorb in the space of a two-day seminar.

Nonetheless, on that weekend in Chicago twenty years ago, I certainly grasped enough of the essentials to understand that William Donald Kelley was one of the most original medical thinkers of the century. Those of us in the audience were mesmerized by the topics he laid before us. And many of us knew from personal experience that they amounted to much more than promising theories.

Over the course of the weekend, two events dramatically changed the course of my life. First, I suddenly realized what I wanted to be doing the rest of my life. I knew I wanted to become actively involved with the science of metabolic typing. It was impossible for me to imagine a more exciting field, or one with more potential to positively affect people's lives.

Then something very unexpected happened. When the seminar was over, Kelley approached me, and to my utter astonishment, asked me if I'd like to go to work as his assistant. Once the real meaning of Kelley's offer had sunk in, it took me all of sixty seconds to make up my mind. I flew back to my hometown of Seattle, closed down my apartment, packed my car, headed for Winthrop, and never looked back.

Advances in Metabolic Typing

During my first two years as Dr. Kelley's clinical assistant, I spent most of my time compiling and writing textbooks, which he used to train other health professionals.

The task of organizing and recording the principles of nonspecific metabolic typing, which had evolved over a thirty-year period, was monumental. But the experience enabled me to develop a very detailed understanding of the science behind the clinical discipline.

Then in 1980 things changed. Kelley asked me to take over as director of his International Health Institute. My primary responsibility in this capacity was to work on the "front line," providing technical assistance to several hundred clinicians around the country who were using Kelley's programs in their practices.

This experience, which was to last six years, gave me a thoroughly unique perspective on the clinical efficacy of the Kelley program, and a chance to evaluate, firsthand, its strengths and weaknesses.

Overall, Kelley's program, with high patient compliance, was quite successful in resolving all manner of chronic health problems. I quickly realized that the experience I'd had conquering my own persistent respiratory problems was no isolated occurrence.

Even more surprising was the fact that Kelley was able to duplicate, over and over again, his personal success in managing his own cancer.

Though there were a fair number of alternative medical practitioners throughout the United States and Europe who were achieving impressive clinical results in terms of extending the lives of people with cancer, Kelley's reputation in this area surpassed just about everyone else's.

Kelley also attracted a large following of people with many other serious degenerative conditions, including cardiovascular disease, diabetes, arthritis, colitis, and a broad range of related problems. Most people were very surprised to learn that we had little concern with their specific clinical problems or diagnoses. Instead, we focused almost exclusively on the specific imbalances unique to their metabolic types.

In many cases people had turned to Kelley and his unorthodox methods only after failing with more conventional medical treatments. And in many instances his was the only therapy they were pursuing.

This meant that Kelley's therapy was really put to the test on difficult and advanced clinical problems, which made the results we were getting all the more remarkable. It also meant that I was in an ideal position to evaluate accurately the real efficacy of the institute's programs.

Though the principles of nonspecific metabolic therapy seemed very logical to me, I still couldn't help being amazed as I observed so many people with very serious ailments regaining their health. The positive results I was seeing seemed to contradict so much of what I'd been conditioned to believe all my life about health and healing and the limits of modern medicine.

This is not to say that Kelley was working miracles. Though there were large numbers of people whom he was helping in a dramatic way, there were also plenty of clinical failures, even among patients who complied faithfully with every aspect of the programs we were developing.

The real essence of my job was to work closely with clinicians who were not getting favorable results with some of their patients. I became troubleshooter-in-chief. Each day I would help clinicians identify possible reasons why some people were not responding, and I would suggest program changes and modifications.

Kelley would often collaborate with me in this role, and together we would closely evaluate the most difficult cases presented to the institute. Sometimes we would come up with program adjustments that worked and turned patients around. And sometimes, no matter what we tried, we just couldn't produce any meaningful clinical results.

It was a very frustrating dilemma for everyone concerned. We desperately wanted to provide effective metabolic typing analyses for all the patients and clinicians who were counting on our help. And we simply couldn't understand why the Kelley model, based exclusively on the autonomic nervous system, worked so well in some cases and not in others. It just didn't seem to make sense.

In fact, in many instances, people reacted exactly opposite to the way they should have according to our clinical model. We were actually making some people worse instead of better. It was at that point I began to cast around for explanations wherever I could.

One day in late 1981, I came across *Nutrition and Your Mind,* a seminal book published in 1972 by a brilliant clinical psychologist named George Watson, Ph.D.

Over many years of clinical practice, Watson had come to the conclusion that biochemical imbalances were at the root of many psychological problems, and this led him to ground-breaking discoveries in nutritional science. He felt it was pointless to try to treat people's emotional problems without addressing any underlying metabolic disturbances.

Watson serendipitously discovered that certain nutrients intensified adverse emotional states in some patients, while in others, the same nutrients could alleviate emotional problems. He recognized that different people have different dietary requirements, so he developed a system for classifying people based on their metabolic differences.

But Watson didn't use the autonomic nervous system as the basis for metabolic classification. Instead he used *cellular oxidation*. He discovered that there is a distinct correlation between people's psychological and emotional characteristics and the rate at which their cells convert nutrients into energy.

Watson observed that some people burned foods and nutrients too slowly, while others burned them too quickly. He also knew that the rate of cellular oxidation, which is determined partly by heredity and partly by environmental influences, could be significantly influenced through diet.

By prescribing foods and nutrients to balance oxidative imbalances, Watson discovered that he was able to quickly resolve many people's clinical problems, including depression, mood swings, agitation, erratic behaviors, and concentration disorders.

In essence, Watson had originated his own unique approach to metabolic typing, and was applying it quite successfully in clinical settings.

On one level, this discovery was very exciting because it corroborated Kelley's belief in the importance of metabolic typing as the basis for effective nutritional therapy. But on another level, it presented me with an enormous problem, because Watson's oxidative model *directly contradicted* Kelley's autonomic model.

According to these two metabolic models, key nutrients act in opposite ways, exerting opposite biochemical effects on the body. Just as one example, according to Watson's model, the essential mineral potassium can be used to alter the body's pH balance by pushing it toward an acidic condition. But under Kelley's model, potassium has an alkalinizing effect.

The contradiction was mind-boggling. Both Kelley and Watson were brilliant researchers with a solid grasp of biochemistry. Kelley's autonomic model had proven itself again and again in clinical settings. Yet Watson's model had also shown equally compelling evidence of its clinical value.

In 1982 I read and reread Watson's extensive writings, searching for some hint that might explain the puzzling reality we were confronting. Initially I tried my best to find flaws in both metabolic models, with the hope of determining which one was right and which one was wrong.

Then one day another explanation occurred to me. Maybe neither model was wrong. Maybe Kelley and Watson were both right.

I began to suspect that in some people an imbalance in the autonomic nervous system was the dominant factor influencing their dietary and nutrient requirements, while in other people just the opposite might be true—imbalances in the oxidative system would dictate their needs for certain types of foods and supplements.

This insight soon led to a major clinical breakthrough. I developed a system for detecting *autonomic dominance* versus *oxidative dominance* in people—and then began to recommend foods and nutrients accordingly. I named this phenomenon "The Dominance Factor."

The results were swift and dramatic. Suddenly I began seeing real progress in those who had not previously responded to nutritional regimens based just on the Kelley autonomic model alone.

But my developmental process did not end there. Even though the autonomic and oxidative systems were clearly of central importance

THE DOMINANCE FACTOR

Within the ANS, one branch, either sympathetic or parasympathetic, is generally dominant. And within the oxidative system, fast or slow oxidation tends to dominate. Similarly, "dominance" exists on a larger systemic level, between the ANS and the oxidative system.

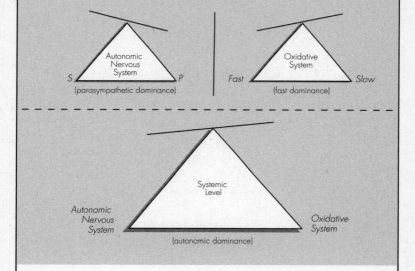

Whether you are "autonomic dominant" or "oxidative dominant" will determine how a food or nutrient behaves in your body, e.g., whether it is alkalizing or acidifying. In order to select an appropriate diet and effectively balance a person's body chemistry, it is essential to first determine which system is dominant.

in determining metabolic individuality, I suspected that they were only pieces of an even larger biochemical puzzle.

Over the course of the next ten years, other pieces of the biochemical "puzzle" fell into place. Today, in addition to autonomic and oxidative factors, we routinely evaluate seven additional physiological parameters, or "homeostatic control mechanisms." As a result, metabolic typing has evolved from a one-dimensional process into a far more precise multidimensional clinical technology.

METABOLIC JIGSAW PUZZLE

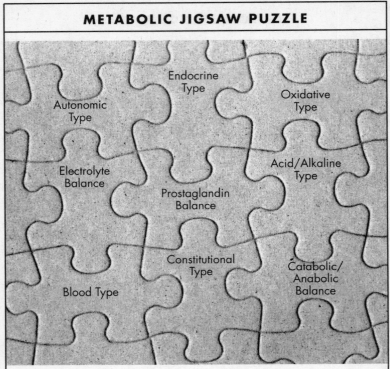

Endocrine
Type

Oxidative
Type

Autonomic
Type

Acid/Alkaline
Type

Electrolyte
Balance

Prostaglandin
Balance

Constitutional
Type

Catabolic/
Anabolic
Balance

Blood Type

The process of metabolic typing involves the evaluation of the interrelationships among the autonomic nervous system, the oxidative system, and seven additional physiological parameters that influence body chemistry.

For example, my technology also incorporates an important homeostatic control system based on aerobic and anaerobic metabolism and membrane permeability. This pertains to catabolic/anabolic balance, a physiological phenomenon discovered by the brilliant researcher Emanuel Revici, M.D.

Chapter 3

PARADIGM SHIFT

Shocking Truths About
Symptom-Based Health Care

When Sarah Hennessey called to introduce herself in the fall of 1996, the first thing I noticed was a sense of profound weariness in her voice. She spoke very softly, in a slow and deliberate cadence, as though she was in pain and our phone conversation was draining her of every ounce of energy she could muster. It was the sound of deep physical and psychological exhaustion, and I had heard it in people's voices at least a thousand times before.

Sarah had spent fifteen years suffering with a health disorder that clinicians today often refer to as "ecological illness," or "EI." She was severely disabled as a result of numerous food and chemical sensitivities. There was hardly any food she could find that would not trigger a cascade of extreme negative reactions: fatigue, arthritic pain, headaches, flulike symptoms, dizziness, bladder infections, depression.

Even a brief exposure to the countless chemicals that permeate our modern environment—the scent of perfume, automobile exhaust, synthetic fibers, detergent, newsprint—was enough to disable Sarah for a long period of time, to send her to bed with a myriad of aches and pains and, in her words, a "toxic hangover."

Like large and growing numbers of people all over the industrialized world, Sarah had become, quite literally, allergic to the twentieth century. Her ability to function normally was so seriously impaired that even simple routine activities—a trip to a department store, a visit to a movie theater, a drive to pick up her child from school, a hairdresser's or doctor's appointment—represented frightening, often insurmountable challenges.

Even worse than the physical suffering was her ongoing inability to find a meaningful solution. Year after year, she consulted practitioners of every conceivable variety. Like so many people with chronic health problems, she started out on an orthodox medical track, seeking out immunologists and other kinds of mainstream physicians.

When that failed, she invested her hope in the alternative medical realm—in physicians practicing "complementary" or "integrated" medicine, in nutritionists, naturopaths, chiropractors, herbalists, iridologists, kinesiologists, and other kinds of professionals and quasi-professionals who seemed like they might have something credible to offer.

After many years of systematic experimentation with endless varieties of diet, nutritional supplements, detox techniques, and other alternative measures, Sarah was able to identify a few remedial approaches that provided a degree of temporary, marginal relief. Her health improved to the point where she could at least look forward to the occasional "good day," or a few hours here and there over the course of a week in which her pain and fatigue would subside, enabling her to forget her problems for a while.

But ultimately it was a meager achievement, especially for someone like Sarah, who had once been a very active, accomplished career woman, occupying executive positions at leading New York ad agencies. Despite the slight improvements she was experiencing, Sarah was still overwhelmingly debilitated, unable to hold a job, venture far from home, or enjoy meals or recreational pursuits or normal interactions with her family and friends.

And after fifteen years of relentless struggle and disappointment, of hoping for a breakthrough that never came, she was running on empty, as burned out emotionally and psychologically as she was physically. The future looked very bleak.

The problem was that nobody seemed to be able to get at the root of Sarah's problems. It was obvious to her that the best dozens of different health professionals had been able to do for her was suppress or alleviate her symptons. But what was causing her chronic immune dysfunction? Why did her illness remain such a mystery? What was the real essence of her disordered physiology? Nobody seemed to know.

All she had left was a long list of partial clues and piecemeal explanations: "a weak liver," a "toxic bowel," a deficiency in this vitamin or that mineral, a "leaky gut" syndrome, a low blood count, an exhausted adrenal system, an enzyme insufficiency, an underactive thyroid, a hormonal imbalance, and on and on.

Yet none of Sarah's clinicians seemed to have a comprehensive, "big picture" grasp of what was wrong, much less a logical and well-integrated strategy to restore her health. It was as though Sarah's illness was a puzzle comprised of a thousand different pieces, but all she had managed to collect was a few dozen—enough information fragments to offer a hint of the total picture, but not nearly enough to bring it into focus.

For a long time Sarah wondered if there might be something peculiar about her case, something unusually complex or out of the ordinary about her physical dilemma that was making it especially difficult for clinicians to find an effective therapeutic solution.

Eventually, it came as little consolation when she realized she was not alone, that her failure to recover was not unique at all, not among allergy or EI patients, and certainly not among people with other forms of chronic illness. Instead, she discovered a rather shocking truth: that there are no "medical solutions" for *any* chronic disease.

Of course there are plenty of ways in which modern medicine can "manage" or "control" or "treat" the *symptoms* of chronic ailments.

But treating symptoms is not the same as addressing the underlying cause of an illness. Delivering a temporary "palliative" remedy is different from eliminating a disease process.

And, surprisingly, as Sarah eventually came to learn, the alternative medical community suffers from the very same limitation as the conventional medical realm.

Conventional practitioners and alternative practitioners are both lim-
ited to treating the outward manifestations of disease, as opposed to
addressing the biochemical processes that set diseases in motion in the
first place.

Think about it for a moment. How many people do you know who have successfully resolved a chronic ailment with the use of a conventional medical treatment—a drug, for example? Similarly, have you ever noticed that people who have turned to clinical nutrition and other alternative modalities are in a perpetual search mode?

The plain fact of the matter is that 80 percent of the patient population—those who suffer with chronic as opposed to acute health disorders—has not been able to find real, lasting solutions at the hands of conventional medical practitioners. And they're not faring much better with alternative medical professionals.

In recent years, people's growing awareness of the dangers and limitations of drugs and invasive medical procedures has precipitated a mad rush toward alternative medicine. People love the fact that alternative practitioners use vitamins and minerals and herbs and other kinds of natural remedies that tend to be much less toxic and far more biologically compatible than synthetic pharmaceutical products.

Growing numbers of health consumers are convinced that natural remedies are not only safer than most drugs, but also that they promote or facilitate the body's own natural healing capabilities. And with each passing year, more and more people become true believers in the value of nutritional science and related areas of alternative medicine.

The problem is that both conventional and alternative medicine are
very limited in their ability to resolve chronic illness because they each
operate on the same symptom- and disease-oriented paradigm—a ther-
apeutic model known as allopathic medicine.

For over a century allopathic medicine has been the dominant medical paradigm in the Western world. It's essentially a philosophy of medicine and an approach to healing that relies primarily on the use of drugs and surgery.

Allopathic medicine is heavily focused on diseases and the symptoms of disease as the targets or focal points of therapeutic strategies. In the allopathic tradition, diseases tend to take on a life of their own. They're often viewed in an externalized way, as foreign entities or invaders, almost separate somehow from the person who is suffering with the disease.

Another key feature of allopathic medicine is its reliance on standardized or "one-size-fits-all" therapeutic protocols. Unlike many therapeutic approaches, drug and surgical treatments can be easily standardized. For instance, let's say an allopathic practitioner sees a patient with depression and prescribes a medication like Prozac. Then let's say this practitioner sees a patient with high blood pressure and prescribes a vasodilator drug, and a third patient with colitis for whom he or she prescribes corticosteroid drugs.

Now let's imagine that lots of other patients with these same kinds of clinical problems consult with this practitioner. The likelihood is very high that this clinician will continue to prescribe the very same kind of remedies, over and over again, to anyone who presents with a given set of symptoms. That's the meaning of standardization.

From a conceptual standpoint, alternative medicine, or holistic medicine, is the opposite of allopathic medicine. Alternative medicine is patient centered rather than disease centered. It tends to de-emphasize the significance of specific diseases, while focusing instead on lifestyle considerations and the constitutional strengths and weaknesses of the individual (the "host").

Allopathic and alternative health practitioners have engaged in competitive struggles for many years. Each side has long distrusted and ridiculed the other's philosophies and clinical capabilities. Alternative clinicians generally view the treatment methods of allopaths as harsh, risky, and ineffective, while allopaths tend to regard alternative practitioners as unfocused, poorly trained, and unscientific.

In the 1800s, before the advent of drugs and breakthroughs in surgical technology, allopathic physicians relied primarily on bloodletting and the administration of toxic minerals like mercury. Then, as now, allopaths had a distinct "battlefield" mentality. They believed that the causative agents of disease were discrete entities that could be targeted and destroyed with the right therapeutic "weaponry."

Meanwhile, herbalists, homeopaths, chiropractors, and other holistic or alternative practitioners maintained a strong belief in subtle, natural, noninvasive treatments—remedies designed to support the body's innate ability to regulate and heal itself.

Unlike allopaths, alternative healers tend not to view diseases as external threats or in simple, clear-cut, cause-and-effect terms. Rather, they see human illness in more complex, multidimensional terms, i.e., they believe that any given health disorder is attributable to a variety or constellation of factors.

OPPOSING PARADIGMS

ALLOPATHIC MODEL	HOLISTIC MODEL
provides the basis of conventional or orthodox medicine	provides the basis of alternative medicine
disease oriented	patient centered
tends to utilize aggressive, technology based treatments, primarily drugs and surgery	utilizes subtle, nontoxic, natural, noninvasive therapies
emphasis on standardized therapeutic protocols	attempts to tailor treatments to individualized needs of patients
most effective for acute health problems	most effective for chronic degenerative illness
tends to focus on single agent causes of disease, e.g., a malfunctioning gene, an infectious microbe	tends to view diseases as "multifactorial," i.e., attributable to a broad range of environmental influences that weaken the body
standardized procedures and patentable drugs provide strong foundation for the growth of heavily institutionalized, heavily regulated, highly successful global industries	wide variety of alternative modalities provide basis for a very diverse, decentralized, deregulated industry, with very limited economic and political strength

On the surface, these two approaches to medicine seem to differ radically, not only on fundamental issues, but in every imaginable way. And in many ways they certainly do, at least in theory. But in reality, a large majority of today's alternative clinicians are actually practicing allopathically, because they are:

1. treating at the symptom level
2. prescribing standardized remedies

Here's an example. If you have insomnia and you go visit a conventional physician, you're likely to get a drug prescription, maybe for an antidepressant or a barbituate. Yet if you go see an alternative practitioner, you're also likely to get a standard insomnia remedy, except in a different form—maybe magnesium or vitamin B_6.

Let's say you have allergies. A conventional doctor would probably give you an antihistamine. But an alternative clinician is just as likely to prescribe a standard allergy remedy of one kind or another—whether it's an herb or a vitamin or a homeopathic remedy. Or, if you have a headache, the tendency among clinicians, whether conventional or alternative, is to rely on some kind of standard "headache remedy."

But this approach simply substitutes natural remedies for drugs—it matches vitamins to symptoms rather than matching drugs to symptoms.

This phenomenon, known as "drug substitution," is also very evident in countless self-help books on alternative medicine. Many of these books are organized, alphabetically, by disease categories: allergies, arthritis, bronchitis, colds, diabetes, influenza, irritable bowel, psoriasis, and so on. Then they list, in reference-book fashion, various natural remedies that people can try when specific symptoms or diseases emerge.

But chronic illness can never be effectively resolved at the symptom level with standardized remedies of any kind.

Most drugs are used for the purpose of suppressing symptoms by inhibiting certain types of chemical reactions within the body. They work by binding to chemical targets known as cellular receptors. One of the chief limitations of drugs currently on the market is that they don't have high enough levels of specificity. In other words, they often interact with more chemical targets than they should, which is why they cause unwanted side effects. And of course drugs are not designed to facilitate the body's innate healing response.

On the other hand, natural remedies like vitamins and herbs do have the capacity to strengthen and support the organs and glands, and thereby enhance the body's own natural regulatory and regenerative processes. Unlike synthetic drug products, natural remedies are biologically compatible, which means that the body can recognize them, break them down, and effectively utilize them. And since they're not foreign chemicals, the liver and other organs of detoxification don't have to work overtime to try to clear them out of the body.

So there's no question that natural remedies can be very beneficial. They're certainly capable of working beyond the symptomatic level to correct chronic health problems. But there's a major problem with the way natural remedies are currently applied.

The problem is that alternative medicine, like conventional medicine, lacks the technology necessary to effectively analyze and resolve the biochemical imbalances that are the underlying causes of chronic illness.

This is the reason people like Sarah Hennessey wander around for years, bouncing from one clinician to the next, unable to find the level of help they really need. Her plight is typical of the plight endured by millions of health consumers.

Many alternative practitioners are every bit as frustrated as patients like Sarah. They'd like to be able to get to the root of people's chronic health disorders, but they don't know how. They'd like to be able to conduct their practices based on the "holistic" paradigm, but in reality they're stuck in an allopathic rut.

Why? Because all chronic diseases have one thing in common: They involve an imbalance in the fundamental homeostatic control mechanisms. These mechanisms regulate all the biochemical reactions taking place in the body at any given moment.

Most clinicians simply lack the knowledge and the tools necessary to address health disorders at this deep a level—the causative level of all chronic illness.

Throughout this book we'll be learning a great deal about the fundamental homeostatic control mechanisms and the very decisive role they play in your health and well-being.

As you may recall from the previous chapter, metabolic typing gives clinicians a reliable way of evaluating and correcting any biochemical imbalances that exist within these essential regulatory mechanisms.

This means that metabolic typing, unlike conventional or alternative medical modalities, has the unique ability to address disease processes at their point of origin.

Homeostasis is what enables every living organism to maintain a normal, healthy equilibrium. It's a powerful and somewhat inexplicable force of nature, an innate biological intelligence that never stops striving to preserve the metabolic integrity of a living system, or to reestablish balance in the event that balance is lost or compromised as a result of physical or chemical disruptions.

In the human body, homeostasis is maintained at every level through the precise orchestration of an infinite variety of biochemical reactions.

Your body's ability to maintain normal blood sugar levels or a normal body temperature or a normal heart rate are examples of homeostasis at work at the systemic level. Your cells' ability to efficiently transport food and oxygen and waste material back and forth across your cell membranes represents homeostasis at the cellular level.

Because of the overwhelming number of biochemical reactions that take place in your body, it would be impossible for clinicians to track them all, much less manage them, in an effort to influence your health.

Fortunately, all biochemical reactions fall under the control of a small handful of regulatory mechanisms—again, the fundamental homeostatic control mechanisms.

Over the years, as metabolic typing has evolved, we have learned a great deal about how these regulatory mechanisms work, how they influence human health and disease, and the many ways in which they're affected by diet and nutrition. We'll get into these topics in detail in subsequent chapters, but for now, here are several key points to keep in mind:

1. *Metabolic typing addresses chronic health problems at the causative level.*
Metabolic typing represents a profound new paradigm shift away from the allopathic medical tradition because it completely bypasses symptoms and standardized therapeutic approaches. It's an advanced nutritional technology that enables clinicians to address chronic ailments on a much deeper level than ever before.

2. *Metabolic typing can be used to prevent illness or repair and rebuild health.*
In its simplest form, metabolic typing provides health consumers with a quick-and-easy method for preventing illness and optimizing their health by tailoring diets to their own unique body chemistry. In its most advanced form, metabolic typing enables clinicians to create in-depth nutritional protocols that are highly patient-specific, for the purpose of restoring the health of people with all manner of chronic ills.

3. *Metabolic typing is highly effective because it balances total body chemistry.*
Unlike most therapeutic approaches, which offer piecemeal solutions by matching remedies to symptoms, metabolic typing resolves health problems in a uniquely comprehensive way. It does this by correcting imbalances within the small number of regulatory mechanisms that manage the vast number of biochemical reactions taking place within the body. Thus, metabolic typing has the ability to address a wide range of physiological problems all at once.

4. *Metabolic typing provides uniquely long-lasting health benefits.*
When chronic health problems are addressed in a symptom-oriented or piecemeal fashion, patients often experience temporary relief. However, the problems never really go away. They frequently shift to other parts of the body or recur before too long. In contrast, metabolic typing can be used to produce enduring health benefits. Rather than sweeping health disorders "under the rug," it is designed

to resolve them completely, by targeting them at the causative level, in a comprehensive manner.

Building Health vs. Treating Disease

As a health consumer, have you ever stopped to consider where your ideas about health and medicine come from? How your medical/scientific knowledge has been shaped? Why you make particular choices with respect to your own or your family's health care?

Most of us have been exposed to an extraordinary degree of "programming" or "conditioning" from a very early age, especially in the modern media culture, where hardly a day goes by when we're not bombarded with messages and information that strongly reinforce prevailing scientific wisdom.

Just think of the huge volume of health-related data that filters into your consciousness from every conceivable direction—from

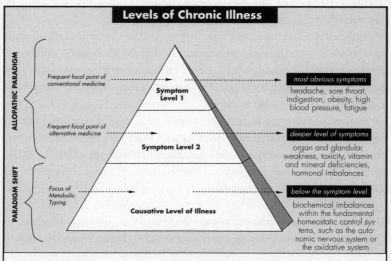

Levels of Chronic Illness

ALLOPATHIC PARADIGM

PARADIGM SHIFT

Frequent focal point of conventional medicine

Symptom Level 1

most obvious symptoms
headache, sore throat, indigestion, obesity, high blood pressure, fatigue

Frequent focal point of alternative medicine

Symptom Level 2

deeper level of symptoms
organ and glandular weakness, toxicity, vitamin and mineral deficiencies, hormonal imbalances

Focus of Metabolic Typing

Causative Level of Illness

below the symptom level
biochemical imbalances within the fundamental homeostatic control systems, such as the autonomic nervous system or the oxidative system

Unlike conventional and alternative approaches to health care, metabolic typing is an advanced nutritional technology that enables clinicians to evaluate and resolve chronic health disorders at their *point of origin*.

newspapers, magazines, books, television and radio news broadcasts, even the perennially popular TV medical dramas.

Over and over we witness extraordinary feats on the part of the medical establishment. Remarkable new inventions: lasers, 3-D scanning devices, computerized diagnostic equipment, and all manner of technological wizardry. People being pulled from catastrophic situations, back from the brink of death, routinely, thanks to fast and effective medical detective work and heroic medical and surgical maneuvers.

This steady stream of words and images creates a very strong impression of modern medicine as a kind of omniscient force, one that has radically improved the quality of life on earth in ways far too numerous and complex for the average person to even begin to comprehend fully.

It's hard not to be impressed with, and thankful for, all that modern medicine has to offer. Yet as health consumers it's often difficult to think for ourselves, to question the judgment of medical authorities, to make decisions that fall outside the bounds of commonly accepted belief systems. At the same time, it's easy to take things for granted, to operate on assumptions, to act reflexively, in a kind of "automatic pilot" mode.

But, as you will see, metabolic typing poses powerful challenges to a great many ideas and assumptions that we as health consumers have somehow adopted, whether consciously or otherwise. Here's just one very basic example: What if I were to ask you to define the meaning of the phrase "good health"?

You may be the most intelligent, well-read, highly educated person in your town, but if you're like ninety-five percent of the health-consumer population, you won't be able to answer the question accurately. Why? Because you've been conditioned all your life with certain kinds of prescribed beliefs or misconceptions about health and disease.

The truth is, most people don't understand the real meaning of good health simply because they've never experienced it. They assume they're in good health as long as they have an absence of disease or an absence of symptoms.

Chronic ailments and substandard levels of health are now so pervasive in our society that most people can't even imagine what it's like to experience robust good health. They've grown very accustomed to functioning below par. They don't know what really good health feels like, and they don't see other people experiencing it. It's simply not part of the societal context in which we live; it's outside our frame of reference.

True good health is *not* a condition that is merely free of adverse symptoms. It's a state of *dynamic well-being*, one that is reminiscent of childhood exuberance and joy. When your body is functioning the way it's designed to function, you should be experiencing boundless energy all the time, a keen awareness of your surroundings, a very strong and positive emotional state, and a natural love and zest for life.

This is very different from most people's experience, which is one of moving through life in a kind of mechanical, often sluggish way, feeling "okay" in between intermittent bouts of colds, headaches, the flu, ennui, and various kinds of aches and pains—that very deficient condition that everyone in modern society has come to think of as normal.

Here's another common misconception I encounter all the time: People automatically assume that age equals infirmity. They're convinced that decline and deterioration are an inevitable part of growing older, and it's very difficult to change their minds on this point. They look around and see the physical breakdowns and diseases that correlate with advancing age in our culture, and they just accept without question that this is the way nature intended things to be.

Yet there's a wealth of evidence to the contrary. Plenty of people in remote cultures are very active and vigorous and able to work and enjoy life to the age of one hundred and beyond. In some cultures it's not unusual for men to father children when they are in their eighties and nineties, and for women to have menopause very late in life. These people simply don't have debilitating senility and arthritis and cancer. When they finally pass away, at very advanced ages, they die of natural causes, not slow degeneration.

When we in modern society see and hear the stories of cultures like these, our first reaction is to attribute these people's remarkable health and longevity to "genes" and "heredity." In other words, we assume that they're built for health and longevity, and we're not. But this is illogical on many levels. Besides, studies show that when long-lived people in isolated cultures relocate and give up their healthful lifestyles, they, too, fall prey to degenerative illness and premature death, just like the rest of us.

The bottom line is, it's not normal to experience progressive physical degeneration as you age. If it seems normal to you, it's only because you're conditioned to think that way. It's your experience and it's what you've come to expect and anticipate. If you're sixty, there's no reason to assume that you should have to endure a dozen more ailments than you had at forty or fifty, or twice as many problems as you had at thirty. In reality, even one chronic ailment is one too many, whether you're twenty-five or fifty-five or eighty-five.

But of all the conditioned thought patterns people exhibit, none is quite as interesting or revealing as a phenomenon I like to call "disease consciousness," or the "allopathic mind-set." I see this constantly with people who are new to metabolic typing.

When people contact my company for the first time to obtain a metabolic profile, or make an initial visit to one of the clinicians for whom I provide metabolic typing services, they almost always come with a very predictable and prescribed set of expectations as to what they came for and how things should proceed.

Of course, on one level they think they're seeking advanced nutritional consulting services, or, where clinicians are involved, "cutting edge" alternative medicine. But what they don't realize is the extent to which their words and actions are actually driven by very conventional medical thinking.

Here's why: Almost every person I meet for the first time is very intently focused on discussing his or her health in terms of the symptoms he or she is experiencing. People expect that we will gather this information, analyze it, and then proceed to offer up a specific diagnosis, and next, provide them with a treatment plan based on the diagnosis. This is always the sequence and the elements they're interested in:

1. symptoms
2. diagnosis
3. treatment

People never fail to be taken aback, even shocked, when I explain that I'm not especially interested in their symptomatic history, and that I have no intention of attempting to "diagnose" or "treat" their condition, whatever it might be. This is true of the clinicians who provide metabolic typing as well.

In fact, the terms "symptom" and "diagnosis" and "treatment" are not even a part of the metabolic typing lexicon. Those of us who provide metabolic typing services use these terms occasionally, but only in reference to other kinds of nutritional and therapeutic approaches, not in reference to ours.

Remember Sarah Hennessey, the chemically sensitive EI patient we've been discussing in this chapter? Sarah was very typical of people new to metabolic typing. At first, her natural inclination was to focus my attention on a list of her symptoms, which in her case happened to be a long one.

She just assumed that an analysis of her symptoms was the logical first step in solving the riddle of her illness, or in characterizing the disease that held her in its grip. In other words, even Sarah, who was a very savvy consumer in the realm of alternative medicine, had a very distinct "disease consciousness" and "allopathic mind-set."

Even she had a hard time letting go of the symptom-disease-treatment orientation. This was, after all, the clinical methodology she'd been taught by scores of health professionals over the course of her fifteen-year odyssey.

So I told Sarah the very same thing I tell everyone who contacts me for a metabolic profile, whether they have allergies or headaches or arthritis or EI or cardiovascular disease or cancer or diabetes or any other kind of chronic health problem.

I explained that metabolic typing is very different from other clinical approaches in many ways, but the most fundamental difference is this:

Metabolic typing is not a diagnostic technology. It's not designed to identify or categorize or "treat" specific kinds of symptoms or health disorders or full-blown diseases. It cannot be used to "treat" anything. It can be used only to build health from the ground up, in a nonspecific way. This is essential to its clinical effectiveness.

The concept of metabolic typing as a health-building technology, as opposed to a disease-treatment technology, sounds simple at first. And in some ways it is. But at the same time, it's a concept so completely foreign to the way we've been conditioned all our lives that it actually takes quite a while for people to comprehend fully.

But here's a good analogy that simplifies this concept considerably: Say you rented a new apartment, a nice big space in a neighborhood you like very much. You got a great deal on the apartment and it has a lot going for it, except for one thing—because it's so big and because of the way it's situated, it's a very dark apartment.

Before you can move in, you'll need to solve this problem. What do you do? Well, you don't stand around and analyze the darkness, you don't curse the darkness, you don't attempt to use magic spells or incantations to vanquish the darkness. In fact, you ignore the darkness. Instead, you go out and buy lots of lamps and set them up in strategic locations. Or you call in an electrician and have him install light fixtures.

By bringing in the light, the darkness just naturally fades away. That's the way it is with your body. To conquer chronic illness, you need to focus all your attention on building health, on implementing health, on installing health. Once good health takes hold in your body, disease can no longer occupy the same space, and illness just naturally fades away.

So the logical question then becomes: How does one go about building health? The first step is to think about the way in which the human body is structured.

The body is organized in a hierarchical fashion. Beginning from the broadest level and moving to the subtlest (or most specific) level, it's comprised of seven basic levels:

1. systemic level (e.g., immune system)
2. organ/glandular level (e.g., thymus gland)
3. tissue level (e.g., membranes, blood)
4. cellular level (e.g., thymus cells, T-cells)
5. nuclear level (nucleus of cell)
6. subnuclear level (chromosomes)
7. genetic level (genes)

Any bodily system (cardiovascular, digestive, immune) is comprised of various organs and glands. These organs and glands are in turn made up of numerous cells of like kind. Here's why this is significant:

> *The efficiency of any system is dependent upon the efficiency of each of its organs and glands, each of which in turn is dependent upon the efficiency of its cells. The cells in turn are dependent upon their capacity for energy production in order to carry out their assigned roles.*

As you may recall from the preceding chapter, your cells can carry out their assigned role in an efficient manner only if they obtain the right "fuel mixture," or the right combination of nutritional substances.

Let's use Sarah's case to illustrate this concept. Since she's suffering with environmental illness (EI), we know that she has a malfunctioning immune system.

But in order for Sarah's immune system to work properly, she's going to need an efficiently functioning thymus gland. In turn, if her thymus gland is going to function correctly, her thymus cells must function properly. And in order for Sarah's thymus cells to function in the right way, to carry out their assigned role in maintaining her systemic immunity, they will first need to generate sufficient energy.

Finally, in order for each of the cells in Sarah's thymus gland to produce an optimum amount of energy, they will need to successfully and completely carry out all the steps involved in cellular oxidation (see illustration on page 19). To achieve this, each of her thymus cells will require the right fuel mixture, or the right balance of nutrients.

So the bottom line is this: *The efficiency of Sarah's immune system is highly dependent on the presence of the proper biochemical or nutritional balance.* But let's not forget that each person has his or her own unique, genetically inherited requirements for nutrition.

In other words, a diet that would support the optimum functioning of Sarah's immune system might have no effect on someone else's immune system, and might in fact retard the immune efficiency of a third person.

As we will see in the section that follows, Sarah didn't need any more "disease treatment." She had spent fifteen years on an intensely concentrated search, seeking out some of the very best "disease treat-ment" available anywhere in the country. She spent vast sums of money and tried countless different therapeutic approaches. None of them worked.

What she needed was a health-building technology—a system that would not only restore integrity and balance within her immune system, but would also do the same for every system, organ, gland, tissue, and cell in her body.

The New Frontier in Foundational Nutrition

All the trillions of cells in your body are like tiny computers pro-grammed to carry out two interrelated, highly specific functions: maintain optimum health at all costs, and work to restore it in the event that it's harmed or weakened in any way.

The genetic material contained in each cell is analogous to an ele-gantly designed computer software program. Genes carry the coded instructions that manage all the physiological activity taking place in your body—including, on a very fundamental level, the care and feeding of each of your cells.

As a result, your cells are "wired" to run perfectly at all times. Like a computerized telephone redial program, the cells are built to perform their assigned tasks in a totally automated and repetitive fashion. They strive continually and relentlessly toward optimum productivity and performance on your behalf.

But before they can fulfill their designated functions, your cells require specific raw materials. Just as a computer program can't be expected to work properly unless the computer operator is familiar with the program and knows how to enter the right commands and follow a specific protocol, your cells can't be expected to function properly with-out the right biochemical input. That's why good health remains out of reach for so many people, even those who pursue a healthful lifestyle.

You might eat all the best and highest-quality organic food, exercise regularly, drink plenty of fluids, get sufficient rest and take the finest supplements money can buy, but you're still not going to feel well or

METABOLIC TYPING
A HEALTH-BUILDING TECHNOLOGY

The Immune System

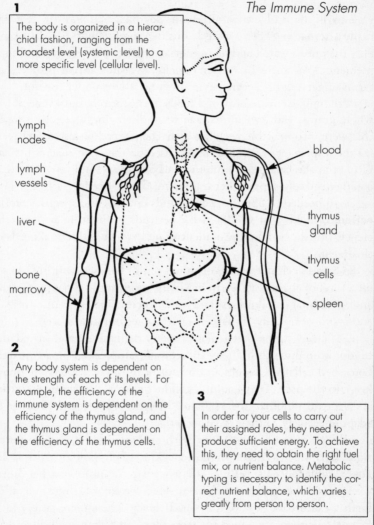

1

The body is organized in a hierarchial fashion, ranging from the broadest level (systemic level) to a more specific level (cellular level).

lymph nodes

lymph vessels

liver

bone marrow

blood

thymus gland

thymus cells

spleen

2

Any body system is dependent on the strength of each of its levels. For example, the efficiency of the immune system is dependent on the efficiency of the thymus gland, and the thymus gland is dependent on the efficiency of the thymus cells.

3

In order for your cells to carry out their assigned roles, they need to produce sufficient energy. To achieve this, they need to obtain the right fuel mix, or nutrient balance. Metabolic typing is necessary to identify the correct nutrient balance, which varies greatly from person to person.

Unlike conventional medicine, metabolic typing is not designed to "treat" any specific symptoms or diseases. Instead, it's designed to build health, from the cellular level on up, in a nonspecific way.

enjoy optimum health unless you regularly obtain the nutrient balance
that's right for you.

This is the problem Sarah Hennessey had. She was eating what many alternative experts would consider an excellent diet, drinking only the purest water, and taking lots of high-quality nutritional supplements. Yet she still couldn't make any substantive progress in terms of getting her severe environmental illness under control.

Although Sarah ate healthful foods in the form of fresh vegetables, whole grains, and lean meats, she was unknowingly selecting foods that were incompatible with her body chemistry. She also didn't realize the importance of eating meals based on the right macronutrient ratio (i.e., the balance of proteins, carbohydrates, and fats), one that could effectively support her unique metabolic needs.

Sarah needed to obtain specific kinds of foods and specific combinations of foods that would enable her cells to function at peak efficiency. But she had no way of identifying her own individual needs in this regard.

So Sarah's cellular metabolism fell out of balance, and in turn set off a kind of chain reaction in her body, resulting in a range of organ and glandular weaknesses and deficiencies and systemic imbalances—most notably, imbalances within her immune system.

Like a car engine that is not properly maintained and fueled and cannot keep up with high-speed freeway traffic, Sarah's inadequately nourished cells and tissues and organs of immunity could no longer keep up the pace. They couldn't conduct normal metabolic activities and in turn mobilize the kinds of defenses people need in order to adapt effectively to their environments.

Like all patients who suffer with chronic disease, Sarah's nutritional deficiencies had set in motion a kind of physiological catch-22. For example, once her cellular efficiency was compromised, her digestive capabilities were weakened. Her weakened digestion then further exacerbated the cellular inefficiency. These increasingly inefficient cells then continued to create more problems, including ever-worsening digestive capabilities.

It's very common for people to get stuck in this kind of downward spiral, with biochemical imbalances and systemic deficiencies multi-

THE DECLINE OF HEALTH

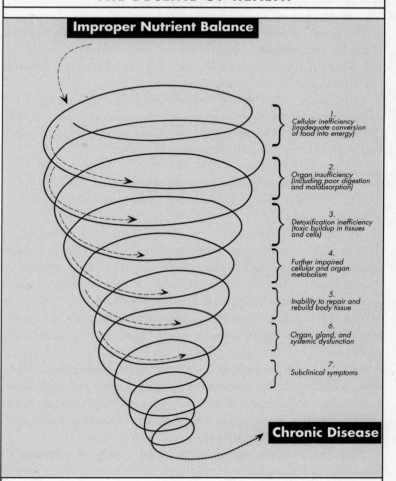

Improper Nutrient Balance

1.
Cellular inefficiency
(inadequate conversion
of food into energy)

2.
Organ insufficiency
(including poor digestion
and malabsorption)

3.
Detoxification inefficiency
(toxic buildup in tissues
and cells)

4.
Further impaired
cellular and organ
metabolism

5.
Inability to repair and
rebuild body tissue

6.
Organ, gland, and
systemic dysfunction

7.
Subclinical symptoms

Chronic Disease

A failure to obtain the kinds of foods and combinations of foods that are appropriate to your metabolic type leads to cellular inefficiency. This triggers a downward spiral, i.e., a whole cascade of biochemical events that lead to weaknesses and deficiencies throughout the body, and ultimately, to chronic disease.

plying and intensifying over time. The only truly effective way to stop the degenerative process and restore health is to start consuming a metabolically appropriate diet.

Of course, the first step is to identify the appropriate diet—which is exactly what we did for Sarah. But to do so we needed to look well beyond her symptoms and explore one very crucial question: What is her body's style of functioning?

Or, in other words, how is her body designed to process foods and utilize nutrients? Another way to ask this same question is simply "What is Sarah's metabolic type?" Or "What imbalances exist within Sarah's fundamental homeostatic controls?"

A person's metabolic type, or "style of functioning," is defined by the imbalances that exist within his or her fundamental homeostatic control mechanisms.

The answers to these questions would tell us what kinds of foods and nutrients Sarah would need to build her health from the cellular level on up. In this way we could do much more than recommend nutritional remedies designed to alleviate symptoms.

Instead, we would know how to provide Sarah with a strong nutritional foundation her body could use to regulate and rebalance and rebuild itself.

Only in this way would she finally be able to move beyond piecemeal solutions to find meaningful, comprehensive nutritional support for her weakened and debilitated body. With a metabolically appropriate diet, she could, at long last, turn the process of degeneration into a process of regeneration.

To find the answers we needed, we used a survey that enabled us to collect all kinds of data pertaining to Sarah's physical, structural, emotional, psychological, and behavioral characteristics—her "metabolic characteristics." All this information constitutes a form of "body language" that has nothing to do with symptoms, but instead reveals a great deal about a person's metabolic individuality or style of functioning.

Since Sarah had a serious chronic ailment, we asked her to complete a very extensive metabolic survey comprised of over three thousand questions. Her responses showed that she had imbalances in three of the nine fundamental homeostatic controls.

Here's a brief summary of the specific roles these regulatory mechanisms play in maintaining health:

FUNDAMENTAL HOMEOSTATIC CONTROLS

HOMEOSTATIC MECHANISM	FUNCTION
oxidative system	intracellular energy conversion
autonomic nervous system	master regulator of metabolism
catabolic/anabolic balance	intracellular oxygen metabolism
endocrine type	influences food selection relative to weight control
acid/alkaline balance	reflects homeostasis through pH
prostaglandin balance	regulates inflammatory and immune responses
constitutional type	links constitutional elements of foods with metabolism
electrolyte balance	regulates circulation and osmotic pressure
blood type	basis for blood type-specific food reactivities

All chronic diseases have one thing in common: They involve an imbalance in one or more of the fundamental homeostatic control mechanisms. These mechanisms regulate all the biochemical reactions taking place in the body at any given moment. Metabolic typing is used to uncover and correct imbalances in these regulatory mechanisms.

Our survey and some additional tests (including a hair analysis) indicated that Sarah had a range of problems—including pH and electrolyte imbalances, a fairly high level of mercury toxicity, an underactive thyroid, a systemic candida infection, and some potential additional toxicity and parasitic problems.

However, the most significant finding by far was a pronounced imbalance in Sarah's oxidative system.

The oxidative system, along with the autonomic nervous system, plays a very central role in managing the body's metabolic activities and, in turn, in maintaining health. It is these two systems more than any other that determine a person's dietary requirements.

We found that Sarah was a fast oxidizer, which refers to the relative speed at which her cells metabolize carbohydrates into energy.

Energy conversion at the cellular level is a multistep process that requires specific nutrients at each step along the way. These requirements vary greatly, in accordance with a person's oxidative rate— whether he is a fast oxidizer, a slow oxidizer, or a mixed oxidizer.

Among other things, fast oxidizers need to obtain increased amounts of protein and fat at every meal. They don't do well on meals high in carbohydrates. Since carbohydrates burn quickly, they can't offer the kind of sustained energy fast oxidizers require.

Sarah never realized she was a fast oxidizer. Though she ate some protein and fat, she wasn't getting nearly enough of these vital macronutrients, and she wasn't eating them in the proportions that make sense for someone with her metabolic style of functioning. Instead, she'd spent years on a diet more appropriate for a slow oxidizer—a diet high in carbohydrates like pastas, grains, and vegetables.

We immediately switched Sarah to a diet appropriate for her metabolic type, one that included liberal amounts of proteins such as red meat, poultry, fish, and eggs.

Unlike slow oxidizers, fast oxidizers can't get sufficient sustenance from lean proteins. They need to emphasize the heavier and fattier proteins, including a specific category of proteins called high-purine proteins.

Purine-rich proteins are an important source of energy for fast oxidizers. They include organ meats and foods such as wild game, anchovies, caviar, sardines, mussels, and herring.

Due to widespread misconceptions about cholesterol, high-purine proteins have long been regarded as unhealthful. But this simply isn't true. For certain metabolic types, high-purine proteins are essential. In fact, they've been a vitally important dietary component in many cultures throughout the world for centuries.

After just a few days on the fast oxidizer diet, Sarah noticed a dramatic improvement in the way she felt. And as the days turned into weeks and then into months, she was very surprised to find herself feeling well on an ongoing basis.

Since chronic illnesses are multifactorial, and since Sarah's problems were severe and of long duration, her dietary shift was not the total solution. She needed to pursue other lifestyle modifications as well, including the avoidance or removal of certain kinds of environmental challenges, various kinds of detoxification measures designed to rid her cells and tissues of accumulated toxins, and nutrient supplementation that could effectively compensate for her unique metabolic imbalances.

Nonetheless, the dietary shift was by far the most important element in Sarah's recovery. Just by eating the right foods in the right proportions at each meal, she immediately regained an enormous amount of strength and energy and motivation. Her chronic depression lifted, and many of her chemical sensitivities and aches and pains subsided.

Sarah was soon able to function at a much higher level than she had in many years. She quickly began to let go of her perception of herself as a housebound victim, a hopeless case, a permanently disabled "patient." At long last, she was actually able to look forward to getting out of bed in the morning, as opposed to thinking of each new day as little more than a painful endurance contest. Within weeks she was even enthusiastically planning what had been unthinkable for well over a decade—a return to the workforce.

The improvement in Sarah's health is very typical of the kinds of improvements we see all the time in people with many different kinds of degenerative illness. It's always amazing to observe what the body is capable of achieving once it starts getting what it needs, once people begin eating according to their metabolic type. Though it's not so amazing when you consider that there's no greater influence on your health than the food you eat several times a day, every single day of your life. That's why it's essential for all of us to heed the ancient adage recommending that we regard food as medicine and choose it wisely, taking care not to make it our poison instead.

It's equally important for you to understand exactly how and why Sarah's recovery came about. It certainly was not by accident. When allopathic nutrition is used, people can and do recover from chronic ailments. But allopathic nutrition is a shot in the dark, a game of roulette. When people get better it's the luck of the draw, not the result of a rational, predictable therapeutic strategy.

So, of course, we did not use allopathic nutrition. Instead, we used metabolic typing to evaluate the real essence of Sarah's physiological problems. Then, to resolve these problems, we used *customized nutrition*, an approach I also like to refer to as *foundational nutrition*. This is exactly what its name implies—a way of giving people the building blocks their bodies need to resolve whatever problems may arise.

Foundational nutrition represents a major breakthrough in medical science because it gives clinicians, for the very first time, extraordinary power and flexibility in terms of addressing chronic health disorders at the causative level. Using Sarah's situation as an example once again, let me briefly explain why this is true.

As you know, Sarah's biggest problem was an imbalance in her oxidative system, one of two primary systems that determine how nutrients behave in the body. But oxidative imbalances are not associated with EI per se, or any other specific disease. Someone else with the very same type of oxidative imbalance as Sarah's could develop an entirely different illness—arthritis, diabetes, colitis, cardiovascular problems, or anything at all.

A given metabolic imbalance can manifest in any number of ways, in any number of different disease states or degenerative processes.

We don't know precisely why the very same kind of metabolic imbalances can cause different kinds of symptoms or disease states in different people. There might be any number of reasons—genetic or environmental factors, or combinations of the two.

What's far more important is that we have the technology that allows us to get to the root of people's unique metabolic imbal-

ances, whether it's a single imbalance or a whole constellation of
imbalances that underlie whatever an individual's health disorder
happens to be.

In the next chapter I'll explain the core principle of metabolic typing and related core principles in greater detail. Through clinical
examples, you'll learn why these concepts hold many profound implications for health consumers and health care professionals alike—and
why we are all poised at the edge of a very exciting and unprecedented new era in science and medicine.

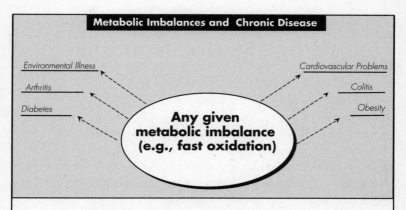

Metabolic Imbalances and Chronic Disease

Environmental Illness

Arthritis

Diabetes

Any given metabolic imbalance (e.g., fast oxidation)

Cardiovascular Problems

Colitis

Obesity

A single type of fundamental homeostatic control imbalance can be a primary
factor in the development of many different types of disease states or degenerative processes in different people. This is a key reason why customized
nutrition or foundational nutrition is far more effective than standardized or
allopathic therapeutic approaches in addressing chronic disease.

Chapter 4

A REVOLUTION IN PATIENT-SPECIFIC NUTRITION

The Hidden Source of Illness

Imagine that you have an apple tree in your backyard that is show-ing signs of illness. Even though it's not autumn, many of the leaves have started to turn brown and fall off. The fruit is not devel-oping properly, and the tree trunk is brittle and lifeless. Perhaps you've noticed that the apple tree has been deteriorating slowly, over the course of many months.

Although you've examined the tree closely, you can't find any indication of what might be wrong. It gets plenty of sunlight and water, and there's no evidence of bugs or microbes or molds. In fact, there does not appear to be any unhealthy environmental influence of any kind, and other trees in your neighborhood are just fine. You're perplexed, so you decide to call in a tree specialist for a consultation.

When the tree expert arrives to evaluate the situation, he studies the tree, scratches his head, and mulls over the problem at some length. But much to your disappointment, it soon becomes clear that he has no readily available diagnosis. Nonetheless, he comes up with a rather unusual recommendation for how to remedy the situation.

He takes out a piece of paper and writes down the name of a product. You assume he's going to send you to a garden supply store to buy something—maybe a fertilizer or bug spray of some kind. But when he hands you the slip of paper, you're more puzzled than ever, because you recognize the product as a popular brand of paint.

At first you assume you must be mistaken, so you ask the tree specialist to clarify his instructions. Much to your surprise, and chagrin, he tells you to go to an art supply store, not a garden supply store. There he wants you to buy spray paint. Green spray paint. As the tree's leaves turn brown, he wants you to paint them green, back to their original color.

It sounds like an utterly ridiculous therapeutic strategy, doesn't it? After all, it doesn't take a horticultural genius to realize that the tree is not going to get better this way, that the leaves are not the source of the problem. It would be obvious to even the most casual observer that the brown falling leaves are merely a symptom of whatever is ailing the tree, not the underlying cause of the dilemma.

Imagine you had a similar situation with ailing house plants. If your plants are drooping and the leaves are turning color or falling off, what's the first thing that comes to mind? You wouldn't attempt to prop up the dried-out, wilted stems with sticks and string, or take out cellophane tape and try to reattach the fallen leaves, would you?

Wouldn't your first inclination be to go to the source of the problem by focusing your attention on the quality of the soil your plants are growing in? Even if you had little or no experience taking care of plants, it would no doubt immediately dawn on you that there must be something wrong with the chemical makeup of your plant soil.

Somehow you'd know that intuitively, even if you'd failed botany and had zero aptitude as a gardener. No one would have to point out where the problem was originating. You wouldn't have to consult with a plant expert. You would just know.

For some reason, however, we as health consumers consistently fail to apply this same type of logic when it comes to managing our own health problems. When chronic illness strikes, our attention almost always gets stuck at one of the symptomatic levels within the body.

We become very focused on the superficial manifestations of

disease—a cough or a cold or an ache or a pain, or, at a deeper symptomatic level, a toxic liver or a weakened adrenal system or a dysfunctional thyroid gland.

The many different symptoms of illness successfully divert our
attention away from the real source of our problems—*the biochemical
imbalances that exist within one or more of the fundamental homeostatic control systems.*

This is understandable simply because we live in such a disease-
and symptom-oriented culture. And because there is still only a small
number of clinicians throughout the world who have learned to
apply the concepts of metabolic typing in their practices. Concepts
such as:

- biochemical individuality
- the importance of building health in a nonspecific way, as
opposed to treating specific diseases
- the essential roles of the autonomic, oxidative, catabolic/ana-
bolic, and other homeostatic systems in maintaining health

No one has ever taught us how or where chronic disease processes
originate, much less how they can be effectively and systematically
resolved. So the tendency among us, clinicians and health consumers
alike, is to do something akin to painting wilted leaves green each
time an ailment emerges.

Remember, if you have a problem like chronic allergies and you
take an antihistamine, or even a natural allergy remedy like vitamin
C, it's really no different from attempting to fix an ailing plant by
attending to problems with its leaves.

Similarly, if you're overweight and you take a drug like Fen-Phen
or adopt some type of generic diet that induces weight loss in an artificial way, i.e., a way that is inappropriate to your metabolic type,
you'll never succeed in resolving the real basis of your problem.

Regardless of what your problem may be—allergies or obesity or
arthritis or colitis or heart disease, or anything at all of a chronic
degenerative nature—you need to move well beyond the superficial
therapeutic strategies that are now widely employed throughout the
health care system, if you expect to regain your health.

Because, in the same way that the chemical makeup of soil is the primary determinant affecting the health of your house plants, the biochemical makeup of your body is the primary determinant that affects your health. In turn, it is the fundamental homeostatic controls that regulate all of your body's biochemical activities.

If these mechanisms are kept in balance with the right kind of nutritional regimen, you can enjoy optimum health. But, as you will see, if they're allowed to fall out of balance as a result of improper nutrition, degenerative processes are the inevitable result.

Reversing Chronic Disease

Metabolic typing provides health consumers with a simple and effective means of keeping the body's essential regulatory systems in balance.

At the same time, metabolic typing is a very powerful but user-friendly technology that enables health professionals to achieve consistent levels of clinical success by escaping the extraordinary limitations of standardized therapeutic protocols.

Here's an example: Imagine that you go to visit your family physician for a checkup. Perhaps you don't have any major aches or pains or other complaints, except that you're twenty pounds overweight, and, because you work long hours and juggle a lot of personal and professional responsibilities, you've been feeling more stress and fatigue than usual of late.

But in the process of running the standard tests, your doctor discovers that you have elevated blood pressure. As you know, this is not a particularly far-fetched scenario, given the fact that high blood pressure, or hypertension, is the most common form of cardiovascular disease (CVD) in industrialized countries, and CVD currently afflicts approximately fifty million people in the United States alone.

For a variety of reasons, you're not at all happy to hear this news. To begin with, you know that hypertension is a serious health risk, a major cause of heart attacks and strokes. Plus, you were really expecting to come away from your doctor's office with a clean bill of health. This adds a new level of complexity and stress to your life that you could certainly do without.

A TREE ANALOGY

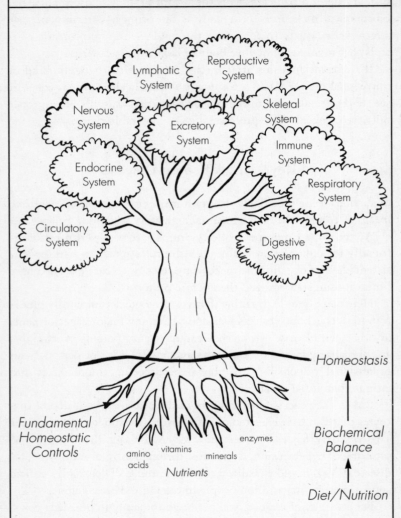

The health of a tree is largely dependent on the chemical makeup of its soil and the influence of the soil through the roots of the tree. Similarly, the health of the human body is dependent on the influence of nutrients on the fundamental homeostatic control mechanisms.

What's more, you're very dissatisfied when your doctor discusses available treatment options. Diuretics, beta-blockers, calcium channel blockers—you know people who take these drugs, so you know they have serious limitations and side effects.

You also recall seeing news reports in which researchers claimed that some hypertensive drugs are suspected of increasing people's risk of heart attack.

Furthermore, you know that many people who take hypertensive drugs end up staying on them the rest of their lives. That's definitely not something you're interested in. What you really want is to find a way to resolve your elevated blood pressure, to make it go away completely so you won't have to rely on artificial means of lowering it.

It occurs to you that if you can just find out what's causing your hypertension, then maybe some effective remedial approach will present itself. You think to yourself that you won't mind adjusting your diet or lifestyle if necessary in order to get your blood pressure back to normal. So you ask your doctor if he can identify the source of the problem.

You're surprised when he tells you that physicians are unable to pinpoint the exact cause of hypertension about ninety percent of the time. Unless it's something obvious, like a kidney malfunction, doctors believe that hypertension may be caused by any number of things—a genetic predisposition, atherosclerosis (plaque buildup inside the arteries), excess consumption of alcohol, dietary fat, salt, even exposure to environmental toxins.

But your doctor hastens to assure you not to worry. All you need to do, he says, is eat more fruits and vegetables and avoid cigarettes, red meat, and a few other questionable dietary items, in addition to taking a drug he's going to prescribe (one with a perfectly good safety profile and the most popular beta-blocker currently on the market), a drug that enjoys favored status among cardiology specialists everywhere.

He pats you on the arm and tells you that everything will be just fine, because he gives this same drug to all his hypertensive patients. When you hear that, you're not sure why, but somewhere in the back of your mind, an alarm bell goes off.

You're ambivalent because this doctor has a good reputation within your community. So you tell yourself that he must know what he's doing. On the other hand, something in your gut is telling you that there's something seriously wrong with his game plan. You leave his office that day with a very uneasy feeling.

As it turns out, your instincts are correct. Why? Well, for a number of reasons, but here are two primary ones:

- This doctor is attempting to treat a chronic ailment at the symptom level, which never works.
- He's using standardized therapeutic approaches, which overlook the importance of a patient's biochemical individuality.

Most important, the doctor is unaware of one of the cardinal principles of metabolic typing, which is simply this:

Any given disease may arise from virtually opposite biochemical imbalances in different metabolic types.

In other words, you and everybody else on your block may all have high blood pressure. You may all exhibit the exact same clinical symptoms, to the point where you can all be considered textbook cases of hypertension. But that doesn't mean you all have the same underlying physiological imbalance.

At the causative level of a chronic degenerative process, you and ten other people with almost identical cases of hypertension could each have a very different metabolic or biochemical imbalance.

My associates and I see this principle at work over and over and over again. It's important for you to understand this concept, because once you do, you'll recognize with utter clarity how futile it is for health professionals to attempt to treat chronic health disorders with standardized therapeutic approaches of any kind.

Whether you go to a conventional doctor to get a drug prescription, or an alternative physician or nutritionist and come away with a vitamin/mineral/herbal regimen, it really doesn't matter. The point is, you cannot possibly resolve a chronic ailment with a "one-size-fits-all" therapeutic protocol.

Since America leads the world in cardiovascular disease, and since it's the number-one cause of death in the United States, the clinicians

I work with encounter many people with elevated blood pressure and related problems. These include atherosclerosis, hypercholesterolemia (high cholesterol), high levels of triglycerides, cardiac arrhythmias, and blood sugar abnormalities.

When we run metabolic profiles on these people, we find different imbalances and combinations of imbalances at the root of their problems.

Of course, this principle applies to every category of chronic illness, not just cardiovascular disease. But hypertension provides an excellent case in point.

The following chart shows how a single disorder like hypertension can arise for different reasons in different individuals. In other words, any given chronic disease can be the result of virtually opposite biochemical imbalances.

As an example, let's compare and contrast two of the individuals in the chart. Subject number two, Nathan, is a man in his mid-fifties who contacted me several years ago in search of a metabolic profile and customized nutritional program.

Nathan's problems were all too typical. His blood pressure and cholesterol levels were elevated well above normal. And at five feet eight inches tall, he weighed 250 pounds, which meant he had a serious obesity problem.

His doctor had prescribed a drug (a beta-blocker) that worked to lower Nathan's blood pressure by interfering with adrenaline stimulation of the heart, thereby slowing down the heart, minimizing constriction of the arteries, and ultimately forcing less blood through his arteries.

The hypertensive drug worked fairly well in terms of keeping Nathan's blood pressure within a normal range. But it also caused a whole host of side effects: drowsiness, headaches, reduced alertness, dry mouth and skin, joint pains, and depression.

In addition, the drug was forcing Nathan's pressure down in an artificial way. And it was designed to work on only a single isolated symptom. Yet it was obvious that he had a whole constellation of cardiovascular problems, not just high blood pressure.

He was also given a generic diet to follow—a low-fat, low-cholesterol, low-protein, low-salt, low-calorie diet.

ORIGINS OF A CHRONIC DISEASE

SUBJECT	DISEASE AND RELATED SYMPTOMS	FUNDAMENTAL HOMEOSTATIC IMBALANCES						
		Autonomic		Oxidative		Catabolic/Anabolic		Electrolyte	
		Sym	Para	Fast	Slow	Catabolic	Anabolic	Excess	Deficiency
Andrew	Hypertension • obesity • elevated cholesterol	✓				✓		✓	
Nathan	Hypertension • obesity • elevated cholesterol		✓	✓			✓		
Sheila	Hypertension • diabetes	✓							
Thomas	Hypertension • elevated cholesterol			✓			✓	✓	
Michelle	Hypertension • atherosclerosis • high triglycerides		✓		✓				

This chart shows how a single disease can be caused by different types of biochemical imbalances in different people. All these people have high blood pressure and related cardiovascular disorders, i.e., virtually identical clinical disorders. Yet, in many cases, they have virtually opposite biochemical imbalances. Note that the hypertension and related conditions are not the real problems. Rather, they are symptoms of deeper problems within these people's homeostatic control systems.

But it was not long before Nathan became extremely discouraged with the drug therapy as well as with the diet. He just couldn't seem to lose any weight regardless of how closely he stuck to the bland, unappetizing food plan, and the drug's side effects were making him miserable.

To get to the real essence of Nathan's problems, we tested him with a standard survey, and found that his metabolic individuality was defined by the following:

1. parasympathetic dominance
2. fast oxidation
3. anabolic imbalance

These findings all pointed to the need for Nathan to obtain a diet high in protein and fatty acids, just the opposite of what his physician had instructed.

But unlike his doctor, we did not use his clinical symptoms as a guidepost in selecting a standardized dietary solution. Instead, we collected a lot of data from him that told us a great deal about his metabolic style of functioning.

Once he began the high-protein/high-fat diet we recommended, Nathan improved quickly. For example, over the course of just a few months, his doctor gradually cut back on the blood-pressure drug until Nathan no longer needed it at all.

Just by getting the right foods and nutrients, Nathan's blood pressure fell from 149/98 to a normal level of 124/83. Within four months his cholesterol plummeted from 346 to 195, and within a year, he shed almost eighty pounds.

In addition, Nathan experienced a tremendous increase in energy—sustained energy that enabled him to awaken feeling refreshed and renewed each morning, and to stay that way all day long. His depression and headaches and joint pains disappeared, and he was able to enjoy vigorous exercise for the first time in over two decades.

Best of all, he didn't have to follow a deprivation diet. Since metabolic-type diets don't involve caloric restriction, Nathan was able to eat normally while choosing from a wide variety of foods he really enjoyed.

Once he was on a metabolically appropriate regimen, he didn't have to endure constant hunger and food cravings. His appetite stabilized naturally as a result of his body getting the right nutrient balance. And since he was not forcing or "tricking" his body into weight loss through a generic or fad diet, when the pounds fell off, they stayed off.

All Nathan needed to do was to be aware of his genetically inherited requirement for specific kinds of foods and nutrients, and to learn how to combine or balance basic food elements in a simple but intelligent way, for meals as well as snacks.

In stark contrast to Nathan's case is that of Andrew, subject number one on the hypertension chart.

Like Nathan, Andrew is a man in his mid-fifties who came to us several years ago seeking nutritional guidance. He also suffered with obesity, and had significantly elevated blood pressure and cholesterol. In other words, his clinical symptoms were virtually identical to Nathan's.

But there was a very important difference between the two men. When we ran a metabolic analysis on Andrew, we found the following imbalances:

1. sympathetic dominance
2. catabolic imbalance
3. electrolyte excess

So, even though Andrew displayed all the same outward manifestations of illness as Nathan, the underlying biochemical imbalances that represented the source of Andrew's problems were entirely different from Nathan's. As a totally different metabolic type, Andrew required a completely different dietary protocol.

We recommended a low-fat, low-protein, high-carbohydrate diet for Andrew, along with some supplemental nutrients that would help to compensate for his metabolic imbalances. This regimen was the exact opposite of what we recommended for Nathan.

Yet Andrew's cardiovascular problems were resolved just like Nathan's. His blood pressure and cholesterol fell to normal levels quickly, and he lost almost fifty pounds over the course of a year. He too had been on a blood-pressure drug before he came to see us, but shortly after Andrew started the nutritional regimen we recommended, his doctor also decided to gradually cut back on the drug dosage until Andrew no longer needed it at all.

Those of us who utilize metabolic typing see this phenomenon at work constantly, with all forms of chronic illness.

In other words, since two people with the same clinical symptoms got better using completely opposite nutritional protocols, it's clear that symptoms can be very misleading. They're not a reliable indicator of anything.

Symptoms don't reveal anything about the real underlying nature of a person's illness, and they can't be used to determine an effective therapeutic response. That's why we need to look beyond symptoms, and focus instead on the unique biochemical origins of any given health disorder in any given individual.

Different people require different nutritional solutions. Everyone needs a nutritional solution that is tailored to his or her own biochemical individuality.

The alternative to this way of thinking results in a kind of "assembly line" approach to health care. And, as we all know, this approach is of limited clinical value where chronic illness is concerned.

So, what have we learned about metabolic typing by exploring the case histories of Nathan and Andrew? What new principles have we covered? Here's a brief synopsis:

1. *Diseases or other health disorders are never the real problems.*
The fact that many different types of imbalance can come into play and result in a single disorder such as cardiovascular disease indicates that hypertension and high cholesterol were not Nathan and Andrew's actual problems. These clinical disorders are merely the reflection, or the symptoms, of deeper metabolic problems. The real problem in each of these individuals was a lack of efficiency or a dysfunction in basic metabolic processes—such as fat metabolism, protein metabolism, or carbohydrate metabolism, to name but a few.

2. *Metabolic typing challenges conventional cause-and-effect relationships.*
Problems like atherosclerosis and elevated cholesterol are generally
considered to be causal factors in other cardiovascular problems such
as high blood pressure. But these conditions are not causes—they're
actually just symptoms of the very same biochemical imbalances that
create problems like hypertension. Similarly, elevated serum cholesterol is generally thought to be caused by excess cholesterol in the
diet. But elevated cholesterol is actually just a symptom of impaired
cholesterol metabolism, which is the result of a metabolically or
genetically inappropriate diet, not a high-fat diet. The real causes of
all these problems—hypertension, atherosclerosis, elevated cholesterol, and other related conditions—are biochemical imbalances
within the body's fundamental homeostatic control mechanisms.
These imbalances create all kinds of disturbances and inefficiencies in
protein metabolism, fat metabolism, carbohydrate metabolism, and
numerous other metabolic processes.

3. *Individualized metabolic protocols offer ideal health solutions.*
Once we provided Nathan and Andrew with the macronutrients and
micronutrients appropriate to their metabolic types, their cardiovascular and obesity problems—all part and parcel of the same underlying
metabolic imbalances—began to automatically correct themselves.
Ironically, Nathan's high-cholesterol problem was resolved only when
he added larger quantities of fat and cholesterol to his diet. That was
the approach that happened to support his particular style of functioning, his body's unique way of utilizing nutrients. It was just the opposite of what Andrew needed. This illustrates the vital importance of
eating according to one's metabolic type.

4. *A single imbalance can result in any number of diseases, and vice versa.*
Any given metabolic imbalance can manifest in any number of different disease states or degenerative processes in different people. For
example, an imbalance in the oxidative system can cause immune
dysfunction, diabetes, colitis, arthritis, cardiovascular disease—anything at all. Conversely, a single disease or health disorder, such as
high blood pressure—can be caused by different types of biochemical

imbalances in different people. For instance, Nathan and Andrew both had high blood pressure, but Nathan had an imbalance in his oxidative system, while Andrew had a significant imbalance in his autonomic nervous system. These two opposing yet complementary concepts are key principles of metabolic typing, or "flip sides" of the same coin.

5. Balancing the body's homeostatic controls has far-reaching effects.
An imbalance in just one of the fundamental homeostatic control mechanisms creates a domino effect in the body, and often leads to a whole constellation of problems and symptoms. This is the reason clinicians are frequently confronted with patients who complain of multiple, seemingly unrelated problems. In other words, people's complaints and health problems frequently do not fit into standard disease categories. Or they exist at the subclinical level, which means they cannot be detected with conventional diagnostic measures, since their problems have not yet evolved into full-blown disease states. As a result, people are told that they're fine, or that their problems are psychologically based, when in reality they have very significant health problems. Conversely, the right type of nutritional protocol can effectively resolve an entire constellation of health problems and symptoms just by correcting an imbalance in one of the fundamental homeostatic controls such as the autonomic or oxidative systems.

6. The pathways of degeneration are infinitely complex and vary greatly from person to person.
The following illustration provides a graphic synopsis of all the afore-mentioned points. The bottom line here is that chronic health problems are rooted in biochemical imbalances. These biochemical imbalances are the result of inadequate nutrition. When a person does not obtain the right balance of nutrients appropriate to his or her metabolic type, he or she cannot properly metabolize proteins, fats, or carbohydrates. Concurrently, multiple other metabolic processes go awry. This leads to any number of subclinical health problems, which gradually evolve into full-blown degenerative processes.

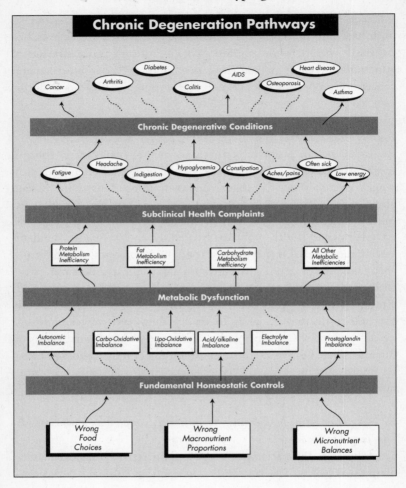

The Failure of Standardized Nutrition

In Woody Allen's futuristic film fantasy *Sleeper*, we are fast-forwarded to the year 2173. In one particularly memorable scene, two scientists are seen discussing a man who has just awakened from a two-hundred-year sleep.

One scientist tells the other that the man has requested a breakfast of "something called wheat germ, organic honey, and tiger's milk."

"Oh, yes," replies the other scientist, "those were the charmed substances that some years ago were thought to contain life-preserving properties."

"You mean, there was no deep fat, no steak or cream pie or hot fudge?" says the first scientist with extraordinary incredulity. To which his colleague replies, "Those were thought to be unhealthy, precisely the opposite of what we now know to be true." "Incredible," answers the disbelieving scientist.

Allen's satiric spoof hardly exaggerates the dramatic shifts and profound uncertainty that have come to define modern nutritional science. In fact, the only certainty in the field of nutrition is change and uncertainty itself.

Actually, the field of nutrition is not unlike the fashion industry, where everything is continually in flux, and trends come and go at fairly predictable intervals. After all, who among us is not interested in the next new and exciting food or nutrient or dietary regimen? Most people I know have more than a passing curiosity about whatever it is that's in vogue in nutritional circles at the moment.

Remember the 1980s, when macrobiotics and megadoses of vitamins and skim milk and margarine and wheatgrass juice and bone meal and brewer's yeast and bran and bee pollen and lecithin and grains and beans and polyunsaturated vegetable oils were very much the "in" thing? And red meat and butter and dairy products and high-protein diets and alcohol were very much in the "out" category?

In the '90s, lots of things changed. Phytonutrients, antioxidants, fish oils, wine, cruciferous vegetables, colloidal minerals, green tea, the "Paleolithic" diet, shark cartilage, algae, and Chinese herbs seized consumer attention and displaced other products in the spotlight. Philosophies and perspectives shifted, and vegetarianism and caloric restriction and low-cholesterol meals and high-carbohydrate diets no longer dominated as they once did.

So, what are we to make of the endless parade of new diets and food supplements that seem to come and go and fall in and out of fashion with such regularity? What is it that sparks the excitement about so many foods and nutrients? And why does the excitement inevitably wear off? Are they all just passing fads—or are they something more?

The answer lies with our own faulty perception of how foods and nutrients are supposed to work. Our expectations and perceptions about the value of these substances are fixed and absolute. We want to be able to identify foods and nutrients that can demonstrate a consistent level of therapeutic activity, regardless of who consumes them.

For example, if a particular nutrient is found to help relieve arthritic pain, we somehow expect this nutrient to have the capacity to work on anyone's arthritic pain. If it doesn't, then we assume there's something inherently deficient about this nutrient as an arthritis remedy. When we don't see a consistent, predictable clinical performance, our hopes are dashed, and we move on in search of something better, a "definitive" arthritic remedy.

The pattern is always the same: a nutritional approach or remedy emerges and looks promising for a time but ultimately disappoints. That's why so many people grow frustrated with nutritional science and often give up on it.

The problem is that we don't understand the rules of relativism that govern the activity of food and nutrients. We're unaware of a very fundamental reality, which is this:

Any given food or nutrient can have virtually opposite biochemical effects on different metabolic types.

Today there are scores of nutrition books on the market that list the beneficial effects of vitamins, minerals, trace elements, and other nutrients. Yet the information is always "nutrient specific," not "patient specific."

In other words, there's never any consideration of the concept that the behavior of a given nutrient may vary significantly from person to person. So we don't realize that the benefits of any particular nutrient do not apply to everyone. We're also unaware that nutrients can make people's health problems worse.

Nutrient-specific benefits will be seen only if a given nutrient is appropriate to a person's metabolic type. Otherwise the same nutrient will have no effect on someone's health condition, or may actually make it worse.

Here's an example: Choline, a part of the B-vitamin complex, is found in liver, egg yolks, sesame seeds, string beans, and spinach. This nutrient plays a key role in the healthy functioning of the liver, the heart, the kidneys, and the brain. It's frequently used as a remedy for conditions like hypoglycemia, asthma, hepatitis, glaucoma, high blood pressure, and hardening of the arteries.

Choline is also frequently prescribed for memory problems, and often works extremely well in improving both memory and mental acuity. However, choline slows down the rate of cellular oxidation in the human body. So, if it's given to someone with a memory problem who also happens to be a slow oxidizer, choline will not only worsen that person's memory, it will also produce depression, fatigue, and a lack of mental acuity.

All nutrients produce different biochemical reactions in different metabolic types. That's why it's vitally important for people to be evaluated and advised on the basis of their metabolic individuality. And why it can be so unproductive and even harmful when people receive generic, "one-size-fits-all" dietary and nutrient recommendations.

Unfortunately, many clinicians in practice today have no substantive ability to develop patient-specific nutritional protocols. They're generally limited to offering "shotgun" or "grab bag" solutions. That's why they get such mixed results with their treatment programs.

What exactly is "shotgun" or "grab bag" nutrition? It's a kind of standardized or formulaic therapeutic approach in which a patient receives a list of recommended nutrients—nutrients that have exhibited (usually in clinical studies) some degree of efficacy in the treatment of a given health disorder.

It's the therapeutic equivalent of directing a lot of ammunition at a target in the hope that some of it hits the bull's-eye by resolving a particular health problem.

Lots of nutrition books also list "shotgun" or "grab bag" solutions for all kinds of chronic health disorders. Some of these generic protocols are comprised mainly of vitamins, minerals, and trace elements, while others include lists of foods and herbs. The specific protocols may vary somewhat from book to book or clinician to clinician, but they're generally pretty similar.

For instance, here's a typical standardized nutritional protocol for high-serum cholesterol:

A "SHOTGUN" OR "GRAB BAG" NUTRITIONAL PROTOCOL		
HIGH SERUM CHOLESTEROL		
niacin	B complex	chromium
choline	coenzyme Q_{10}	carnitine
inositol	vitamin E	beta-carotene
vitamin C	arginine	

All the substances listed in this chart have excellent therapeutic properties or nutrient-specific characteristics.

But here's the catch: Like any nutrient, every single one of these nutrients has a very specific and precise effect on the body's fundamental homeostatic control mechanisms. In general, nutrients influence the homeostatic controls in one of the following ways:

• They either stimulate or inhibit one side or another of a control mechanism, e.g., a given nutrient might stimulate the sympathetic side of the ANS, while inhibiting the parasympathetic side.

• They produce either an alkaline or acidic effect in the body.

In subsequent chapters you'll learn more about the specific stimulatory/inhibitory or acid/alkaline influence of nutrients. But for now, it's sufficient to understand that a single nutrient can exert completely different biochemical influences on different metabolic types, even those who may exhibit identical symptoms or diseases.

This means there are all kinds of opportunities for any given nutrient to *worsen* a person's health condition by creating *new* biochemical imbalances or exacerbating existing imbalances. How a nutrient behaves depends on the underlying source of the health problem, i.e., the specific imbalance in a given homeostatic control mechanism.

In other words, nutrients simply can't be taken at face value or judged in absolute terms; they have to be evaluated in terms of the broad physiological context in which they're expected to work. They can't be expected to produce positive clinical benefits unless they're tailored to someone's unique biochemical status.

That's why it's never a good idea to toss a fistful of nutrients at a clinical problem, like throwing a handful of dirt at a wall, based on the notion that some of it is likely to stick. Yet, hard as it may be to believe, this is the clinical strategy upon which much of modern nutritional science is currently based.

Using elevated cholesterol as an example, let me briefly describe why standardized, "grab bag" nutrition is at best unreliable, and at worst ineffective and detrimental.

One of the most commonly prescribed nutrients for elevated cholesterol is niacin, also known as vitamin B_3. Niacin can be either helpful or harmful for high cholesterol, depending on the metabolic type of the person who consumes it.

For instance, niacin helps to normalize the biochemical imbalances of people who are sympathetic dominants or slow oxidizers. So, for people with high cholesterol who happen to fall into one of these categories, niacin is beneficial because it works to resolve the underlying cause of high cholesterol—dysfunctional cholesterol metabolism.

On the other hand, niacin exacerbates imbalances within the fundamental homeostatic control mechanisms of people who are parasympathetic dominants or fast oxidizers, especially in the large quantities typically recommended for elevated cholesterol. In doing so, niacin *further disrupts cholesterol metabolism in these individuals*, thereby worsening rather than improving the clinical problem it's supposed to treat.

Clinicians who utilize metabolic typing in their practice observe the variability of nutrient effects over and over, with virtually every nutrient, in virtually every chronic disease category. That's why it's impossible to apply metabolic typing for any length of time without coming to the rapid conclusion that standardized nutritional protocols are of extremely limited value.

Just as niacin behaves differently in different people, so too do all the other nutrients listed in the high-cholesterol "grab bag" chart.

A STANDARDIZED "GRAB BAG" NUTRITIONAL PROTOCOL		
OSTEOPOROSIS		
arginine	magnesium	vitamin D
boron	phosphorus	zinc
calcium	sulfur	
lysine	vitamin A	

To give you a more in-depth understanding of how this works, let's look at a typical standardized nutritional protocol for osteoporosis, a disease that causes bones to become thin and fragile.

As you know, osteoporosis is a very widespread problem in today's society, due in part to the aging of the baby-boom generation. Since it's associated with hormonal imbalances, it's especially common among postmenopausal women.

Osteoporosis is also associated with calcium deficiency. In fact, calcium supplements are the very first thing most nutritionists prescribe for women at risk of bone loss. As a result, women today are buying up calcium supplements like mad.

Say you're a woman who's showing signs of osteoporosis. Is calcium the thing you ought to be taking? Well, the answer is—yes and no. Yes if it's appropriate to your metabolic type, and no if it's not.

But here's a crucial point you need to understand: Contrary to conventional wisdom, osteoporosis is not a calcium deficiency per se. It's actually a dysfunction or an inefficiency in calcium metabolism and bone metabolism, along with estrogen/progesterone imbalances.

For some metabolic types, such as fast oxidizers or parasympathetic dominants, this dysfunctional calcium metabolism is the result of an actual lack or quantitative deficiency of calcium in the body. So there are some people with osteoporosis who do need to obtain calcium, and plenty of it.

Then there are other people with osteoporosis who have entirely different biochemical imbalances at the root of the problem. For these people, dysfunctional calcium metabolism is actually the result of a relative excess of calcium. This calcium excess exists relative to synergistic nutrients, i.e., the other nutrients that calcium requires in order to be properly utilized.

So, for some metabolic types, taking more calcium only worsens osteoporosis, by accelerating deficiencies in synergistic nutrients. This in turn accelerates the rate of calcium loss from bone tissue, where it should be held.

Now let's go further by looking at a broader spectrum of bio-chemical imbalances that could potentially lead to osteoporosis.

Note that the following chart references four of the fundamental homeostatic control systems:

- the autonomic nervous system
- the oxidative system (aka the "carbo-oxidative" system)
- catabolic/anabolic balance (aka the "lipo-oxidative" system)
- electrolyte balance

An imbalance in one or more of these systems could cause calcium and bone metabolism to go awry and cause osteoporosis.

Each of these homeostatic controls is dualistic, meaning it's comprised of opposing biochemical imbalances: sympathetic/parasympathetic, fast oxidation/slow oxidation, and so on.

What's important to realize is that every nutrient has a stimulating effect on either one side or the other of these dualistic homeostatic controls.

As just one example, calcium has opposite effects on the two opposing sides of the autonomic nervous system. It has a stimulatory effect (S) on the sympathetic branch of the ANS, while it inhibits (I) the parasympathetic branch.

The following chart shows the highly specific effects of ten different nutrients (nutrients that represent a typical standardized protocol) on four of the body's nine different fundamental homeostatic controls.

Note that not every nutrient influences every control. Calcium, for example, influences each of the four homeostatic controls, while lysine influences only one.

THE STIMULATORY/INHIBITORY EFFECT OF NUTRIENTS

NUTRIENT	AUTONOMIC		CARBO-OXIDATIVE		LIPO-OXIDATIVE		ELECTROLYTE	
	Sympathetic	Para-sympathetic	Fast Oxidation	Slow Oxidation	Catabolic	Anabolic	Excess	Deficiency
	Acid	Alkaline	Acid	Alkaline	Acid	Alkaline		
Arginine	S				S			
Boron	S	I	I	S	I	S		
Calcium	S	I	I	S	S	I	S	
Lysine					S	I		
Magnesium	I	S	S	I	S	I	I	S
Phosphorus	S	I	S	I	I	S	S	I
Sulfur					S	I		
Vitamin A			S	I	S	I	S	
Vitamin D	I		I	S	S	I	S	
Zinc	I	S	I	S	I	S	I	

This chart is designed to show four things:

1. The fundamental homeostatic controls, such as the autonomic nervous system, the oxidative system (also known as the carbo-oxidative system), and catabolic/anabolic balance (also known as lipo-oxidative balance) are "dualistic," i.e., they're comprised of opposing yet complementary influences.

2. All nutrients tend to strengthen or stimulate (S) one side or the other of the homeostatic controls, while inhibiting (I) the opposite side.

3. The specific strengths or weaknesses (i.e., imbalances) within these controls are what define a person's biochemical or metabolic individuality.

4. Any given chronic disease can be caused by any one or more of these influences.

Depending on the control imbalance that lies at the base of the illness in question, a given nutrient will either correct the imbalance, worsen the imbalance, or have no effect; and in turn it will improve the condition, worsen the condition, or have no effect.

The variable effects of the ten different nutrients on the various metabolic imbalances provide a stark illustration as to why "shotgun" or "grab bag" nutrition doesn't work. Let me give you a brief clarification of this point, using the following chart—one that's almost identical to the previous chart, with one exception, as you'll see.

But first, imagine that you have osteoporosis and you go to an allopathic clinician who attempts to "treat" your "condition" rather than address your underlying imbalances—by prescribing the ten standard nutrients in the osteoporosis "grab bag."

Now imagine that the cause of your osteoporosis is an imbalance in the sympathetic branch of your autonomic nervous system (ANS). This would mean that you're sympathetic dominant, i.e., your sympathetic system is too strong and overactive by comparison with your parasympathetic system.

If you're a sympathetic dominant, you need to obtain foods and nutrients to strengthen your parasympathetic system—since the goal is to create balance within the ANS.

But if you take calcium—what happens? Look at the preceding chart and see. Calcium stimulates or strengthens the sympathetic branch and inhibits the parasympathetic branch—just the opposite of the balancing influence you need. So, as the following chart indicates, taking calcium would make your osteoporosis worse (W) instead of better (B).

Now look again at the preceding chart and notice what would happen if you have osteoporosis and you happen to have a parasympathetic imbalance, i.e., you happen to be a parasympathetic dominant. This would mean that your parasympathetic system is too strong and overactive by comparison with your sympathetic system.

To establish balance in the autonomic nervous system, your sympathetic system would require nutritional support. And since calcium stimulates or strengthens the sympathetic system, you'd be in luck. Because calcium helps normalize parasympathetic imbalances,

THE FAILURE OF STANDARDIZED NUTRITIONAL PROTOCOLS

NUTRIENT	AUTONOMIC		CARBO-OXIDATIVE		LIPO-OXIDATIVE		ELECTROLYTE	
	Sympathetic Acid	Para-sympathetic Alkaline	Fast Oxidation Acid	Slow Oxidation Alkaline	Catabolic Acid	Anabolic Alkaline	Excess	Deficiency
Arginine	W				W			
Boron	W	B	B	W	B	W		
Calcium	W	B	B	W	W	B	W	
Lysine					W	B		
Magnesium	B	W	W	B	W	B	B	W
Phosphorus	W	B	W	B	B	W	W	B
Sulfur					W	B		
Vitamin A			W	B	W	B		
Vitamin D			B	W	W	B	W	B
Zinc	B	W	B	W	B	W	B	B

This chart is designed to show five things:

1. The nutrients listed in the far left column represent a fairly typical standardized nutritional protocol for osteoporosis.

2. The eight other columns represent various kinds of fundamental control imbalances that could potentially lead to dysfunctional calcium and bone metabolism, and in turn lead to osteoporosis.

3. Due to the variable ways in which nutrients either stimulate or inhibit opposite sides of these homeostatic controls, any given nutrient may either benefit (B) or worsen (W) a given health problem such as osteoporosis.

4. Since different people (metabolic types) who share the identical health problem may have completely different imbalances at the root of their health disorder, it makes no sense for clinicians to recommend a standardized or generic "grab bag" of nutrients.

5. Unless a person obtains nutrients that have been tailored to his or her own unique underlying disturbances, a "grab bag" protocol can succeed only by chance. Or, in many cases, a generic protocol like this will either have no effect at all on a given health problem, or might actually worsen the problem.

your osteoporosis would improve or get better (B) if you happened to be a parasympathetic dominant.

Are you beginning to see how standardized nutrition can be a real "toss of the dice" from a biochemical standpoint? The examples are endless.

Look at magnesium, for instance. It too is a typical component of standardized osteoporosis nutritional protocols, but it behaves very differently from calcium. For example, if you have osteoporosis and you happen to be a sympathetic dominant, you'd get better (B) with magnesium. But if you happen to be a parasympathetic dominant, magnesium could make your osteoporosis worse (W).

Just by glancing at the two charts we've been discussing here, you can see how nutrients behave differently in different metabolic types, regardless of what type of imbalance lies at the root of someone's health problem—whether it's an ANS imbalance, an oxidative imbalance, a catabolic/anabolic imbalance, or an imbalance within one of the other homeostatic controls.

For instance, if you happen to have an oxidative imbalance, the stimulatory/inhibitory effect of various nutrients is even more straightforward and plain to see.

If you're a fast oxidizer, calcium would work to inhibit (I) your fast oxidative rate. Common sense dictates then that calcium would help make you better (B), whereas some other nutrient, such as magnesium, would stimulate (S) your already fast oxidative rate. Here again, common sense tells us that magnesium would make you worse (W).

The point is that standardized nutritional protocols are by definition hit-or-miss solutions. A nutrient that works to correct one type of imbalance or help one person's metabolic type is not necessarily going to correct some other type of imbalance or help someone else who is a different metabolic type.

As you can see, it makes little or no sense for a health professional to recommend a batch of nutrients to someone just because each of the nutrients in the batch happens to have demonstrated some degree of clinical efficacy in relation to a given health problem. It's an uncertain approach at best, and the results are purely a matter of chance.

For some people the protocol will neutralize itself due to opposing effects of various nutrients, and very little will change for a patient; or others will be lucky and experience clinical benefits; or some people's biochemical imbalances and related health problems will get worse. But, realistically, there's no way to determine in advance who will improve and who won't.

Here's a related problem: The uncertainty involved with the use of standardized nutrition is so great that even when clinicians do luck out and get good results with someone, they don't know why they're getting good results.

They may assume it's due to the collective value of the nutrients in the protocol—but this can't explain why they get neutral or bad results in other patients so much of the time with the very same protocol.

How do we know this to be the case? Because today there is not a health practitioner anywhere using clinical nutrition who would not have to admit that what works on one person who comes through his door doesn't work on the next person. It's not that today's nutritionists aren't extremely bright, talented, able clinicians. It's just that they lack a systematic means of obtaining consistent, predictable, reproducible results.

Fortunately, metabolic typing is a highly evolved scientific discipline that enables clinicians to predict accurately how specific nutrients will affect a person's unique metabolic imbalances.

Unlike standardized nutrition, which lacks specificity and precision due to the fact that it's "nutrient specific" rather than "patient specific," metabolic typing addresses people's underlying biochemical imbalances on a case-by-case basis, with a high degree of precision and specificity.

It's also important to keep in mind that everything we've discussed here in relation to nutrients also applies to foods. Foods have highly specific effects—and variable effects—on the body's fundamental homeostatic controls, in the same way nutrients do.

For instance, any given vegetable can either stimulate (S) or inhibit (I) a given homeostatic control—just as calcium or magnesium or niacin or any other nutrient exerts these kinds of precise and specific effects.

With respect to the autonomic nervous system, for example, parasympathetic dominants do better on root vegetables, whereas sympathetic dominants do better on leafy vegetables. This is due to the fact that some vegetables contain more potassium than others, and potassium either stimulates or inhibits one side or the other of the ANS, depending on the quantity of the mineral that is present.

Vegetables also exert specific influences on people with oxidative imbalances. This has to do with the way in which different vegetables produce different pH shifts in the body. Using oxidative imbalances as an example, the chart below shows why some vegetables are beneficial for certain metabolic types, while others are not.

METABOLIC INFLUENCES OF SELECTED VEGETABLES

VEGETABLE	FAST OXIDIZERS	SLOW OXIDIZERS
Beans	B	I
Broccoli	I	B
Carrots	B	I
Cauliflower	B	I
Lettuce	I	B
Onions	I	B
Peas	B	I
Potatoes	I	B

Vegetables are good for everyone. But not all vegetables are for all metabolic types. This chart lists a few common vegetables, along with their very specific influences on the oxidative types. For example, carrots and cauliflower help to balance (B) fast oxidizers, but tend to imbalance (I) slow oxidizers. Specifically, these vegetables produce an alkaline shift in blood pH in oxidizer dominants—just what the fast oxidizer with his acid blood pH needs, but the last thing the already overly alkaline slow oxidizer should have.

Conventional Wisdom Turned Upside Down

Over the last decade or two the medical establishment has come under heavy attack by an increasingly assertive and health-conscious public. One commonly heard criticism is that doctors have little or no training in diet and nutrition, and that patients today tend to be far better informed than their doctors in this vital area.

The average medical school curriculum consists of about four thousand hours of medical education. Yet for years medical students have typically received less than five hours of training in the clinical application of foods and nutrients. And this is frequently in the area of "dietetics," a food discipline that's not really comparable to nutritional science.

In recent years this situation has begun to change, but it's happening much too slowly for a restless public that wants solutions and wants them now. That's why growing numbers of consumers are pulling away from conventional medicine and each year spending billions of their own discretionary dollars in search of effective alternatives to drugs and surgery.

Is the medical establishment really as out of touch as its critics seem to think? If not, why have so many physicians been so slow to embrace nutrition, so resistant to integrating it into their practices?

Do doctors have a deep philosophical commitment or ego attachment to the therapeutic modalities they learned in medical school? Have they been too heavily conditioned by the drug industry? Is it that they're too busy or they can't be bothered to tackle a new subject area? Or because clinical nutrition can't provide adequate financial incentives?

These are the kinds of cynical thoughts one frequently hears expressed by a disaffected public. But these explanations are really quite simplistic and overlook one very fundamental reality, which is this: Nutritional science is an area of staggering complexity—one that could not be more inhospitable or inaccessible to health practitioners.

Think of how difficult it is as an individual consumer to try to figure out a nutritional solution to some problem you may have. How confusing and even futile it can be to try to sort through the overwhelming volume of information available to you. Now multiply your own personal challenge by a factor of ten or fifty or one hundred, and you may start to get an inkling of what it's like these days for a physician trying to offer nutritional therapy.

One of the problems is that we live in an age of hyper-specialization, which means that every individual food and nutrient and dietary supplement has been analyzed and investigated to an unimaginable extent.

In the last decade alone, billions have been spent on nutritional research, by the public sector as well as pharmaceutical companies and other commercial entities that recognize the growth potential in this area.

Now more than ever, research is conducted at a blistering pace, and in many cases there are literally hundreds of separate research studies devoted to a single nutrient—studies that attempt to evaluate a nutrient's usefulness in an almost limitless range of clinical applications.

This means that physicians are regularly inundated with a tidal wave of very complex, difficult-to-digest information—articles and journals and studies and symposia proceedings and abstracts and endless new findings and data on a mind-numbing array of arcane and hyper-specific scientific topics.

How does a clinician with an interest in nutrition keep pace with all of this, or even begin to absorb a small fraction of the information? More important, how does one begin to utilize all this data, to translate all kinds of disparate infobits into some type of practical, usable, coherent therapeutic approach?

The truth is that for years now, plenty of doctors, even conventional doctors, *have* understood the value of nutrition. They *have* wanted to integrate it into their practices. But their hands have been tied, for two primary reasons:

1. Without some type of technology or system or at least a cohesive theoretical framework, it's virtually impossible for doctors and other health professionals to tap into the avalanche of available nutritional data and apply it in clinical settings in a logical or meaningful way.

2. An even bigger problem for today's clinicians is the contradictory nature of the data itself, because clinical studies in virtually every area

of nutritional science are notoriously inconclusive. For every study you can find that demonstrates some type of clinical benefit for a given nutrient, you'll find just as many studies to show just the opposite effect.

Here's an example: An article in the fall 1993 *Journal of the Neuro-musculoskeletal System* cites five separate clinical studies that examined the effect of calcium on hypertension (high blood pressure). Of the five studies, two found that calcium lowers elevated blood pressure, while the other three studies found that calcium has no beneficial effect on high blood pressure.

This same article also references seven other studies that investigated the role of potassium on high blood pressure. Here again, results were split right down the middle. Three of the seven studies found that potassium helps reduce elevated blood pressure, while the four remaining studies found that potassium has no effect on hypertension.

This "dueling studies" phenomenon can be seen over and over again in the medical/scientific literature. It's a problem frequently addressed by Dr. Guy Schenker, a Pennsylvania-based chiropractor, nutritional expert, and highly innovative researcher in the area of metabolic individuality.

In his *Nutri-Spec Newsletter* for physicians, Schenker has observed that virtually all research in clinical nutrition today is seriously flawed and largely useless because it overlooks the critical importance of biochemical individuality.

Dr. Schenker correctly asserts that nutritional studies rarely yield valid or meaningful results—simply because foods and nutrients are almost always tested on heterogeneous patient populations rather then homogeneous patient populations.

In other words, the patient population in any given study is invariably composed of a random mix of different metabolic types. That's just the way the studies are designed. Many clinical researchers are simply unaware of the significance of biochemical individuality. And those who are aware of the importance of this concept don't necessarily have the practical knowledge or the tools necessary to differentiate study participants on the basis of their metabolic type.

Naturally, any food or nutrient being tested in a given study is going to behave differently in different metabolic types. This means that the study cannot possibly gauge the real clinical efficacy of the food or nutrient in question.

Unless the biochemical baseline in a nutritional study is held constant, i.e., unless everyone in the study is the same metabolic type, the results will be hopelessly skewed and, therefore, as Dr. Schenker points out, of little or no real value.

Can you imagine what the "dueling studies" phenomenon would mean if you were a health practitioner trying to offer nutritional therapy? You couldn't get straight answers to simple questions. If you wanted to know whether calcium benefits hypertension, for instance, some researchers would say yes, others would tell you no, still others would say maybe. You'd be stuck in an endless loop of uncertainty.

Virtually all nutritional studies today use heterogeneous patient populations, i.e., they fail to differentiate people on the basis of their metabolic type. This prevents researchers from obtaining accurate assessments of the clinical value of a given food or nutrient. The results of any given study then become a matter of chance dependent upon the metabolic types that happened to be included in the study.

The confusing and ultimately inconclusive nature of current nutritional data is what discourages so many clinicians from offering nutritional therapy. But metabolic typing can resolve this problem by enabling researchers to develop patient-specific clinical studies, as opposed to disease-specific or nutrient-specific clinical studies.

Patient-specific research—and, in turn, patient-specific therapy—is very much the wave of the future, not just in nutritional science, but in many other areas of medicine as well.

Many drug companies and conventional health care provider organizations (e.g., hospitals, clinics, HMOs) are beginning to understand the vital importance of tailoring their products and services to the highly individualized needs of patients. As a result, many mainstream corporations within the health care industry have begun to look for effective ways to develop customized solutions of one kind or another.

For instance, pharmaceutical companies are hoping that future breakthroughs in molecular biology (such as the effort to decipher or "decode" the chemical instructions contained in the "human genome," the sum total of all the genes in the human body) may one day yield effective methods for providing patient-specific drug therapy.

There can be little doubt that medical thinking is about to undergo a profound shift, as more and more health professionals become aware of the extreme limitations of "one-size-fits-all" therapeutic solutions. A revolution is definitely beginning to take shape, and the science of metabolic typing is at the forefront.

Chapter 5

THE ONE AND ONLY YOU

The Limits of Conventional Diagnostics

Have you ever heard the joke about the hypochondriac who passes away after living to a ripe old age? His tombstone reads "Do you believe me now?"

People who obsess over imaginary ailments have long been a favorite target of comedy writers, though they're no laughing matter within the medical profession. Doctors are understandably frustrated by cases in which they can't find physical evidence of a patient's maladies. And by all accounts, this happens all the time.

A 1998 article in *Psychiatric Times* reports that anywhere from four percent to twenty percent of Americans suffer with persistent delusions of ill health and spend an estimated $20 billion a year on unnecessary doctor visits and medical tests. Hypochondriasis, according to the medical literature, is a very real and very widespread clinical problem, one that absorbs an inordinate amount of time and energy on the part of many a doctor on any given day.

Health disorders that doctors consider to be "all in the mind" are believed to be rooted in anxiety, depression, and other kinds of psychological disorders. That's why you're likely to be given a tranquilizer or antidepressive drug in the event that you've got health complaints your physician can't explain.

The important question is: How often are people's unexplained ailments real, and how often are they figments of someone's imagination?

Or, when standard diagnostic techniques fail to pick up evidence of a health problem, does that mean the problem doesn't exist?

Clinicians who utilize metabolic typing have very different perspectives from most doctors and other practitioners on these sorts of questions. One reason for this is that metabolic typing involves testing approaches that are radically different from the kinds of conventional testing methods that have become such an integral part of all our lives.

Metabolic type testing techniques are designed to evaluate a person's nutritional status, not to diagnose illnesses. But, as you will see, they reveal a wealth of essential, practical information that conventional medical tests cannot.

We all know what it's like to visit a doctor's office and be poked and prodded and tested and screened—with electrodes and tongue depressors and stethoscopes and needles and X-ray equipment and various kinds of scanning devices. And certainly a lot of this can be very useful in many instances.

Yet many of the standard diagnostic procedures to which we all routinely submit—particularly laboratory tests such as blood tests and urinalyses and hair mineral analyses—are of little or no value in a vast number of clinical situations. It may sound hard to believe, but it's true, for two primary reasons.

First, lab tests are mainly useful to confirm the presence of health problems that have already progressed to an advanced stage—once an organ, gland, or body system has reached a serious state of malfunction or collapse. They're generally not very useful in detecting the presence of health disorders in their early or developmental stages ("subclinical" conditions), or those that fail to exhibit all the earmarks of a commonly recognized "diagnosable" disease.

For example, if high levels of the enzymes GGTP and SGTP are found in your blood, it most likely indicates liver damage or liver disease. But these enzymes are just markers of the result of a degenerative process. They can't reveal anything about the months and years of chronic degeneration that led up to your liver dysfunction.

Second, even if traditional lab tests were more effective in detecting chronic health disorders in progress, they're limited because they don't provide the kind of physiological data that can be used to pinpoint the source of a given health problem. This means lab tests can't shed any light on what someone can do to restore or rebuild his or her health.

With respect to chronic illness, blood tests and other standard laboratory tests have surprisingly limited clinical value. They're not very useful in identifying the source of a health problem or a "subclinical" condition, i.e., the early stage of a disease. And unlike metabolic type testing procedures, conventional diagnostic tests cannot provide a blueprint for effective nutritional therapy.

Despite the serious limitations of laboratory tests, both conventional and alternative clinicians use them all the time in an attempt to determine their patients' nutritional imbalances and to design nutritional protocols. Using blood tests as an example, let me briefly explain just how ineffective this approach really is.

As you know, blood tests are typically used to identify organ weaknesses or dysfunction or to look for deficiencies or excesses in various kinds of enzymes and nutrients.

For instance, if a blood test reveals a deficiency in a specific nutrient, the general assumption is that all a clinician needs to do is prescribe that nutrient to compensate for the deficiency.

But in the real world of day-to-day clinical practice, this simplistic approach rarely works and has no real scientific validity. If it did, there would be far fewer sick people walking around and far more health professionals producing dramatic clinical successes.

The routine use of blood tests to identify nutrient deficiencies is an example of how medical procedures are often accepted on the basis of blind faith.

The truth is that neither scientific research nor clinical practice has ever demonstrated that making diet and nutrient recommendations on the basis of "nutritional deficiencies" found in standard blood analyses has ever provided effective, repeatable, reliable results.

Here's one reason blood tests are so limited: The blood is a transport and homeostatic mechanism, meaning that its job is to keep all its constituents at a certain level (in balance) in order to transport whatever is needed, wherever it is needed in the body.

As an example, let's imagine that your body is deficient in calcium. Then let's say you have your blood tested, but when the test results come back, the level of calcium in your blood appears to be within the normal range. This is actually a very typical occurrence, particularly with calcium.

Why? Because your body would most likely react by robbing your teeth and bones of calcium in order to compensate for the deficiency in your system, just to keep the calcium in your blood at a normal level.

If your blood level of calcium were allowed to get too far out of whack, you'd get very ill and might even die. To prevent this, to keep things stable, your body would "rob Peter to pay Paul." That's the way homeostasis works.

Yet a blood test has no way of showing this kind of regulatory process at work. So, even though you might have a chronic calcium deficiency that represents a serious "subclinical" health problem, it would go undetected because your blood would seem normal.

Attempting to peer into the body's biochemical machinery through the "window" of standard blood analyses is a little like trying to stand outside a house and look inside through windows that are covered with mud. In other words, you can't tell with any degree of precision or certainty exactly what's going on inside.

You might be able to spot overt disease processes, but more subtle biochemical activities such as nutrient balances will be misleading and difficult to discern. In many instances you simply won't know whether you're looking at the actual status of a nutrient or the body's defense against a nutrient excess or deficiency.

Here's another reason blood tests are limited: They don't tell you the level of any given nutrient inside your cells. Yet the interior of your cells is where all the "action" takes place, where nutrients are converted into that all-important life-sustaining energy.

Standard blood analyses provide information concerning your nutritional status at the systemic level, and that's what most clinicians focus on. But nutrient levels outside the cells may or may not be equivalent to nutritional levels inside the cells.

Remember, the bloodstream and the intracellular environment are separate levels within the body, with separate roles to play.

Clinicians frequently overlook the status of the intracellular environment. Yet your body's ability to function properly is largely dependent on having specific combinations of nutrients that are appropriate for your metabolic type available to your cells, in the right place, at the right time.

For instance, someone who is a fast oxidizer (e.g., an Eskimo who needs plenty of meat and fat) has high intracellular levels of potassium relative to calcium. What this person needs is a diet that will raise their intracellular calcium level, to bring it into balance with their potassium level.

A slow oxidizer (e.g., a person from the tropics) typically has just the opposite situation—high intracellular calcium relative to potassium. That's why a slow oxidizer requires a diet that will elevate their potassium level—a diet high in fruits, vegetables, and other carbohydrates.

Of course there are specialized blood-cell analyses that clinicians can use to measure the intracellular level of nutrients.

But, here's yet another problem: In actual clinical practice, it doesn't help to know the level of a given nutrient inside someone's cells unless you also know that individual's metabolic type.

One of the fundamental benefits of metabolic typing is that it provides a context or frame of reference through which nutrient deficiencies or excesses can be accurately identified and understood.

As you will see in this and subsequent chapters, nutrient deficiencies or excesses have no real meaning in and of themselves.

So, trying to evaluate nutrient imbalances independently of a person's metabolic type is like trying to assess the overall status of an entire ecosystem by zeroing in on some of the chemical constituents in a pond or a lake, i.e., the individual components or sublevels within the ecosystem. It's much too narrow a focus.

But if you first understand the mechanisms or principles that keep an ecosystem in a healthy, balanced condition, you'll have the frame of reference you need to understand all its component parts—trees and plants and rocks and soil and air and water and fish and insects and other living things.

That's the way it is with your body. You can't expect to get an accurate, "big picture" understanding of your body's style of functioning—and its related nutritional requirements—just by measuring the concentrations of nutrients at various sublevels within the body. The results will be misleading, for two reasons:

1. Nutrients behave differently at different levels within the body. In other words, systemic behavior is different from tissue behavior is different from cellular behavior, and so on.

2. In addition to providing an incomplete picture of what is going on at a physiological level, standard laboratory data is of limited value because clinicians are forced to evaluate it in absolute terms.

A New Frame of Reference

An ancient Chinese proverb, which dates back to the fourth century B.C., goes like this: If we say that a thing is great or small by its own standard of great or small, then there is nothing in all creation which is not great, nothing which is not small.

Since the dawn of civilization, people have understood that we live in a relative universe, meaning that it's pointless to try to characterize or quantify things in absolute terms. Throughout history, scientists and other observers have recognized that we need reference points to discriminate or make judgments about virtually anything, that measurements or values of any kind are meaningful only in relation to some specified frame of reference.

For instance, if you earn a six-figure income and have a range of impressive assets—a stock portfolio, a large home, a sports car or two, should I assume you're rich? The answer would depend on my frame of reference. If I have a minimum-wage job and live in a dingy apartment, then to me you might seem as rich as Bill Gates. On the other hand, if

I were a billionaire industrialist, I'd probably think of you as a pauper.

One of the most fundamental problems with nutritional science is that it lacks a logical system of reference points—a system with enough flexibility to accommodate all the biological diversity among people. The only reference points it has are "normal ranges," i.e., fixed values that are supposed to represent optimal, healthy levels of nutrients.

Yet these so-called "normal ranges" are actually just averages of nutrient levels typically found within the population, and they're problematic on many levels.

As an example, let's say your doctor prescribes a blood-cell analysis for you, and when the lab report comes back, it indicates that the level of calcium in your cells is above the "normal" range. For purposes of discussion, let's say that the normal range for intracellular calcium is between 8.5 and 10.3, but you're showing a calcium score of 10.5.

In the realm of conventional nutrition, that 10.5 score on your lab report would be viewed in absolute terms, which means you'd be viewed as high in calcium, regardless of other considerations, and therefore *not* a candidate for calcium supplementation.

But in the realm of metabolic typing, this kind of "absolute" laboratory data has virtually no practical value. Because if you're simply going to be categorized as "high" or "low" in a given nutrient, two critical questions remain unanswered:

1. high or low compared to whom—the general population?
2. high or low compared to what—what's the median point for each nutrient?

Comparing your test value to the "normal" reference range won't work, because you can't be compared to the general population. You're a unique metabolic type with unique needs for specific kinds and quantities of nutrients.

But the general population is a heterogeneous mix of all different kinds of metabolic types, including many people with needs that are very different from yours. For instance, as Roger Williams pointed out, it's not unusual to find as much as a hundredfold difference in nutrient level requirements from one person to the next.

Furthermore, the way in which "normal ranges" are established is rather arbitrary. They're supposedly based on the laboratory data of "healthy" and "average" people. But these concepts are very hard to define with any degree of precision. Not all clinicians agree on what constitutes good health versus poor health.

In fact, the medical profession has had to keep "shifting the goalposts" on the so-called normal reference ranges. The ranges keep expanding to accommodate "average" individuals because the health of people in modern culture is on the decline. Just as one example, diseases that used to be thought of as conditions of the aged have become commonplace in younger and younger people over the last few decades.

Additionally, there is no way to establish a "median point" or "ideal level" for any given nutrient. The ideal level of each nutrient is different in different metabolic types.

The good news is that the limitations of laboratory data ultimately don't matter, because metabolic typing very effectively "fills in the blanks," and tells us what we need to know about what specific kinds of foods and nutrients people need to optimize their health.

For instance, let's revisit the example we were just discussing about your being found to have high levels of calcium in your cells.

If you're high in calcium and we know your metabolic type is that of a slow oxidizer, we would know right away that you don't need any calcium supplementation.

Why? Because we already know that slow oxidizers have high concentrations of calcium in relation to potassium and other nutrients, regardless of the *absolute* calcium level found either in the blood or in the cells.

Or, alternatively, if your lab tests indicate you're high in calcium and we also know you're a fast oxidizer, we would know right away that you need more calcium through diet and supplements. So we would give you more calcium, no matter how high your calcium level might be in "absolute" terms.

Why? Because if you're a fast oxidizer, your level of calcium is low relative to your level of potassium and other nutrients.

ABSOLUTE VS. RELATIVE NUTRIENT LEVELS

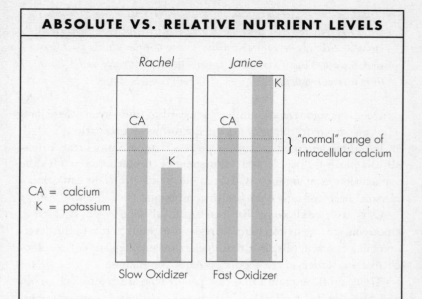

Here's an example of why "absolute" laboratory data can be very misleading, and of limited value for prescribing nutrients—without metabolic typing as a frame of reference.

In absolute terms, both these individuals have high levels of calcium in their cells.

Rachel, as a slow oxidizer, also has high levels of calcium relative to potassium and other nutrients. Thus she would not require calcium supplementation.

But as a fast oxidizer, Janice is actually low in calcium relative to potassium and other nutrients. For this reason, she requires additional calcium, despite the high absolute value of calcium in her cells.

Discovering Your Biochemical Individuality

Here's one of the most common complaints I hear from people who are seeking nutritional guidance (the exact words may vary from person to person, but the core message is always the same). . . .

"I just had a complete physical, including blood tests and all the usual lab work. All the tests came out normal. My doctor gave me a clean bill of health. He says there's nothing wrong with me that a good two-week vacation won't cure. But I don't feel well at all, and I know there's something wrong."

Does this sound at all familiar? It's hard to find anyone these days who can't relate to this very typical doctor/patient scenario.

In our modern medical culture, "stress" has become a great "catch-all" diagnosis for people with all manner of chronic ailments. It's the explanation most frequently trotted out when clinicians can't find a physical basis for someone's health complaints.

Of course, we all know that "stresses" of all kinds—physical stress, emotional stress, environmental stress—are causal factors in the development of chronic ills. But that doesn't mean there are not real biochemical disorders at the root of patients' complaints.

Time and time again I find that people who are given a "clean bill of health" by the medical establishment actually have very real physical problems—biochemical or nutrient imbalances that generally escape detection through traditional diagnostic methods.

So I tend to dispute the widespread clinical perception that holds that there are lots of patients out there these days with overactive imaginations or hypochondriacal tendencies or problems that are purely psychosomatic.

And as you might imagine, the clinicians whom my organization assists with metabolic profiling services don't believe it's sufficient to simply send patients home with sedatives and upbeat assurances and recommendations for vacations and the like.

Because even if people could go home and wave a magic wand and suddenly remove all the stresses in their lives, more likely than not there's already a pathological process in place that needs to be actively addressed with a nutritional solution.

Fortunately, today's savvy health consumers are increasingly less likely to accept the notion that their problems could be "all in their mind." If they can't get satisfactory explanations within the conventional medical realm, they typically go running to the alternative medical realm.

Of course, there can be no doubt that alternative medicine, or complementary medicine as it's now often referred to, is an area very rich in valuable healing options.

But in terms of the diagnostic approaches that are used to establish patients' nutritional regimens, alternative medicine tends to suffer from the very same limitations as conventional medicine.

If you're among the millions of Americans who routinely pursue alternative therapies of one kind or another, you're probably familiar with diagnostic approaches such as kinesiology (muscle-strength testing), iridology (mapping the markings in the iris of the eye), live-blood-cell analysis, hair mineral analysis, pH tests of saliva and urine, and so on.

These kinds of tests can and do provide provocative evidence of organs and body systems that are weak and dysfunctional. But what these tests can't do is provide a comprehensive or "big picture" understanding of the underlying source of a person's health problems—in other words, why the body is imbalanced from a biochemical perspective and, in turn, why its homeostatic systems are faltering.

As a result, these tests cannot provide a plan or a blueprint that is tailored to someone's highly individualized needs, i.e., what specific diet/nutritional regimen a person should pursue in order to rebuild or optimize their health.

The problem might best be described as "tunnel vision,"meaning that many if not most of the diagnostic approaches used by alternative clinicians today are too narrowly focused on the status of one level or another within the body.

In contrast, metabolic type testing approaches are never focused on one level of the body. They're always geared toward a multidimensional assessment of the body's overall style of functioning.

At its introductory level, metabolic typing uses body language—a vast lexicon of anatomical, physiological, and even psychological data—to identify people's inherited capabilities for transforming foods and nutrients into life-sustaining energy.

Metabolic type testing approaches may seem unconventional at first, or "fluffy" or less "scientific" than many of the standard diagnostic methods with which we're all so familiar. But, as you will see, just the opposite is true.

The methods we use to evaluate people's metabolic individuality are all firmly grounded in "hard" science—in disciplines that include biochemistry, physiology, endocrinology, and neuroendocrinology.

However, before I describe more about metabolic type testing and why it's so effective for the development of individualized nutritional protocols, let me give you a few additional examples of the profound limitations of standard diagnostic procedures—in this case, the standard testing approaches used by alternative clinicians.

For instance, alternative clinicians are often interested in testing the pH value of both saliva and urine for the purpose of making dietary recommendations.

As you know, the pH value of any given solution refers to its acidity or alkalinity. And, in order for your cells, tissues, and organs to function properly, they need to maintain specific levels of acidity or alkalinity. For example, all the chemical and metabolic activity inside your cells is made possible by enzymatic reactions, and the efficiency of these reactions is heavily influenced by the pH level of the cellular environment.

Alternative clinicians tend to be very aware of the crucial role that proper acid/alkaline balances play in your health. Since pH balances in your body are heavily influenced by your diet, clinicians are naturally interested in monitoring your pH levels and prescribing nutrients to keep you from becoming either too acid or too alkaline.

It's commonly believed that if a pH test shows that your system is too acid, then so-called "alkalinizing" foods should be eaten. And, conversely, if your pH values are too alkaline, then so-called "acidifying" foods should be eaten.

Yet here again we have a clinical approach and way of thinking that is far too simplistic, and that simply doesn't work, except by chance. For instance, you may recall that one of the core principles of metabolic typing is that any food or nutrient can have opposite biochemical influences in different metabolic types.

This means that the very same food that produces an alkaline condition in one person can produce an acidic condition in another person.

VARIABLE pH EFFECT OF FOODS

	AUTONOMIC-DOMINANT TYPE	OXIDATIVE-DOMINANT TYPE
vegetables	alkalinize	acidify
meats	acidify	alkalinize

One important way in which foods or nutrients affect your health is by influencing your body's acid/alkaline balance. The proper pH balance is essential to the maintenance of good health.

But contrary to conventional wisdom, foods and nutrients have no fixed or inherent acid/alkaline qualities.

The very same food that can produce an alkaline shift in one metabolic type can produce just the opposite (acidic) shift in another metabolic type.

According to conventional dietary wisdom, there are some foods that are inherently acidic, meaning they will acidify the body no matter what. And then there are foods that are inherently alkaline, meaning they will alkalinize the body no matter what.

But the truth of the matter is that we live in a relative universe, so the pH effect of any given food cannot be viewed in "absolute" terms. Contrary to conventional wisdom, no food or nutrient has an acid or alkaline effect on the body because of some quality inherent in the food or nutrient. Rather, the acid/alkaline effect of foods and nutrients on the body are determined by their variable and highly specific effects on the various fundamental homeostatic controls in different metabolic types.

The body's pH balance or acid/alkaline balance is a very important factor in the maintenance of good health, and is largely determined by the types of foods and nutrients a person consumes. Yet the way in which any given food or nutrient affects a person's biochemistry is always relative to that individual's metabolic type.

Hair tissue mineral analysis is another very popular tool among alternative health practitioners, and is widely used for the purpose of determining nutritional protocols.

Yet your hair is a tissue-level substance and, like your blood, represents just one level within your body. Since your body is a complex physiological system comprised of many levels, nutrient values found in the hair can be misleading if they are interpreted or analyzed in "absolute" terms.

Outside the context of metabolic typing, our experience is that hair tissue nutrient levels alone are simply not a reliable indicator of what a person needs in terms of a nutritional protocol.

The two charts on page 119 provide an excellent case in point. These hair analysis charts are taken from actual client files. They show the results of two people's hair tests, in this case a husband and wife. Note that these two individuals show almost identical patterns and levels of nutrient excesses and deficiencies.

Based on these test values alone, a clinician would have to conclude that both these people are low in potassium and high in calcium, and since potassium tends to lower calcium, they should therefore both receive potassium supplementation.

But here's the catch: These two people are actually opposite metabolic types. And they each have intracellular oxidative imbalances: Kitty is a slow oxidizer and George is a fast oxidizer.

This means that Kitty has metabolic imbalances that can be resolved only with a high-potassium/low-calcium protocol. In Kitty's case, this would seem to be the logical conclusion just by glancing at her hair analysis chart.

In George's case, however, just the opposite is true. Even though his laboratory data makes it seem as though he has the exact same nutritional needs as Kitty, and that it would be logical to cut back on his calcium and increase his potassium, we couldn't make that assumption without knowing his metabolic type.

Since George happens to be a fast oxidizer, what we actually did was decrease his potassium intake while increasing his calcium intake.

Thus, we recommended opposite nutritional protocols for these two people, based on their metabolic types, despite the extraordinary similarity of their lab tests.

Even though they both began with high calcium levels, we cut Kitty's calcium intake while actually increasing George's calcium

METABOLIC TYPING:
AN ESSENTIAL FRAME OF REFERENCE

Kitty

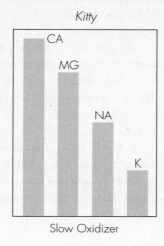

Slow Oxidizer

George

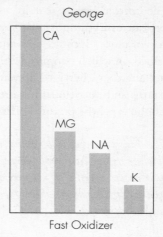

Fast Oxidizer

CA = calcium
MG = magnesium
NA = sodium
K = potassium

The above hair analysis chart shows two people with almost identical nutrient excesses and deficiencies. Thus they would appear to require the same kind of nutritional protocol. But in reality, these people required opposite nutritional protocols. As a slow oxidizer, Kitty resolved her chronic health problems with a high-potassium/low-calcium protocol. And as a fast oxidizer, George was able to resolve his problems with a low-potassium/high-calcium protocol.

This shows why a tissue level substance (hair) is not a reliable indicator of cellular nutrient requirements, and why metabolic typing provides a crucial frame of reference for interpreting nutrient levels found in the body, and in turn establishing correct nutritional protocols.

Because Kitty was a slow oxidizer, we know her cellular calcium levels are high and we know her tissue levels are high from the hair analysis. Thus we know she has a quantitative excess of calcium. But because George is a fast oxidizer, we know his cellular calcium levels are low. And because his hair tissue calcium levels are high, he has a qualitative insufficiency, meaning that there is enough calcium present in his body, but qualitatively, it is neither where it should be (in the cells) nor is it being used properly.

intake. With this approach, each saw their calcium levels fall, their potassium levels rise, and their health problems improve.

The bottom line is that in nutritional science, as in every other area of life, everything is relative, nothing is absolute.

For instance, I could cite endless examples like the one I just described, in which two people's lab results look just the same on the surface and they, therefore, appear to have the same kind of biochemical status and nutritional requirements. But when we identify their metabolic type, the picture shifts dramatically.

> *The body's biochemical status cannot be effectively evaluated in absolute terms. Two people might have identical levels of nutrients in their tissues or cells, yet the very same nutrient balance that indicates good health in one metabolic type can indicate pathology in another metabolic type.*

Body Language Holds the Key

If you asked many different types of professionals—a clergyman, a philosopher, a microbiologist, a surgeon, a sculptor, a geneticist, a psychologist, a painter, an athlete—to describe the human body, you'd get many different perspectives. All would have validity, yet none would be definitive.

Likewise, if you had a health problem and you sought out clinicians or healers from different cultures around the globe—Indian or Chinese or Middle Eastern or Native American—you'd surely get a wide variety of opinions on the nature of your condition.

There is a strong tendency in every culture and within every branch of the health profession for people to assume that its way of seeing and understanding human health and disease is the best and most accurate way.

In the West in particular it's often difficult for us to fully appreciate what other healing traditions have to offer, especially in diagnostics, where our technical prowess is quite spectacular. There is no tissue or cell or atom or molecule or strand of DNA that is outside our grasp, our range of vision, our dissection capability.

We have endless arrays of tools—electron microscopes and ultrasound and radioisotopes and magnetic resonance imaging and ultrasensitive chemical assays and highly sophisticated genetic probes—that enable us to analyze efficiently the farthest reaches, the deepest levels, the smallest constituents of the human body.

To many, these approaches represent the ultimate in terms of scientific advancement and objectivity. But not everybody would agree. Practitioners within Eastern medical traditions see enormous limitations in modern Western medicine's methods of diagnosing and treating illness. They're generally mystified by, and critical of, what they view as modern medicine's mechanistic approach to health care, and its excessive reliance on machines and testing equipment and computers and data.

In our drug and surgically oriented system, we tend to see the body itself as a biochemical machine comprised of interchangeable parts. As scientific iconoclast Fritjof Capra has observed, modern medicine has adopted an "engineering approach to health in which illness is reduced to mechanical trouble and medical therapy to technical manipulation."

Holistically oriented systems such as Chinese medicine, Ayurvedic medicine, and homeopathy, which are among the world's oldest and most sophisticated healing traditions, are radically different. They see the body as a highly integrated system, and have very little use for modern technology of any kind. In fact, their diagnostic methods are esoteric and impossible to define in quantitative or objective terms.

For instance, to get to the root of a problem, classical homeopathic or Chinese physicians first seek to identify the unique essence of each patient, not just in physical terms but in metaphysical terms as well. They evaluate all sorts of psychological, emotional, behavioral, and personality-based traits and characteristics, along with more tangible factors like physical symptoms and traits.

In other words, unlike Western medicine, which has a reductionist orientation, meaning that its approach to scientific understanding is to break everything down into even smaller units (atoms and molecules and genes), traditional healing systems seek to evaluate the body and physical ailments in broader, more expansive, "bigger picture" terms.

As an example, if you develop an eye problem, and you live in the United States, you'd most likely consult an eye specialist, since our mainstream health-care system is organized entirely around medical specialties. Your ophthalmologist would no doubt focus entirely on your eye and its inner workings and component parts.

But in traditional Chinese medicine there are no specialists, since all health problems are perceived to be interrelated. An eye problem, for instance, is viewed as a symptom of liver dysfunction. And in turn, liver dysfunction is interpreted as a sign of broader systemic or physiological imbalances, which could be the result of energy blockages, or any number of environmental, dietary, psychospiritual, or other irregularities.

As a means of evaluating human health problems, metabolic typing has elements in common with both modern medicine and traditional healing systems. It represents a kind of synthesis or convergence of concepts and information drawn from both areas.

For example, Dr. Francis Pottenger, M.D., and Dr. Royal Lee, D.D.S., the scientific investigators who did some of the earliest developmental work in the field of metabolic typing in the 1930s, utilized a great deal of mainstream medical knowledge in key areas such as endocrinology and neuroendocrinology. And in the years since, other scientists who have contributed to the evolution of metabolic typing have made very extensive use of the modern science of biochemistry.

But at the same time, metabolic typing is conceptually similar in many ways to Eastern or ancient healing traditions.

Metabolic typing is holistically oriented and focuses on identifying the "big picture," the constitutional essence of each person. In fact, metabolic typing practitioners see individuality as far more significant than any given disease or set of symptoms, in the very same way that ancient healers did.

In the fourth century B.C., the great Greek physician Hippocrates, the father of medicine, said, "It's more important to know what kind of patient has a disease than what kind of disease a patient has." He even came up with a rudimentary system for categorizing patients according to "type."

Chinese and Ayurvedic medicine also use "typing" as a primary means of evaluating people and determining an appropriate dietary regimen or other kind of therapeutic course of action. The Chinese use a typing system based on the "five elements"—fire, wood, water, metal, and earth.

Like the Chinese, Ayurvedic practitioners, the traditional healers of India, also use a system that identifies three basic constitutional types known as "doshas." Both these medical systems are extremely sophisticated even though they're thousands of years old.

Homeopathy is another very advanced medical discipline that categorizes people according to constitutional types. Although homeopathic principles date back to ancient times, the clinical discipline was organized and formalized in the 1700s by the brilliant German physician Samuel Hahnemann.

It was not until the twentieth century that American scientists and physicians began to recognize the potential clinical usefulness of differentiating people according to type.

But by that time, even as early as the 1920s and '30s, scientists had a tremendous advantage: Modern biochemical research and food science were burgeoning, and researchers had begun to discover, isolate, and map out the constituents of foods—such as vitamins, minerals, and enzymes.

In ancient times, healers were limited to empirical observations about the effects of foods and physiological processes. They had no way of knowing about things like cellular oxidation or the role of the autonomic nervous system or macro- or micronutrients.

Thus, over the course of the twentieth century, the tools and technologies and products of modern research finally enabled scientists to understand, in precise scientific detail, why people are different from a biochemical standpoint, and exactly why specific nutrients affect the metabolism and the health of different individuals in different ways.

In the hands of highly skilled practitioners, Chinese medicine, Ayurvedic medicine, and homeopathy are very effective healing arts. Yet they're considerably more abstract than the modern science of metabolic typing. For example, they make heavy use of concepts like "prana" and "qi" and "life force"—concepts that refer to the roles that energy or the spirit or other intangible forces play in human health.

Metabolic typing is a more tangible or "hard" science or clinical discipline, heavily based on the contemporary science of biochemistry. Though it's philosophically analogous to the ancient healing traditions, metabolic typing is also a new branch of nutritional science that is very much a product of the twentieth century.

Here's an analogy that clarifies how metabolic typing differs from the other types of medical disciplines I've described here: Think of a flower as if it were a focal point of clinical interest. Modern Western medicine, which is specialty driven, would tend to focus on the individual component parts of the flower: the stem, the leaves, the petals, the stamen, the pistil, and so on. Eastern holistic disciplines would tend to see the flower as a unified botanical organism, and to utilize a wide range of clinical arts to assess the health of the flower and its environmental conditions.

In contrast, practitioners of metabolic typing have a more specific focus—they would zero in on the biochemical balance of the sap that runs through the flower to provide its nourishment, and the quality and the mix of nutrients the flower obtains from sunlight or the soil in which it grows.

The modern science of metabolic typing utilizes a variety of methods and a very systematic approach to identifying peoples' biochemical individuality.

One method is the interpretation of "body language," or the evaluation of any number of the hundreds of different traits and characteristics that make one person distinct from another in terms of:

- physical appearance
- anatomical or structural traits
- psychological characteristics
- personality and behavioral traits
- food reactions and dietary preferences

Believe it or not, all your highly individualized characteristics have biochemical correlates. In other words, they are a direct result of

A Synthesis of Old and New,
A Convergence of East and West

Modern Western Medicine

- Product of 20th century
- Based on advanced academic disciplines, including biochemistry, physiology, endocrinology, and neuro-endocrinology
- Faclitated evolution of nutritional science, including discovery of vitamins

Eastern Healing Traditions

- Centuries old
- Holistically-oriented as opposed to specialty-driven
- Emphasis on constitutional differences between people
- Utilize "typing" systems based on physical, psychological, and other characteristics

Metabolic Typing

Metabolic typing combines aspects of both modern Western medicine and classic Eastern healing traditions such as Chinese and Ayurvedic medicine. It is philosophically aligned with Eastern medicine, yet grounded in many of the academic disciplines of Western medicine.

the unique way in which your regulatory (homeostatic) control systems are designed.

We all have genetically inherited strengths or weaknesses or differences in our:

- autonomic nervous system
- oxidation rate
- catabolic/anabolic balance
- endocrine system

These are the key systems that determine your metabolic type.

As you may recall, your autonomic nervous system manages all the involuntary activity in your body—your heartbeat, your breathing, your digestion, reproductive functions, immune activity, and so on.

The oxidation rate and catabolic/anabolic balance are concerned with the quantity and quality of energy production, and your endocrine system exerts all kinds of influences on your metabolism through the secretion of hormones, the chemical messengers that manage the activity of tissues and cells.

There are countless readily observable clues that help reveal how these systems function for you.

For example, if you're tall and have good concentration but weak digestion, these are traits that suggest something about the way your autonomic nervous system influences your metabolism. Your body may be more influenced by the sympathetic branch of the ANS, relative to the parasympathetic branch.

Or if you have a poor appetite and have low energy but function well on sugar or starches, you might be a slow oxidizer.

Maybe you suffer with insomnia or are prone to digestive disturbances such as diarrhea, an indication that your catabolic influences may be more dominant than your anabolic influences. Or perhaps you have a small skeletal frame with fine bone structure. This might mean that your thyroid gland is your dominant energy-producing gland.

There are endless possible variations in your traits that indicate the nature of the "imbalances" within your regulatory systems and, in turn, define your metabolic individuality.

These traits or clues tell us a great deal about the efficiency with which all your organs and glands function, the kinds of health disorders you're subject to, and the effect that different foods and nutrients have on your health.

Most important, your "body language" in all its dimensions can provide a road map or a blueprint for developing a nutritional regimen that can be used to balance your body chemistry and thereby optimize your health.

However, "body language" is never absolutely clear cut. In other words, there are no "pure types"—people who have traits that reflect only specific imbalances, such as sympathetic dominance versus parasympathetic dominance or fast oxidation versus slow oxidation, and so on. You're more complex than that, like an extraordinarily complex mosaic comprised of countless facets arranged in a highly unique configuration.

So what we need to do is look for patterns among your traits and characteristics that can tell us something about your dominant tendencies.

Think of it this way: If you're lost in the wilderness at night and want to find your way home, you have a good chance of doing so if it's a cloudless night and you have some understanding of astronomy.

What does astronomy do? It makes sense and gives meaning to the infinite number of stars visible in the night sky. It organizes them into recognizable patterns called constellations that can be used to determine direction.

If you can locate the Big Dipper, you can find the North Star and identify the four directions. Using that as your reference point, you can determine the proper direction to find your way home.

Metabolic types are like constellations. They're patterns that organize the infinite minutiae of your physiological and biochemical makeup, enabling you to know what nutritional path to follow in order to balance your body chemistry.

THE MOSAIC THAT IS YOU

		Traits	Jane	Mary	Sally
Auto-nomic	Parasym-pathetic	short	X		X
		moist/oily skin		X	
		rashes			X
		depression	X		
		fast digestion	X	X	
	Sympa-thetic	tall		X	
		dry skin	X		X
		acne	X		
		anxiety		X	X
		poor digestion			X
Carbo-Oxidative	Fast Oxidation	hyper but exhausted	X	X	
		craves salt		X	
		strong appetite	X		
	Slow Oxidation	weak appetite		X	X
		does well on sugar			X
		low energy			X
Lipo-Oxidative	Anabolic	tachycardia	X		
		somnolence			X
		constipation	X		X
	Catabolic	bradycardia		X	
		diarrhea		X	
		insomnia		X	X
Endocrine	Thyroid	small, fine-boned	X		
	Adrenal	thick musculature		X	
	Gonad	small rib cage; wide hips			X
	Pituitary	large head	X		

Here are a few examples of the different kinds of traits that reflect imbalances in the homeostatic control mechanisms and in turn define someone's metabolic type. Note that the "mosaic" of individual metabolism is infinitely varied. No person is a "pure type," manifesting characteristics of only one side of one homeostatic control. Rather, we all have a mixture of traits arising from varied influences of all the homeostatic controls. Yet these traits always fall into patterns that can be identified as a metabolic type.

Chapter

6

IDENTIFYING YOUR
METABOLIC TYPE

A New Plateau of Self-awareness

Are you overweight or out of shape? Do you find it difficult to lose weight or keep it off? How's your energy level? Do you spring out of bed each morning with vim and vigor and feel strong, vibrant, and alert all day long? Or do you frequently drag yourself out of bed and suffer intermittent bouts of fatigue, irritability, or poor concentration?

What about your overall level of health? Are you free of aches and pains and nagging ailments of any kind? Or are you more typical of most of us in modern society, with a chronic disorder of one sort or another that just doesn't seem to go away . . .

- allergies
- arthritis
- headaches
- low blood sugar
- indigestion
- cardiovascular problems
- depression
- recurrent infections

If you have problems like these, or you're simply not functioning well or feeling up to par, chances are you're suffering from malnutrition.

Remember, there are many forms of malnutrition, not just the kind that afflicts starving children in third-world countries. Here in America, for instance, malnutrition is very common, even among the affluent, and others generally thought of as "well fed."

Believe it or not, obesity is a sign of malnourishment. Overweight people are literally starving for the right kinds of foods and nutrients to satisfy their hunger and normalize their metabolism.

Even if you're consuming only the highest quality and most heathful foods and food supplements available, it's entirely possible you're very deficient in the vital nutrients your body needs to function properly.

Fortunately, your body always lets you know when you're not feeding it correctly. The symptoms you experience are the signals that your body sends you, alerting you to the fact that it needs to be more effectively supported with "body fuel" that's well suited to your particular "engines of metabolism."

Even if you're currently slim and trim and symptom free, it's still critically important for you to find out how your body processes foods and utilizes nutrients, and why your body is unique on a biochemical level.

Whether you're seeking to optimize or maintain your health, there's simply no substitute for eating according to your metabolic type.

Regardless of your current physical status, discovering your metabolic type is the critical first step in moving to a much higher plateau of self-awareness, and, in turn, enjoying a life full of vibrant health and fitness, free of the degenerative ailments that burden most people in modern society.

The self-test provided in this chapter is a very simple means of identifying your metabolic type.

It takes approximately thirty minutes to answer all the questions, tally your score, and immediately identify your "basic," or "general," metabolic type category. The three metabolic type categories are:

- the Protein Type
- the Carbo Type
- the Mixed Type

Each of these general metabolic type categories corresponds to a specific diet. But keep in mind that your general category is simply a starting point.

Once you've identified your metabolic type and the diet that's right for you, you can use a variety of simple techniques (the techniques for added precision that I'll describe in subsequent chapters) that will enable you to fine-tune or customize your diet to your own highly individualized needs.

After all, there's a tremendous amount of biological and biochemical diversity among people, so there are far more than three metabolic types. You may be in the same general category as someone else, yet your dietary needs could be distinctly different.

For example, you and a friend might both be Protein Types, which means you don't function well on vegetarian-oriented diets or on meals and snacks centered mainly around carbohydrates. But even though you both need to emphasize protein and restrict carbohydrates to a certain extent, your friend might require heavier proteins on a more consistent basis throughout the day, and be more sensitive and reactive to carbohydrates (i.e., sugars and starches) than you.

In addition, your metabolic type is not something that's carved in stone. Although you were born with a specific set of dietary requirements dictated by your genetic heritage (your Genetic Type), your needs can shift for any number of reasons, such as illness or stress or nutrient deficiencies or excesses.

Your Functional Type refers to the way your metabolism is functioning today, or what your dietary needs are at the moment. But a month or six months or a year down the road, your needs could potentially shift, maybe back toward your actual genetic type.

Where metabolism is concerned, everything is highly individualized and everything is constantly in flux. That's why testing your metabolic type and fine-tuning your diet are techniques you'll want to employ on an ongoing, intermittent basis.

When you determine your metabolic type and fine-tune your diet,

you'll learn exactly what kinds of foods are compatible with your particular body chemistry. This means you'll discover what foods can
energize you and make you feel great right away, in addition to supporting your health over the longer term.

Just as important, you'll discover the secrets of how to combine
macronutrients (protein, carbohydrates, and fats) in the specific proportions that are just right for you.

*Learning exactly what foods to choose and exactly how to combine them
is of fundamental importance for eating according to your metabolic
type.*

The chart on page 133 gives you a brief synopsis or preview of the
three general metabolic type categories and the diets that correspond
to each category.

If you find that you're a Protein Type, it means one of two things—
either your cells tend to metabolize carbohydrates too quickly and you
are overly reliant on glycolysis for energy (meaning you're a fast oxidizer), or the parasympathetic branch of your autonomic nervous system is stronger and more dominant than the sympathetic branch.

In general or simplistic terms, Protein Types require a high protein
intake in order to strengthen the sympathetic system, thereby acidifying their too-alkaline metabolism. Or they need high protein (especially the high purine proteins) to slow down their too-rapid cellular
oxidation rate, thereby alkalinizing their too-acid metabolism.

If you're a Carbo Type, just the opposite is true. In general, you
need a higher percentage of carbohydrates in your diet in order to
strengthen the parasympathetic branch of your nervous system,
which is weaker than your sympathetic system, and thereby alkalinize your too-acid metabolism. Or you need more carbohydrates in
your diet in order to speed up your naturally slow cellular oxidation
rate, thereby bringing it into balance by acidifying your too-alkaline
metabolism.

If you're a Mixed Type, it means you're somewhere in the middle
of the other two types, which have more pronounced or clear-cut
metabolic imbalances. You *need* to eat a mixture of foods that will
support both sides of your autonomic nervous system—both your

HIGHLIGHTS OF THE METABOLIC TYPE DIETS

METABOLIC TYPE	DIET	METABOLIC IMBALANCE
Protein Type	• high protein • heavy, fatty, high-purine proteins • high fats and oils • low carbohydrates	fast oxidizer *or* parasympathetic dominant
Carbo Type	• low protein • light, lean, low-purine proteins • low fats and oils • high carbohydrates	slow oxidizer *or* sympathetic dominant
Mixed Type	• mixture of high-fat, high-purine proteins *and* low-fat, low-purine proteins • requires relatively equal ratios of proteins, fats, and carbohydrates	neither fast *nor* slow oxidizer neither parasympathetic *nor* sympathetic dominant

The three general metabolic type categories provide an effective starting point that will enable you to customize your diet.

sympathetic system and your parasympathetic system. The same principle applies to your oxidative system, since your cellular oxidation rate is neither fast nor slow, but somewhere in the middle. You'll want to be sure to eat a mixture of foods so that you will not create a one-sided or pronounced effect in terms of either speeding up or slowing down your cellular oxidation rate.

Even though the self-test you're about to take is quite short and simple (only sixty-five questions), it has a very high degree of accuracy. It's a distillation of my twenty years of working in the research and development of the science of metabolic typing.

Since metabolic typing is a complex science, and since you have countless traits that are indicative of your metabolic individuality, there are literally hundreds of highly detailed questions we could ask about your physical, psychological, and behavioral traits. Of course, that's just what many health professionals do when they're assessing people in clinical situations, using extremely in-depth metabolic typing evaluation procedures.

Nonetheless, the brief self-test contained in this chapter is a remarkably advanced and powerful tool that can provide you with a comprehensive understanding of what your unique dietary needs are all about. Especially if you take your time and answer each question as carefully as you can.

Remember, though, no test designed to gauge metabolic individuality, no matter how long or detailed, can ever be totally foolproof and completely accurate in one hundred percent of cases.

There is a very small percentage of people for whom questionnaires of any kind may not be enough. If you're one of these people, never fear.

In addition to fine-tuning techniques that you will find in Chapter 9, there is a very simple troubleshooting technique in Appendix A that you can use either to verify the accuracy of your self-test results, or to resolve any potential problem that might arise as you implement your diet.

The bottom line is this: The following chapters are loaded with very simple tools and instructions that will ensure you get off on the right foot, are eating the correct foods for your metabolic type, and can easily adjust your dietary regimen if the need should arise.

In the meantime, answer the following questions as best you can, and follow the simple scoring instructions that will reveal your general metabolic type category.

And remember, learning about your own metabolic individuality is a fun and interesting process. So don't forget to enjoy yourself on the road to self-discovery.

THE METABOLIC TYPE SELF-TEST

Instructions

For each of the following questions, please circle the one response (A, B, or C) that best applies to you.

If for any given question you are certain that none of the responses applies to you, simply leave that question unanswered.

However, in some cases you may find that none of the responses to a given question describe you exactly. In these instances, don't worry about the fact that a given response may not describe you with absolute precision. Just choose the answer that best describes your general tendencies.

Remember, we're looking for your general metabolic patterns or tendencies, so there's no need to get hung up on the exact details or specific wording of each question or response.

Please answer all questions in terms of how you are now, not how you used to be or would like to be or think you should be. Try to be as thoughtful and honest as you can, but remember that there are no right or wrong answers!

You may be surprised to realize that you really don't know the answers to some of the questions. For example, you may not know offhand how you would react to a specific type of food or combination of foods. If this is the case, what you should do is simply put the self-test aside for a little while until you can test your reaction to the foods in question.

Though you should not have to struggle with any question or aspect of this test, accuracy is important, so it's best to take your time and not rush through it.

Note that you can always take the test again at any point in the future. This is something you'll want to do periodically anyway, to see if your body chemistry has shifted, which can occur.

1. Anger and Irritability

Sometimes we all get angry "for good reason." But for some people, feelings of anger or irritability occur frequently or even daily, and are specifically influenced by what is—or isn't— eaten. Skip this question if you do not experience anger or irritability that is affected by food.

A. When I feel angry, eating meat or fatty food seems to make it worse.

B. Sometimes eating relieves my anger and it doesn't really matter what I eat.

C. I often notice that feelings of anger or irritability have abated after I eat something heavy and fatty like meat.

2. Anxiety

Some people have a tendency to be anxious, apprehensive, or worried. In many cases these feelings are increased or lessened by the kinds of foods that are eaten. Don't answer this question if you do not experience anxiety that is influenced by food.

When I feel anxious

A. fruits or vegetables calm me down.

B. eating almost anything helps alleviate my anxiety.

C. heavy, fatty food improves the way I feel and lessens my feelings of anxiety.

3. Ideal Breakfast

Some people say that breakfast is the most important meal of the day. But this simply isn't true from a metabolic perspective. Actually, every time you eat *anything*, what you eat is very important, because your ability to function depends on the kind of fuel you provide your "engines of metabolism." What kind of breakfast gives you the greatest energy, sense of well-being, peak performance, and satisfies your hunger the longest?

A. either no breakfast or something light like fruit; and/or toast or cereal; and/or milk or yogurt

B. egg(s), toast, fruit

C. something heavy like eggs, bacon or sausage, hash browns, toast; or steak and eggs

Page Tallies

A = _____   B = _____   C = _____

4. Meal Preference

Pretend it's your birthday and all rules and restrictions for dieting and (supposed) good health are thrown out the window. You're ready to cut loose and treat yourself to your favorite foods and just have a good time. If you went to a sumptuous buffet dinner tonight, what kinds of food would you choose?

A. I would choose lighter foods such as chicken, turkey, light fish, salads, vegetables, and I'd sample various desserts.

B. I would choose a combination of foods from answers A and C.

C. I would choose heavy, rich, fatty foods: roast beef, beef Stroganoff, pork chops, ribs, salmon, potatoes, gravy, few vegetables, or maybe a small salad with vinaigrette or blue cheese dressing; cheesecake or no dessert

5. Climate

Climate, temperature, environment—all can make a big difference in a person's sense of well-being, energy levels, productivity, and moods. Some thrive in the heat, while others wilt. Some come alive when it's cold, while others retreat and "hibernate." For others, temperature and climate don't seem to make much difference. Please select the choice that best describes how temperature affects you.

A. I do best in warm or hot weather. Can't take the cold.

B. Temperature doesn't matter that much. I do pretty well whether it's hot or cold.

C. I do best in cool or cold temperatures. Can't take the heat.

6. Chest Pressure

Some metabolic types commonly experience "chest pressure," a distinct sensation of pressure in the chest area. It often makes people feel as though a weight is on their chest, and tends to inhibit the ability to breathe.

C. I have a tendency to get or have problems with chest pressure.

Page Tallies

A = _____   B = _____   C = _____

7. Coffee

Coffee, when organically grown, properly prepared, and not misused, is an acceptable beverage for some metabolic types. Of course, anything that is overdone can be bad for you, even water. Nonetheless, coffee affects different people in different ways. Please indicate how coffee affects you.

A.   I do well on coffee (as long as I don't drink too much).
B.   I can take it or leave it.
C.   I don't do well with coffee. It makes me jittery, jumpy, nervous, hyper, nauseated, shaky, or hungry.

8. Appetite at Breakfast

Appetites vary dramatically from person to person, from ravenous to normal to very little. Of course, your appetite can vary from day to day to some degree, but what is being asked about here is your overall tendency. A "normal" appetite is to feel hunger around regular mealtimes (morning, noon, and evening), but not to a noticeable extreme in either direction.

My appetite at breakfast is typically
A.   low, weak, or lacking.
B.   normal. Don't notice it being either strong or weak.
C.   noticeably strong or above average.

9. Appetite at Lunch

For many people, appetites can change from breakfast to lunch to dinner. For others, it remains pretty much the same throughout the day. Please circle the answer that best describes your typical *tendency*—the way you are most of the time.

My appetite at lunch is typically
A.   low, weak, or lacking.
B.   normal. Don't notice it being either strong or weak.
C.   noticeably strong or above average.

10. Appetite at Dinner

For many people, their strongest appetite is at dinner. For others, it's just the reverse. How does your appetite at dinner compare to your appetite at other times of the day? Choose the answer that best describes your usual appetite around dinnertime.

My appetite at dinner is typically
A.   low, weak, or lacking.
B.   normal. Don't notice it being either strong or weak.
C.   noticeably strong or above average.

Page Tallies

A = _____   B = _____   C = _____

11. Concentration

Concentration or intense mental activity actually uses up a lot of energy and thus requires
sufficient fuel. But it also requires the right
kind of fuel—to enable individuals to maintain
mental clarity and stay focused. The wrong kind
of fuel can make your mind hyper, causing a
flood of uncontrollable thoughts. Or you could
feel spacey or sleepy, or experience thoughts that
seem to dissipate as soon as they arise. What
foods worsen your ability to concentrate?

A. meat and/or fatty food
B. No particular kind of food seems to be disrupt my concentration.
C. fruits and vegetables and grain-based carbohydrates

12. Coughing

Usually we think of coughing as something
associated with illness. But some people naturally cough, easily and often, and do so every
day, even when they aren't sick. Typically, the
cough will be a "dry" cough, and usually short
in duration. It often worsens at night or soon
after eating. If you're one of these people, circle answer C to the right.

C. I tend to cough every day.

13. Cracking Skin

Some people have a problem with their skin
cracking for no apparent reason. This typically
occurs on the fingertips or on the feet, especially on the heels. The problem can show up
any time of year, but tends to happen more
often in the winter.

C. I have a tendency to have problems with skin cracking.

14. Cravings

Some people do not have food cravings, so
answer this question only if you do. Sugar is
intentionally not listed as a choice here
because most people, when low on energy, will
begin to think of something sweet. Please
indicate any other kinds of food cravings you
might have besides sugar.

A. vegetables, fruits, grain-based products (bread, cereal, crackers)
C. salty, fatty foods (peanuts, cheese, potato chips, meats, etc.)

Page Tallies

A = _____   B = _____   C = _____

15. Dandruff

Dandruff is the exfoliation, or shedding of skin, on the scalp in the form of dry white scales. If you have a tendency to have dandruff, please circle the answer to the right.

C. I tend to have problems with dandruff.

16. Depression

Like other emotional issues, depression can arise from many possible causes. Yet depression is often alleviated or worsened by what you eat. If you suffer from depression and have noticed a connection to food, select the appropriate choice on the right.

A. I seem to feel more depressed after eating meats and fatty foods (and less depressed after eating fruits and vegetables).

C. I seem to feel more depressed after eating fruits and vegetables (and less depressed after eating meats and fatty foods).

17. Desserts

Foods provide various combinations of the six tastes: sweet, sour, salty, bitter, astringent, and pungent. We like to experience each of these effects from time to time, and they all have beneficial roles to play in our health. For example, everyone likes sweet foods, but not to the same degree and in the same quantity. What's your general feeling or attitude toward having desserts after meals?

A. I really love sweets, and/or I often need something sweet with a meal in order to feel satisfied.

B. I enjoy dessert from time to time, but can really take it or leave it.

C. I don't really care for sweet desserts that much; I may like something fatty or salty instead (like cheese, chips, popcorn) for a snack after meals.

Page Tallies

A = _____   B = _____   C = _____

18. Dessert Preference

What are your favorite kinds of desserts? Which would you choose most often? Even if you don't particularly like desserts, if you were forced to choose, which kinds would you gravitate toward?

(NOTE: Ice cream is purposefully not listed in the choices, as almost everyone likes ice cream, regardless of their metabolic type!)

A. cakes, cookies, fruit pies, candies
B. Truly no preference. I'd choose different kinds each day.
C. heavier, fatty types like cheesecakes, creamy French pastries

19. Ideal Dinner

The right kind of food at dinner can provide great energy and well-being for the entire evening. Whereas the wrong dinner for your type can leave you feeling exhausted, and initiate a strong case of couch potatoitis. What kind of meal works best for you at dinnertime?

A. something light like skinless chicken breast, rice, salad, maybe a little dessert
B. Most foods work fine for me.
C. I definitely do better with a heavier meal.

20. Ear Color

This query is concerned with blood flow to the ears. In some Caucasians, the ears are bright red, while in others, they're noticeably pale. Darker or lighter ears can also be seen in people of color. Please select the response that best describes your ear color.

A. My ears tend to be pale, lighter than my facial skin tone.
B. My ears tend to be the same shade as my face.
C. My ears tend to be pink, red, or darker than my facial tone.

Page Tallies

A = _____   B = _____   C = _____

21. Eating Before Bed

Eating before bed helps some people sleep better, while it clearly disrupts other people's sleep. For some, it depends on what they eat. For others, eating anything at all is a problem. This question concerns the latter.

Eating just about anything before going to bed:

A. disrupts or worsens my sleep.

B. doesn't seem to make a difference; I can take it or leave it.

C. usually helps me sleep better.

22. Eating Heavy Food Before Bed

Please indicate what reaction you would typically have to eating heavy foods before bedtime. "Heavy food" refers to protein foods or fatty foods like meat, fowl, and cheese.

A. It prevents or disturbs my sleep.

B. It's usually okay, as long as it isn't too much.

C. It improves my sleep.

23. Eating Light Food Before Bed

Please indicate what reaction you would typically have to eating light foods before bedtime. "Light food" refers to carbohydrates like bread, toast, cereal, or fruit—perhaps accompanied by small amounts of foods like milk, yogurt, or nut butter.

A. I usually don't do well eating before sleep, but I definitely do better with lighter food.

B. I can take it or leave it.

C. It's better than nothing, but I do better with heavier food.

24. Eating Sweets Before Bed

People have quite a range of reactions to sweets and sugars. Some can eat sugar before going to sleep and note no ill effect; it does not keep them from sleeping or disturb their sleep in any way. For others, sweets can cause insomnia, prevent them from sleeping soundly, or cause them to wake up, needing to eat something in order to go back to sleep. (Skip this question if you know you have candida overgrowth problems or are diagnosed as hypoglycemic or diabetic.) How do sweets affect your sleep?

A. Sweets don't interfere with my sleep at all.

B. Sweets sometimes bother my sleep.

C. I clearly don't do well eating sweets before sleep.

Page Tallies

A = _____   B = _____   C = _____

25. Eating Frequency

How often do you eat each day? The answer to this question should reflect your *need* to eat. For maximum energy and performance, some people need to eat more than three times a day. For others, twice is plenty. How often do you need to eat in order to maximize your well-being and productivity?

A.	2 to 3 meals a day and either no snacks, usually, or light snacks
B.	3 times a day and no snacks, usually
C.	3 meals or more a day and snacks, often something substantial

26. Eating Habits

Different types of metabolizers have different feelings toward food. Some people are very focused on food. They think about it a lot. They imagine what they'll be eating long before mealtimes. They enjoy talking about food, particularly about their likes and dislikes, or recounting stories of great meals or restaurants. These are the "live to eat" types. For others, food is almost the last thing on their minds, even to the point of forgetting to eat. They tend to view food more as one of life's unavoidable necessities, as compared to one of life's real pleasures. Having to eat is bad enough, but talking about food is an uninteresting waste of time. They're the "eat to live" types. What's your attitude toward food?

A.	I'm unconcerned with food and eating; may forget to eat; rarely think about food; eat more because I have to than because I want to.
B.	I enjoy food, enjoy eating, rarely miss a meal, but don't really focus on food in any way.
C.	I love food, love to eat, food is a big or central part of my life.

27. Eye Moisture

Like most functions in the body, eye moisture is something we really don't notice unless it's out of balance. Everyone's eyes at some point will feel too dry, or perhaps produce excessive moisture and tearing. But some people have a *noticeable tendency* in one direction or the other. Which of the following best describes your eyes?

A.	My eyes tend to be dry.
B.	I don't notice one way or the other.
C.	My eyes tend to be very moist, even to the point of tearing.

Page Tallies		
A = _____	B = _____	C = _____

28. Skipping Meals

Some metabolic types hardly notice when they haven't eaten. They often just happen to look at their watch and realize that it's long past their mealtime. But other metabolic types don't do well at all if they miss a meal. Their bodies let them know in no uncertain terms that it's time to eat. If *they* miss a meal, their performance drops dramatically. What happens to you when you go four hours or more without eating or skip a meal altogether?

A. Doesn't really bother me. I can easily forget to eat.

B. I may not be at my best, but it doesn't bother me, really.

C. I definitely feel worse, getting irritable, jittery, weak, tired, low on energy, depressed, or other negative symptoms.

29. Facial Coloring

The combination of thickness of the skin along with blood-flow level can produce variability in facial coloring. Increased blood flow can produce a pink, red, flushed, ruddy appearance, while decreased flow can produce a noticeably pale look. How would you characterize your facial coloring?

A. I'm noticeably on the pale side.

B. I have average coloring.

C. I'm noticeably darker (not from sun) or pink, flushed, ruddy.

30. Facial Complexion

Some people simply have a very bright look to their face. The skin may appear noticeably clear, translucent, shiny. Others can have the opposite look: noticeably pasty, chalky, unclear, dull. Most fall somewhere in between. How would you characterize your facial complexion?

A. more dull or pasty

B. average

C. bright, radiant, clear

31. Fatty Food

Contrary to popular opinion these days, fatty foods are not bad for everyone. They're actually beneficial for certain metabolic types. How do you feel about fatty foods? Remember, don't respond by indicating how you think you're supposed to feel. Value judgments aside, how much do you like or dislike fatty foods in general?

A. I don't really like fatty foods.

B. They're fine in moderation.

C. I love them or crave them and would like them often if I knew they were good for me.

Page Tallies

A = _____   B = _____   C = _____

32. Fingernail Thickness

Fingernails have a lot of properties: size, shape, moon or no moon, ridges or smooth surfaces, and so on. They can even develop troughs or they can curl. But this question pertains only to thickness. How would you characterize the thickness of your fingernails?

A. My nails tend to be thick, strong, hard.
B. Seem average in thickness
C. I definitely tend to have thin and/or weak nails.

33. Fruit Salad Lunch

How would you tend to feel after eating a (large) fruit salad with a little cottage cheese or yogurt for lunch?

A. It satisfies me; I do well on it and don't get hungry until dinner.
B. I do pretty well, but usually need a snack before dinner.
C. Pretty bad result. I usually get sleepy, tired, spacey, depressed, anxious, irritable and/or hungry as a result and definitely need to eat something else before dinner.

34. Gaining Weight

When you eat foods that are wrong for your metabolic type, what usually happens is that the food does not get fully converted to energy but gets stored as fat instead. Which of the following options best describes your tendency to gain weight?

A. Meats and fatty foods cause me to gain weight.
B. No particular foods seem to cause me to gain weight, but I'll gain weight if I eat too much and don't get enough exercise.
C. I tend to gain weight eating too many carbs (bread, pasta, other grain products, fruits, and/or vegetables).

Page Tallies

A = _____   B = _____   C = _____

35. Gag Reflex

No one likes to gag, but everyone has a gag reflex. However, sensitivity to the gag reflex varies dramatically. Some people gag often and very, very easily—at the dentist's, while brushing teeth and tongue, even from eating. Others rarely, if ever, gag, and it takes a lot for them to gag when they do. How would you describe your gag reflex?

A. I rarely, if ever, gag; it's hard to make me gag.
B. I probably have a normal reflex.
C. I easily gag and/or often gag.

36. Goose Bumps

The formation of goose bumps is a reaction produced by the nervous system. They often appear on the arms and legs as the result of fright, or a sudden chill, or light brushing or touching of the skin. Some people form goose bumps very easily and often, while others rarely, if ever, seem to form them. Are you prone to goose bumps?

A. I often get goose bumps.
B. I occasionally get goose bumps.
C. I rarely, if ever, get goose bumps.

37. Energy Boosters

Food is our fuel for life. But different foods have different energy-boosting effects on different metabolic types. Most people know how to bolster their energy using either wholesome foods or quick pick-me-ups like sugar or caffeine. What kinds of foods generally boost your energy—and give you lasting energy?

A. Fruit, candy, or pastry restores and gives me lasting energy.
B. Just about any food restores lasting energy.
C. Meat or fatty food restores my energy and well-being.

Page Tallies

A = _____   B = _____   C = _____

38. Heavy-Fat-Meal Reaction

Liking fat is one thing, but how you react to it is another. Let's find out here. Note that this question concerns how you *feel* after eating fat, *not* whether you think fat is good for you. Please choose the option that best describes how you would react to a high-fat meal.

A. decreases my well-being and energy, or makes me sleepy, or too full, or causes indigestion

B. causes no special reaction one way or the other

C. increases my well-being; makes me feel good, energetic, satisfied, like I "had a good meal"

39. Hunger Feelings

Getting hungry can produce a variety of symptoms, ranging from occasional thoughts of food, to all-out hunger pangs, even to the point of nausea. What kind of hunger signals do you typically get from your body?

A. I rarely get hungry or feel real hunger, or have weak hunger feelings that pass quickly, or can easily go long periods without eating, or can forget about food altogether

B. I have pretty normal hunger around meal-times or when I'm late for meals.

C. I often feel hungry; need to eat regularly and often; may get strong hunger sensations.

Page Tallies

A = _____   B = _____   C = _____

40. Energy Drain

What kinds of foods take your energy level down a notch or two instead of giving you the boost you're looking for?

A. Meat or fatty food generally makes me more tired, lowers my energy even more.
B. No foods in particular seem to take me down on a regular basis.
C. Fruit, pastry, or candy makes me worse, usually giving me a quick lift, then a crash.

41. Insect Bite or Sting

No one likes to get stung by a bee or bitten by a mosquito. But reactions can be extremely varied, ranging from a very small or mild reaction that disappears quickly to a very strong reaction (nonallergic) involving itching, pain, bruising, or welts that take a long time to go away, sometimes leaving discoloration for weeks or months. How do insect bites or stings affect you?

A. Reactions tend to be mild or weak and go away quickly.
B. Average reaction.
C. Clearly strong reaction, stronger than most (can involve above-average swelling, pain, itching, bruising, redness), and can take a long time to go away, even leaving discoloration afterward.

Page Tallies
A = _____   B = _____   C = _____

42. Insomnia

There are many kinds of insomnia. But with a certain type of insomnia, people routinely wake up in the middle of the night for reasons other than having to use the bathroom. Typically with this type of insomnia, people need to eat something in order to fall asleep again. With that in mind, do any of the following choices apply to you?

A. I rarely or never get this kind of insomnia.

B. I occasionally wake up and need to eat in order to go back to sleep.

C. I often wake up and need to eat in order to go back to sleep. Eating something before going to sleep helps this problem or shortens the time that I'm awake.

43. Itching Eyes

From time to time, everyone experiences itching eyes. This can happen when you have a cold, or hay fever, or candida overgrowth, or allergies. But for many people, itching eyes can be a common occurrence even when the above conditions are not present. This is the focus of this question.

C. I tend to get itching eyes often, even though I don't have a cold, allergy, or candida problem.

44. Itching Skin

This question concerns itching skin that is not due to bites or stings. Everyone's skin itches occasionally. But some people find that their skin itches on a regular daily basis, typically the scalp, arms, or calves. Because they're so used to it, they may not even be conscious of their frequent scratching.

C. My skin tends to itch often.

Page Tallies

A = _____   B = _____   C = _____

45. Meal Portions

Most everyone eats at least three meals a day. But the amounts at each meal can vary dramatically. Some people eat a lot of food, and may even have two or three helpings. Others eat very little but still feel full as a result. If you're not sure, think of it this way: When you eat out, do you usually eat less than others, more than others, or about the same as others?

A. I don't eat that much. Definitely less than average. Doesn't take much to get me full.

B. I don't seem to eat more—or less—than other people.

C. I generally eat large portions of food, usually more than most people.

46. Nose Moisture

Normally, we're not aware of the moisture content of the skin inside our nostrils. It's only when the nose becomes too dry or too moist (runny, watery) that we're likely to think about it at all. Please select the option that best describes the way you are when you're not ill or not suffering from an allergic reaction.

A. My nose often seems too dry.

B. I don't notice my nose being too dry or too moist.

C. My nose often tends to run.

47. Fruit Juice Between Meals

If you're hungry, say between meals, how does drinking a glass of orange juice (or other fruit juice) affect you? Overall, is it a good effect or a bad effect? Does drinking fruit juice satisfy your appetite and leave you feeling well until your next meal? Or does it result in some kind of adverse reaction?

A. It energizes me, satisfies me, works well to nourish me until my next meal.

B. It's okay, but isn't always the best snack for me.

C. Overall bad result. Can make me lightheaded, hungry soon after, jittery, shaky, nauseated, anxious, depressed, etc.

Page Tallies

A = _____   B = _____   C = _____

48. Personality

People have distinctly different personality traits, and many of these traits are related to, or heavily influenced by, one's biochemical makeup. Which of the following choices best describes your natural tendency in social gatherings, or your preference with respect to day-to-day interactions with other people?

A. I tend to be more aloof, withdrawn, a loner, or introverted.
B. I'm pretty average, neither introverted nor extroverted.
C. I tend to be more social, a "people person," or extroverted.

49. Potatoes

Potatoes are a wonderful food and they have many excellent nutritional attributes. But they aren't the best food for all metabolic types. Whether or not you think that potatoes are good for you, how do you feel about potatoes?

A. I don't really care for them that much or don't like them at all.
B. I can take them or leave them.
C. I really love them, could eat them almost every day.

50. Red Meat

Contrary to conventional wisdom, red meat is a healthy food choice for some metabolic types. When you eat red meat—like steak or roast beef—how do you normally feel afterward? Here we are seeking your *reaction* to red meat, *not* your belief as to whether or not you think it's good or bad for you.

A. It decreases my energy and well-being. Can make me depressed or irritable.
B. I don't notice one way or the other.
C. I definitely feel good or better when I eat red meat.

51. Pupil Size

Your pupils are the black, center portion of your eyes. The iris is the colored portion that surrounds the pupil. This question concerns the size of the pupil relative to the size of the iris. Average means the pupil and iris are basically the same size. Larger means the width of the pupil is clearly larger than the width of the iris. To answer, first look in a mirror, but do so in an average-lighted room—not dark, not bright.

The size of my pupil tends to be
A. Larger than my iris.
B. Average. The same size as my iris.
C. Smaller than my iris.

Page Tallies

A = _____   B = _____   C = _____

52. Salad for Lunch

If you eat the wrong foods for lunch, you're likely to tank in the afternoon. Instead of being productive, you may find that you can barely keep your eyes open, or that you need coffee or candy to try to stay alert and focused. If you ate a large vegetarian salad for lunch, what effect would it have on your productivity through the afternoon?

A. I do pretty well with that kind of lunch.
B. I can get by, but it isn't the best type of food for me.
C. Bad result. Makes me feel either sleepy, tired, lethargic, or hyper, nervous, irritable.

53. Saliva Quantity

Many people have had the experience of their mouth becoming very dry when frightened or nervous, such as when they're about to give a speech. In contrast, most of us have experienced our mouth's "watering" when we encounter the aroma of good food. However, for some people, these conditions are their natural tendency for no apparent reason. Please select the option that most accurately characterizes your saliva.

A. My mouth tends to be dry a lot of the time.
B. I don't notice that I have too little or too much saliva.
C. I tend to have a lot of saliva, or I have a tendency toward drooling.

54. Salty Foods

Salt, like sweet, is one of the six tastes. And like sweet, people have a varied reaction to and interest in salt. Some people salt their food heavily and seem to crave salt. Others really aren't that interested in it and actually find that many prepared foods taste too salty. Whether or not you feel that salt is good for you, how do you feel about salt?

A. Foods often taste too salty, or I like my food salted only lightly.
B. I don't really notice salt one way or the other. Rarely seems like too much or too little. Just use an average amount on foods.
C. I really love salt, or crave it. Like a lot of salt on foods, to the point that others think my food is too salty.

Page Tallies

A = _____   B = _____   C = _____

55. Snacking

Assume for this question that you eat three meals a day. If this is the case, do you typically need to snack, or to eat something between meals? Or are those three meals all the food you need for peak performance?

A. I rarely if never want or need snacks.

B. I occasionally want or need to snack between meals.

C. I often want or need to snack between meals.

56. Snack Preference

A good snack should provide you with lasting energy and improve your emotional well-being, in addition to satisfying your hunger. It should also not produce a negative effect, such as a craving for sweets. With this in mind, which of the following choices best describes your preference for snacks?

A. I generally don't need snacks, but if I do have one, I usually prefer and do well on something sweet.

B. I sometimes need snacks and do well on pretty much anything.

C. I definitely want and need snacks in order to be at my best. Do poorly on sweets, but do well on protein and fat (meat, chicken, cheese, hardboiled egg, nuts).

57. Sneezing

We usually think of sneezing in connection with colds or allergies. But some people sneeze daily as a matter of course, even when they're not sick or plagued with allergies. For example, some people sneeze routinely after eating. This question pertains to brief sneezing attacks composed of just one or two sneezes—not continuous, prolonged sneezing attacks. With that in mind, please select the option that best describes you.

A. I almost never sneeze unless I'm sick or have allergies.

B. I do sneeze from time to time when not sick or allergic, but not regularly.

C. I often regularly tend to sneeze and/or usually sneeze a little after eating.

Page Tallies

A = _____   B = _____   C = _____

58. Sociability

Many people believe that social tendencies are learned behavior. But one need only look at siblings in a family to see that people have innate tendencies with regard to sociability, even though these tendencies are influenced to a degree by life experiences. How would you describe your natural, innate tendency toward sociability, apart from the way your family or friends may have influenced you in this regard?

A. I tend to be a little "antisocial," in that I enjoy being alone, feel awkward at social gatherings or parties, and usually prefer to leave quickly or not to go at all.

B. I'm in the middle—not really antisocial, but also not particularly compelled to be with others.

C. I tend to be very social, a "people person," and love company and to be with others, prefer not to be alone.

59. Sour Foods

Sour, like sweet and salty, is one of the six tastes. Some people really like, love, or even crave sour foods like pickles, sauerkraut, vinegar, lemon juice, or yogurt. Others have an aversion to sour foods, or just don't like them all that much. Which of the following best describes your reaction to sour foods?

A. I generally don't care for sour foods.

B. I don't feel one way or the other, particularly. Don't like or dislike them much more than any other food.

C. I definitely like (some) sour foods or crave them.

60. Physical and Mental Stamina

Stamina refers to physical endurance, or the ability to persevere or work long hours without exhaustion. This capacity is greatly dependent on what we eat. Some foods optimize physical and mental stamina, while other foods noticeably reduce it. What type of foods best support your stamina?

My stamina is better when I eat:

A. lighter foods like chicken, fish, fruit, vegetables, grains.

B. pretty much any wholesome food.

C. heavy foods, fatty foods.

Page Tallies

A = _____   B = _____   C = _____

61. Consuming Sweets

There's hardly anyone who doesn't like sweets from time to time. But this question is not concerned with whether or not you like sweets. Rather, how do you react when you eat something sweet all by itself (e.g., cake, cookies, candy, etc.)?

A. Sweets don't bother me even when I eat them by themselves. Generally sweets satisfy my appetite and don't produce bad reactions.

B. I'm sometimes bothered when eating sweets by themselves, and often they don't satisfy my appetite.

C. I usually don't do well eating sweets by themselves. They usually produce some manner of bad reaction and/or create a desire for more sweets.

62. Meat for Breakfast

In this question, meat refers to flesh proteins like ham, sausage, bacon, steak, hamburger, and salmon. How do you feel after consuming meat for breakfast—as opposed to going without it? Remember, this question does not include eggs, milk, or cheese as a substitute for the other animal proteins listed above.

A. I don't feel as well as I do without it. Tends to make me feel more tired, sleepy, lethargic, angry, irritable, thirsty, or causes me to lose my energy by midmorning.

B. I can take it or leave it, varies.

C. I feel much better with it: more energetic, have good stamina, keeps me going without getting hungry before lunch.

Page Tallies

A = _____   B = _____   C = _____

63. Red Meat for Lunch

In this question, red meat refers to flesh proteins like beef or lamb. How do you feel after consuming some red meat at lunch, as opposed to going without it? This question does not include eggs, milk, or cheese as a substitute for the other animal proteins listed above.

A. I don't feel as well as I do without it. Tends to make me feel more tired, sleepy, lethargic, angry, irritable, thirsty, or causes me to lose my energy by midafternoon.

B. I can take it or leave it, varies.

C. I feel much better with it: more energetic, have good stamina, keeps me going without getting hungry before dinner.

64. Red Meat for Dinner

In this question, meat refers to flesh proteins like beef or lamb. How do you feel after consuming some red meat for dinner, as opposed to going without it? This question does not include eggs, milk, or cheese as a substitute for the other animal proteins listed above.

A. I don't feel as well as I do without it. Tends to make me feel more tired, sleepy, lethargic, angry, irritable, thirsty, or causes me to lose my energy.

B. I can take it or leave it, varies.

C. I feel much better with it: more energetic, have good stamina, keeps me going without getting hungry before bedtime.

Page Tallies

A = _____   B = _____   C = _____

65. Dinner Preference

Pretend you're on vacation in the American West. It's nighttime and you're driving across the Death Valley Desert. You just spotted a sign that says DINER AHEAD. 10 MILES. NEXT EATING PLACE, 150 MILES. You're hungry, so you decide to pull into the diner. There you find that there are only three choices on the menu—Dinner Plates 1, 2, and 3. Since you have a long drive ahead of you, it's essential for you to eat the kind of food that will keep you awake and energized. Which dinner plate would you choose to give you the best stamina, energy, and alertness?

A. Dinner Plate 1— skinless chicken breast, rice, salad. Apple pie.

B. Dinner Plate 2—a combination plate including a little of everything from Plates 1 and 3.

C. Dinner Plate 3—pot roast cooked with carrots, onions, and potatoes, served with biscuits and gravy. Cheesecake.

Page Tallies

A = _____   B = _____   C = _____

SCORING YOUR TEST
AND IDENTIFYING YOUR TYPE

Congratulations on completing your self-test! You're about to identify your metabolic type!

All you need to do now is tally your score. It's very simple. Just follow the three easy steps below:

1. On each page of the self-test, add up the number of times you circled choices A, B, and C and write each subtotal at the bottom of the page in the Page Tallies box.

2. Then add up the subtotals on each page and write them in this scoring box:

> Total A answers = _____
>
> Total B answers = _____
>
> Total C answers = _____

3. Next, refer to the scoring box above and select your metabolic type classification, using the following criteria:

- If your number of A answers is 5 or more higher than *both* B *and* C, then you are a Carbo Type (example: A=25, B=20, C=15)
- If your number of C answers is 5 or more higher than *both* A *and* B, then you are a Protein Type (example: A=15, B=20, C=25)
- If your number of B answers is 5 or more higher than *both* A *and* C, then you are a Mixed Type (example: A=20, B=25, C=15)
- If *neither* A, B, *nor* C are 5 or more higher than *both* of the other two, then you are a Mixed Type (example: A=18, B=22, C=20)

Now you're ready to learn all about the diet for your metabolic type:

- If you're a Protein Type, turn to page 164.
- If you're a Carbo Type, turn to page 187.
- If you're a Mixed Type, turn to page 211.

tain your body's uni
be—easy and enjo
Imagine the
the first time
well inform
purchases
work a

EAT ACCORDING TO
YOUR METABOLIC TYPE

The End of Dietary Roulette

There are few things in life as liberating as discovering your metabolic type, few things as enlightening as finally coming to understand exactly what foods and food combinations will enable you to enjoy your life thoroughly and live it to the fullest.

Most of us have been slaves to food in one way or another all our lives. Quite literally, what we eat controls every aspect of our existence—how we look and feel, our range of productivity and performance, the quality of our emotional experiences, whether we stay well or fall prey to disease, even the quality of our sleep and the nature of our dreams.

When we don't understand how specific foods affect us, eating becomes a daily struggle. We struggle to feel satisfied, to fight the battle of the bulge, or just to feel decent from one hour to the next.

Once you recognize your metabolic individuality, however, everything changes. The balance shifts, the tables are turned—suddenly you're the one in control of food, it's not in control of you. Eating right is no longer a complex challenge and food is no longer your adversary. When you know how to choose foods that effectively sus-

que style of functioning, eating is what it should
yable.

sense of excitement and empowerment you'll have
you go to the supermarket and select groceries in a truly
ed and targeted way, rather than being forced to make
in a random, haphazard fashion, based largely on guess-
out what might or might not be good for you or your family.
nink of the freedom you'll experience once you're able to identify,
h certainty, what kinds of meals or snacks will make you feel great
nd give you high levels of energy and endurance for hours at a time.

Won't it be exhilarating to know exactly what you can eat anytime
you need to be at your best for a business presentation or a tennis
match, to take an exam or embark on a long road trip? What's more
important than knowing how to choose just the right sustenance to
enable you to put in a long day at the office, enjoy your kids, pursue
your hobbies, write a novel, or burn the midnight oil doing any one
of a thousand different things?

It's not an exaggeration to say that once you identify your metabolic type and begin to eat accordingly, your life will never be the
same. It's literally like having a blindfold removed and experiencing
a whole new dimension in life. You'll wonder how you managed to
function for so long without this kind of fundamental self-awareness.

Health and Fitness Benefits for Every Type

When you start to eat correctly, you'll experience lots of positive
changes that will sharply improve the quality of your life. Some of
these benefits will occur right away, others will take a while longer.

Here are the kinds of improvements you can expect in the *short term:*

• Your food will be efficiently converted to energy rather than
stored as fat.

• You'll enjoy plenty of physical and mental energy following
meals and snacks.

• You'll feel full and hunger free, four to five hours after meals.

• You'll lose your cravings for sweets and starchy foods.

- Digestive problems—indigestion, gas, bloating—will subside.
- You'll have sustained energy and endurance throughout the day.
- You'll be capable of improved athletic performance.
- Your ability to concentrate will be significantly enhanced.
- You'll enjoy a renewed sense of well-being and positive mental outlook.
- Irritability, anxiety, depression, and hyperactivity will fade away.

There are plenty of long-term benefits you can expect as well, although they're different for everyone, since people have different kinds of metabolic imbalances and an almost infinite assortment of related health problems.

In general, however, here are the kinds of *long-term* health benefits you can expect if you stick to a diet that's tailored to your metabolic type:

- natural weight loss without dieting or restricting calories
- permanent weight loss without struggle, deprivation, or hunger
- achievement of your ideal weight, whether you're overweight or underweight
- prevention of chronic disease
- enhanced immunity
- improved resistance to colds, flu, recurrent infections
- reversal of chronic or degenerative health disorders
- slowing of the aging process

A customized diet will provide you with much more than symptom suppression, a quick fix for common ailments, a temporary energy boost, or a way to help you shed a few pounds in the short term—only to have your health problems and your weight reappear again soon. It's a process that enables you to optimize your health in a permanent way by balancing the homeostatic mechanisms that control all aspects of your metabolism.

When you consistently consume the right fuel mixture, you're providing your body with the raw materials it needs to regulate and repair and regenerate itself on an ongoing basis. That's the essence of real health and real healing, and the reason people are very successful when they use metabolic typing to prevent and reverse chronic illness. You'll be amazed at the kinds of results you can achieve with customized nutrition, especially if you apply a little time and perseverance.

Food as Medicine

What's essential to understand is that food is the ultimate medicine. There is no drug or vitamin pill or herb or other nutritional supplement that can influence your health as profoundly as your diet.

In this day and age, with nutritional supplements so widely available, many people make the mistake of thinking they can eat what they want as long as they take vitamins and minerals. But this is definitely *not* the case. Supplements are just what their name implies— a supplement to your diet, not a substitute for it.

To a limited extent, supplements may compensate for a diet that is inadequate for your metabolic type. But of the two—diet and supplements—your diet is the more important. It's the foundation upon which your health is built.

Remember, your body is designed to sustain itself on the same core dietary building blocks (in the form of proteins, carbohydrates, and fats) that were available to your ancestors, not on products that come in a bottle or a box.

You may take very high quality supplements, perfectly well suited to your metabolic type. But if you're not eating the right diet, it's like trying to run in opposite directions at the same time. In that case, the best you can hope for is that your supplements will offset some of the adverse influences of the foods you're consuming.

The best way to balance your body chemistry, increase your metabolic efficiency, and, in turn, improve your health is to eat a wide variety of the foods that are right for you and avoid all the foods that are wrong for you.

In the following diet section (see the section that applies to your particular metabolic type), I'll give you very simple and focused instructions for doing just that.

As you go forward, keep in mind that it's important to fine-tune your diet by listening to your body. I'll show you very simple techniques for this as well. It's very easy to do, and the payoffs are enormous.

Fine-tuning your diet from time to time is essential, because your metabolism is subject to occasional shifts. All you need to do is to pay attention to, and learn to interpret, the multiple messages your body is continuously attempting to send you.

People in today's society tend to be out of touch with their own bodies, and many people are not even conscious of what genuinely good health feels like. Our diets have been so seriously deficient for so long that many of us have either forgotten what robust good health is all about, or we've simply never experienced it at all.

As a result of substandard nutrition, most people fail to live up to their true, genetically endowed health potential. Someone may have the built-in design capacity for excellent health, but without the right body fuel, it simply never materializes. Fortunately, customized nutrition enables us all to claim our natural birthright.

Characteristics of Your Metabolic Type

Many Protein Types share similar characteristics. However, if you're a Protein Type, that doesn't mean you're like everyone else in your metabolic category in the way you react to foods, your strengths and weaknesses, your energy level, the strength of your appetite, and so on. After all, you're unique on a metabolic level!

Nonetheless, here are some typical tendencies you may have in common with other Protein Types:

Strong Appetites

Protein types tend to have strong appetites to the point of being ravenously hungry a great deal of the time. You may feel the need to eat frequently, though you're also likely to have a hard time feeling satisfied with meals and snacks. In addition, you probably have a tendency to overeat sometimes, perhaps even stuffing yourself to the bursting point, only to find that you're still hungry.

Cravings for Fatty, Salty Foods

Protein types typically gravitate toward rich, fatty, salty foods like sausages, pizza, and roasted and salted nuts. However, if you stray too far from these heavier foods and consume too many carbohydrates, you may quickly find yourself craving sugar. The likelihood is that the more you eat anything sweet, the stronger your cravings become. And sugar most likely causes your energy to drop or makes you feel nervous and jittery.

Failure with Low-Calorie Diets

You may have tried to lose weight by cutting calories, only to find your weight either increased or stayed the same. Or perhaps you've had the willpower to try radical measures like fasting or the "grapefruit diet," but were astonished to find that your weight actually increased despite these severe deprivation approaches.

Fatigue, Anxiety, Nervousness

Characteristically, those with your metabolic type have energy problems of one kind or another—either lethargy or a "hyped-up" kind of superficial energy. In other words, you might have low, "flat" energy, and be prone to feeling apathetic, depressed, listless, and sleepy. Or you might feel "wired" or "on edge" on the surface of things, while feeling exhausted underneath. When you feel anxious, nervous, jittery, or shaky, eating probably makes you feel better.

If any of these situations describes you, it's a clear indication that you're pumping the wrong kind of "body fuel" into your "engine of metabolism."

Dietary Emphasis for Protein Types

As a Protein Type, what you need is a diet comprised of relatively high amounts of protein and fat compared with carbohydrates.

But, all proteins are not created equal. You need to focus on certain kinds of proteins—those high in fat and high in purines. As you'll see in the food list I've prepared for you, there are many types of foods that are rich in purines.

More than any other kinds of foods, purine-containing foods are oxidized (converted to energy) at the proper rate for your metabolic type.

At the opposite end of the spectrum from purine proteins are carbohydrates. People with your metabolic type need to minimize the consumption of carbohydrates, since they're converted to energy too quickly. The heavier proteins and fatty foods effectively slow down the too-fast oxidative rates of most Protein Types.

For many years, popular wisdom has held that red meat and high-fat diets are bad for human beings. But this is simply not true. The truth is, any food can be good for you and any food can be bad for you. Everything is dependent on your metabolic type.

If you happen to be a Protein Type, you definitely need a high-protein, high-fat diet in order to lose weight, feel energized both physically and mentally, and stay on an even keel emotionally. Over the longer term, this same diet, if properly followed and tailored to your metabolic individuality, can prevent you from developing all kinds of serious degenerative diseases—cardiovascular problems, immune deficiency, blood sugar abnormalities, osteoporosis, arthritis, digestive disorders, and many other chronic illnesses—all of which are rooted in metabolic imbalance.

THE PROTEIN TYPE DIET ALLOWABLE FOODS CHART

PROTEINS[1]			CARBOHYDRATES			OILS / FATS	
MEAT/FOWL	SEAFOOD	DAIRY	GRAIN	VEGETABLE	FRUIT	NUT/SEED[4]	OIL/FAT
high purine	high purine	whole fat	whole grains only	nonstarchy	avocado	all are okay	all are okay
organ meats	anchovy	low purine	high starch	asparagus	olive	walnut	butter
pâté	caviar	cheese	amaranth	beans, fresh	not fully ripe—	pumpkin	cream
beef liver	herring	cottage cheese	barley	cauliflower	apple (some)	peanut	ghee
chicken liver	mussel	cream	brown rice	celery	pear (some)	sunflower	oils:
medium purine	sardine	eggs	buckwheat	mushroom	high starch	sesame	almond
beef	medium purine	kefir	corn	spinach	banana	almond	coconut
bacon	abalone	milk	couscous	high starch		cashew	flax
chicken[2]	clam	yogurt	kamut	artichoke		Brazil	olive
duck	crab	LEGUMES	kasha	carrot		filbert	peanut
fowl	crayfish	low purine	millet	pea		pecan	sesame
goose	lobster	tempeh	oat	potatoes, fried		chestnut	sunflower
kidney	mackerel	tofu	quinoa	in butter, only		pistachio	walnut
lamb	octopus	medium purine	rye	squash, winter		coconut	
pork chop	oyster	beans, dried	spelt	LEGUMES		hickory	
spare rib	salmon	lentils	triticale	nonstarchy		macadamia	
turkey[2]	scallop	NUTS	sproutedgrain bread is the only bread allowed[3]	tempeh			
veal	shrimp	all are okay		tofu			
wild game	snail			high starch			
	squid			beans, dried			
	tuna, dark			peas, dried			
				lentils			

1. Every meal should contain a protein from these sources, but dairy, legumes, or nuts are not a substitute for meats at main meals.
2. Dark meat is best.
3. Sproutedgrain breads such as Ezekiel or Manna brands are listed from highest to lowest protein content.
4. Nuts are listed from highest to lowest protein content. Higher protein is preferable.

Important Tips on Your Allowable Foods

Eat Protein at Every Meal.

Eating sufficient protein at every meal will maximize your energy, trim your waistline, and assure peak performance. Failure to do this can lead to chronic fatigue, diminished well-being, and emotional imbalances such as depression, anxiety, and melancholy. Many people make the mistake of eating carbohydrate alone at a meal or snack. *This is especially undesirable for your metabolic type.* It will only worsen your imbalance, tend to increase your fat stores, and intensify any food cravings, particularly for sugar or other sweets.

Emphasize High-density, High-purine Proteins.

Purines are special substances derived from a class of proteins called nucleoproteins, which play an important part in the energy-producing processes in body tissues. They have particular benefit for protein-type metabolizers and directly contribute to balancing their body chemistry. Note that any animal, fowl, and seafood protein is permissible in your diet. As higher-density proteins, animal proteins are preferable to the vegetable proteins. But due to the special needs of

P R O T E I N S [1]		
MEAT/FOWL	SEAFOOD	DAIRY
high purine	*high purine*	whole fat
organ meats	anchovy	*low purine*
pâté	caviar	cheese
beef liver	herring	cottage cheese
chicken liver	mussel	cream
medium purine	sardine	eggs
beef	*medium purine*	kefir
bacon	abalone	milk
chicken[2]	clam	yogurt
duck	crab	*LEGUMES*
fowl	crayfish	*low purine*
goose	lobster	tempeh
kidney	mackerel	tofu
lamb	octopus	*medium purine*
pork chop	oyster	beans, dried
spare rib	salmon	lentils
turkey[2]	scallop	*NUTS*
veal	shrimp	*all are okay*
wild game	snail	
	squid	
	tuna, dark	

1. Every meal should contain a protein from these sources, but dairy, legumes, or nuts are not a substitute for meats at main meals.
2. Dark meat is best.

your metabolic type, you fare better on high- and medium-purine proteins. These are all the foods listed in the meat/fowl and seafood columns in your Allowable Foods Chart. Most people in your metabolic type category require a higher purine protein with every meal. Lower-purine or lower-density proteins like dairy, legumes, and nuts are not a substitute. You should notice that if you eat low-purine, low-density foods as the primary protein source at any meal, you won't feel as satisfied, nor will your performance or energy be optimal. On the other hand, incorporating the higher-purine, higher-density proteins into two or three of your meals on a daily basis will supercharge your diet with the ideal fuel mixture for your engines of metabolism.

Snack as Needed.

If you snack, be sure to include a protein food. It's best for your metabolic type to never eat carbohydrate alone. Any protein can be used for a snack, but stick with what works best for you. You may find that nuts or dairy work well for snacks but are not adequate protein sources for main meals. On the other hand, if nuts or dairy snacks leave you hungry or craving something sweet, or cause a drop in energy or mood, you likely will need heavier proteins for snacks as well. Learn to listen to your body!

Be Cautious with Carbohydrates.

All plant-based foods—grains, vegetables, or fruits—are carbohydrates. But there are different kinds of carbohydrates and they don't all affect your metabolism in the same way. For example, some carbohydrates are higher in starch and some carbohydrates are lower in starch. Starchy carbohydrates break down easily into sugar, which means they hit your bloodstream quickly. This can cause a strong insulin response from your pancreas, which can lead to increased fat storage and blood sugar problems like hypoglycemia. Over time, excess insulin secretion can contribute to more severe disorders such as: allergies, asthma, alcoholism, atherosclerosis, cancer, carbohydrate addiction, heart disease, chronic fatigue, depression, diabetes, insulin resistance, glucose intolerance, hypertension, obesity, and peptic ulcers. Carrots, potatoes, squash, bananas, and all grains tend to be high in starch and must be carefully regulated. Thus, grains, starchy vegetables, and fruits are your "caution carbs." For this reason, Protein Types do best limiting starches and need to emphasize the nonstarchy vegetables as their primary source of carbohydrates.

CARBOHYDRATES		
GRAIN	*VEGETABLE*	*FRUIT*
whole grains only	nonstarchy	avocado
high starch	asparagus	olive
amaranth	beans, fresh	not fully ripe—
barley	cauliflower	apple (some)
brown rice	celery	pear (some)
buckwheat	mushroom	high starch
corn	spinach	banana
couscous	high starch	
kamut	artichoke	
kasha	carrot	
millet	pea	
oat	potatoes, fried in butter, only	
quinoa	squash, winter	
rye	*LEGUMES*	
spelt	nonstarchy	
triticale	tempeh	
sprouted-grain bread is the only bread allowed[1]	tofu	1. Sprouted-grain brands such as Ezekiel or Manna breads
	high starch	
	beans, dried	
	peas, dried	
	lentils	

Beware of Bread.

Limit bread intake, both in quantity and frequency, as much as possible. If possible, opt for sprouted-grain breads like Ezekiel or Manna brands. Unlike regular breads, sprouted-grain breads won't inhibit calcium absorption, thereby disrupting your calcium balance—a critical consideration for your metabolic type. When you do eat bread, always use butter, as it will minimize any potential adverse blood sugar fluctuations.

Go Easy with Grains.

Use only whole-grain products. Do not consume *any* refined grain products made with white flour or enriched flour. All baked foods should contain only whole grain flours. However, avoid wheat and wheat products as much as possible, since wheat breaks down into sugar faster than any other grain and therefore has a disruptive influence on insulin metabolism. But don't worry—most any other grain is fine for your metabolic type. Here's a tip: Try using spelt instead of wheat, since spelt shares many of wheat's desirable attributes for baking but not wheat's influences on insulin. Keep in mind, though, that all grains are starches, which means they readily break down into sugar, so they should be used sparingly. For this reason, cooked whole grains are preferable to products like breads and crackers. The worst offenders for your metabolism are refined grains of all kinds.

Closely Monitor Fruits.

Because Protein Types tend to be fast oxidizers or parasympathetic dominants, they're predisposed to low blood sugar problems. This means you're not likely to do well on fruits, which are high in potassium and sugar. However, most Protein Types do well on avocados and olives, and limited amounts of apples, pears, and bananas that are not fully ripe. But you're likely to run into big problems if you attempt to eat fruit by itself.

Use Juices Judiciously.

Vegetable juices, as long as they're freshly made, are allowed in moderation—but don't have more than one glass, three to four times per week. It's best to use a combination of starchy and nonstarchy vegetables such as carrot, celery, and spinach. Use a reduced proportion of starchy vegetables like carrots, since they're too sugary. Do not consume fruit juices at all. Fruit juices, or even excessive amounts of vegetable juice, will strongly imbalance your metabolic type and lead to weight gain, food cravings, blood sugar fluctuations, energy disruptions, and a desire for sugar. Avoid canned juices of any kind.

Freely Use Fats and Oils.

The subject of fats and oils and their effects on human metabolism has been extensively researched and documented. An in-depth discussion of them is beyond the scope of this book (for a complete discussion, see *Fats and Oils*, an excellent book by Udo Erasmus). In general, what you need to know is that fats and oils in their natural state are not bad for you and eating them will not produce high cholesterol or heart disease any more than any other natural food. Fats contain fatty acids that are essential for good health, efficient immune func-

OILS / FATS	
NUT/SEED[1]	OIL/FAT
all are okay	all are okay
walnut	butter
pumpkin	cream
peanut	ghee
sunflower	oils:
sesame	almond
almond	coconut
cashew	flax
Brazil	olive
filbert	peanut
pecan	sesame
chestnut	sunflower
pistachio	walnut
coconut	
hickory	
macadamia	

1. Nuts are listed from highest to lowest protein content. Higher protein is preferable.

tion, normal hormonal production, cellular respiration (energy production), proper cell membrane permeability—in short, for life itself. Whether a food is good or bad depends both on the quality of the food and on the metabolic type of the person consuming the food. Fats are no exception. Unlike other types, Protein Types need to support their metabolisms by consuming liberal amounts of natural oils and fats. But never consume margarine, hydrogenated oils, or fat substitutes, as research is uncovering the fact that these substances can have a serious negative impact on your health! If you must buy packaged foods, read the labels to make sure they do not contain these substances. Use only real butter (organic if possible) and natural cold-pressed oils that have been properly manufactured. Recommended brands are Omega, Flora, or Bio-San, widely available in health food stores. Other good sources from which to derive your quota for fatty acids are from nuts, nut butters, and the animal-based foods listed in your Allowable Foods Chart.

Foods to Avoid

Certain foods really aggravate your metabolic imbalances and should be avoided. You may have strong adverse reactions to these foods, or if your metabolism is less sensitive, the reactions may be slight or even nonexistent. Or your reactions to these problem foods could vary from time to time. All these possibilities are common and reflect yet another facet of metabolic individuality

Keep in mind that the effects of nutrition are cumulative. The more you ingest a food, the stronger the effect becomes. So even if you don't display any noticeable adverse reactions, it's still best to minimize your intake of the following foods whenever possible.

In short, stick to your allowable foods. But, if you simply must eat something not on that list, be aware that the following foods are particularly undesirable for your metabolism.

Alcohol.

In any form (beer, wine, hard liquor), alcohol is a form of poison to your body. When you consume it, your body must detoxify it and neutralize its adverse effects. From this standpoint, it really isn't good for anyone. But as a simple sugar, alcohol is also the worst kind of fuel for Protein Types, particularly if you're a fast oxidizer. Instead of providing a steady and prolonged conversion to energy, ingesting alcohol is akin to throwing gasoline on your metabolic fire—it produces a quick energy burst but is followed by an energy crash. Similarly, if you're a parasympathetic Protein Type, you might experience a temporary lift from drinking alcohol, but the result will be only a worsening of your metabolic type's natural inclination toward low blood sugar, along with excessive insulin secretion and increased fat storage.

Allergenic or Reactive Foods.

Your Allowable Foods Chart provides recommendations for foods that will specifically support your metabolic type. This means that they contain the right balance of nutrients for your type. Whether or not you are currently reactive or allergic to any of these foods is a completely different issue. If you have known reactions to any recommended foods, leave them out of your diet temporarily, but try them from time to time. As your chemistry changes, so too may your food reactivities. This is the experience of many individuals who have properly customized their diets to match their metabolism.

Caffeine.

Avoid caffeine products as much as possible, including coffee, black teas, caffeine-containing herbs, and soft drinks. If you do insist on drinking coffee, make sure it's organic and limit it to no more than one to two weak cups per day. Also, when drinking caffeinated beverages, make sure to eat some protein, as protein will, to a degree, help combat caffeine's adverse effects on your type. Bottom line: Caffeine is counter-productive for your metabolism, whether you are a fast oxidizer or a parasympathetic dominant. In fast oxidizers, coffee directly worsens the imbalances in their cellular oxidative processes, increasing their oxidation rate even further. In parasympathetics, the caffeine stimulation to the adrenals is akin to whipping a tired horse, as most parasympathetics have weaker adrenal function to begin with. Short term, this stimulation is pleasurable, but long term it only worsens the problem by further exhausting the adrenals.

Fruit Juices/Citrus Fruits.

Fruit juices in general, and citrus fruits specifically, are best avoided. Fruit juices are too high in sugar for Protein Types. Devoid of fiber, the concentrated juice has a particularly powerful negative impact on your type. The flooding of sugar into your bloodstream causes a strong insulin surge that rapidly lowers blood sugar and increases fat storage. And next to alcohol, citrus fruit is probably the poorest choice of any food for you—whether you are a fast oxidizer or a parasympathetic dominant. Because citrus fruit is high in potassium, sugar, and citric acid, it directly accelerates fast oxidative processes, worsening the imbalances of fast oxidizers. In parasympathetics, citrus has the most powerful alkalinizing effect of any food and thus dramatically worsens their already too-alkaline body chemistry, leading to increased lethargy, depression, and fatigue.

Sugar.

In significant quantities, sugar is not good for anyone. However, sugar is particularly bad for your metabolic type, so avoid or minimize it as much as you can. Be especially watchful for hidden sugars in processed packaged foods. Sugar is added to a great many commercial foods, and it can really add up if you're not careful, secretly sabotaging your best intentions to follow your dietary recommendations. By the way, by "sugar" I mean all forms of sugar—processed and natural—including beet sugar, cane sugar, brown sugar, molasses, honey, fructose, maltose, dextrose, corn syrup, maple syrup, etc.

Foods High in Oxalic Acids.

Oxalic acid is a naturally occurring acid in some foods that interferes with the absorption of calcium. Because calcium is particularly important for your metabolic type, you should avoid or minimize foods high in oxalic acid. These include black tea, blackberry, beets, beet greens, chard, chocolate, cocoa, cranberries, currants (red), endive, gooseberries, grapes, green peppers, plums, raspberries, rhubarb, strawberries, tomatoes. Apples, asparagus, and spinach are exceptions. The good news is that cooking destroys the oxalic acid, so items such as beets, beet greens, chard, cranberries, green peppers, rhubarb, asparagus, and spinach are all best eaten when cooked.

High-Glycemic Foods.

All carbohydrates—fruits, vegetables, grains—are converted to glucose in the body. Carbohydrates are categorized according to the rate or speed at which they hit the bloodstream as glucose, and are ranked accordingly in what is known as the glycemic index (GI). High-glycemic foods such as grains and starchy vegetables hit your bloodstream much more rapidly than low-glycemic foods like proteins and fats. That's why you need to carefully regulate high-glycemic foods and place much more emphasis on those foods that are lower on the GI. Your metabolic type simply can't handle large amounts of foods that convert rapidly to glucose in your bloodstream. Whenever you do eat high-glycemic foods, be sure to eat plenty of protein and fat at the same time to help slow down the rate at which high-glycemic foods are converted to sugar. (Note: Check Chapter 9 for the complete glycemic index. It's very important for all metabolic types to become familiar with the GI, but it's particularly critical for your type.)

Foods High in Phytates.

As Sally Fallon and Mary Enig point out in their wonderful book *Nourishing Traditions* (Mega Distributing, 1-877-707-1776 or www.newtrendspublishing.com), in every traditional culture in the world, for thousands of years, whole grains have been prepared by soaking or fermenting them prior to cooking. Modern science has revealed the wisdom of these traditions by discovering that all grains and legumes contain substances called phytates. Phytic acid is a chemical found in the bran portion of grains and the skins of legumes. It binds with calcium (and iron, magnesium, phosphorous, and zinc) in the intestinal tract, thereby preventing absorption of these minerals. When consumed excessively, phytates can cause serious mineral deficiencies, allergies, intestinal distress, and bone loss. Since you're a Protein Type, with an increased need for calcium, phytate products are particularly problematic for you. All grains contain phytates, but wheat, oats, soy, and soy milk have the highest concentration. What to do? Simply soak any grains (such as oat, millet, rye, barley, and quinoa) overnight before you cook them. You can also liberally use miso, soy sauce, and tempeh, since these are fermented products, and fermentation destroys phytates. However, tofu, soy milk, and soy protein powders are not fermented and do contain phytates, so you should limit consumption of these food items.

Sprouted-grain breads, and sourdough bread with its long fermentation process, are also almost entirely free of phytates. All other breads are full of phytates and should be limited or avoided.

Foods High in Gluten and Enzyme Inhibitors.

Grains contain hard-to-digest proteins like gluten. Insufficient digestion of such proteins has been linked to problems such as allergies, celiac disease (sprue), mental illness, indigestion, and yeast overgrowth (candida albicans). But here again, soaking and fermentation renders such proteins more digestible and their nutrients more readily available. So, sourdough breads and sprouted breads (like Ezekiel and Manna brands) are preferable to other varieties. Soybeans also contain potent enzyme inhibitors that need to be neutralized through fermentation or soaking.

Your Macronutrient Ratio

This diet is easy! There are only two things you need to remember:

1. Eat the right kinds of foods for your type and avoid the wrong foods for your type—in other words, stick to your allowable foods.
2. Eat the right proportions of macronutrients (proteins, fats, carbohydrates) at each meal.

If you think of your food as *fuel*, then the proportions of proteins, carbohydrates, and fats can be viewed as your fuel mixture. If you get the right fuel for your type and the right fuel mixture, you'll have a powerful force at work. Your food will be efficiently converted to energy rather than stored as fat.

Here's your general macronutrient ratio:

PROTEINS	&	FATS	CARBOHYDRATES
70%			**30%**
(approx. 40% proteins)		(approx. 30% fats)	
Higher Amounts of Proteins and Fats			*Lower Amounts of Carbos*
red meats, fowl, seafood, dairy, legumes, nuts		fatty meats, fowl and seafood, dairy, nuts, seeds, oils, butter	fruits, vegetables, grains

Stick to your seventy percent/thirty percent food ratio whenever you eat, getting approximately thirty percent of your calories from carbohydrates, and about seventy percent of your calories from proteins and fats. Note that more of your calories should come from protein than from fat.

It's not necessary to be perfectly precise in terms of your percent-

ages. When combining your food, just try to approximate as best you can.

It's unnecessary to measure out by weight everything you eat, or to calculate the number of calories in a meal. When you get the right balance for your metabolism, your appetite will naturally be satisfied, and the calorie issue will eventually take care of itself. So it doesn't matter whether you eat a small meal or a large meal or something in between. What is important is eating the right foods for your type and in the right proportions for your type every time you eat.

If you happen to be especially concerned with weight loss, or if you need to lose a significant amount of weight, I will explain issues regarding calories and food quantities in the chapter on weight management. However, it's very important to realize that:

Your weight will begin to normalize just by eating the right foods in the right combinations. When you balance your macronutrients properly, you'll lose weight if you're overweight and gain weight if you're underweight.

Try to eat at regular intervals and stick to the same mealtimes every day if at all possible. It's also important to eat when you're hungry, preferably before you get hungry, so snack if you need to. This will keep you from overeating and will keep your blood sugar on an even keel.

A helpful way to think about your macronutrient percentages is in terms of a plate of food. The majority of food on your plate should be protein and fat (two thirds) and the rest should be carbohydrate (one third), primarily of the nonstarchy variety.

A lot of people are very confused about how to eat a meal composed of thirty percent fat. But you'll notice that most of the proteins listed in your Allowable Foods Chart are also sources of natural fats and oils. This means that your requirement for fats can easily be met just by eating your protein foods and making liberal use of butter and oils on your foods.

HOW TO COMBINE YOUR FOOD AT MEALS

Plate of food

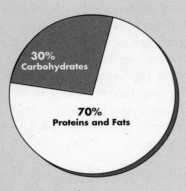

30%
Carbohydrates

70%
Proteins and Fats

example:
- broiled steak
- buttered peas and corn
- sliced avocado marinated
  in olive oil and vinegar

Each time you eat, the majority of your food should be a source of protein. Most Protein Types require heavier sources of protein (meat, poultry, or seafood) two to three times per day. Eating carbohydrates alone, even for snacks, is not recommended. Note that your protein foods are *also* sources of natural fats and oils. This means your requirement for fats can be met just by eating your allowable protein foods and making liberal use of butter and oils on your food.

Note that the 70%/30% ratio is just a general guideline for protein types. You will need to follow the twelve steps on page 184 to identify the specific macronutrient ratio or "personal fuel mix" to meet your highly individualized needs.

Sample Menus

The following are *suggestions only* for possible meal plans. These are not intended as receipes, but are provided as ideas for good ways to use your allowable foods. Feel free to create your own menus, combining your allowable foods in any manner that suits your taste at any given meal. Your metabolic type *needs* to make sure you *get protein every time you eat.* Refrain from eating carbohydrate all by itself. Note that snacks should always contain proteins. *Bon appétit!*

MEAL	DAY ONE	DAY TWO
BREAKFAST	bacon, scrambled eggs, small serving of potatoes fried in butter	2 poached eggs, Canadian bacon, 1 slice of spelt toast with butter
LUNCH	dark meat chicken, raw carrots, celery, and cauliflower with olive spread or mayonnaise/yogurt dip	tunafish salad with celery and natural mayonnaise, 1 piece spelt bread, small lentil soup
SNACK	full-fat cottage cheese mixed with flax oil, ½ sliced green apple	peanut butter or almond butter on celery sticks
DINNER	broiled salmon, steamed green beans, quinoa and butter, spinach salad with sliced olives, vinaigrette dressing	broiled lamb chops, steamed asparagus, baked winter squash with butter

MEAL	DAY THREE	DAY FOUR
BREAKFAST	pork, turkey, or chicken sausages, buckwheat cereal (whole grain) with butter	vegetable omelette, smoked salmon, sprouted rye bread with butter
LUNCH	hamburger patty, steamed corn with butter, spinach salad with artichokes and mushrooms, olive oil, and lemon juice	shrimp salad with celery and mayonnaise, avocado with olive oil and lemon, small serving of wild and brown rice
SNACK	full-fat cheese with either ½ pear or Rye-Krisp crackers	½ banana with almonds
DINNER	broiled steak, buttered peas and corn, sliced avocado marinated in olive oil and vinegar	chicken thigh and drumstick, steamed artichoke with butter or mayonnaise, buttered string beans and slivered almonds

MEAL	DAY FIVE
BREAKFAST	2 fried eggs, 3 mini sausages, small serving of oatmeal with butter or cream
LUNCH	pot roast with small serving of potatoes and carrots
SNACK	full-fat yogurt with sunflower seeds and cashews
DINNER	roast beef, steamed cauliflower, barley, spinach salad with bacon, mushrooms, vinaigrette dressing

Finding Your Personal Fuel Mix

It's important to keep in mind that the seventy percent/thirty percent macronutrient ratio is a general guideline for Protein Types. Think of it as a starting point or a first step. It provides you with the general parameters you need to follow in order to be at your best. Due to metabolic individuality, however, different people within the protein-type category have different macronutrient requirements.

As an example, some Protein Types can get by on less protein and tolerate larger amounts of carbohydrates, even those with a higher sugar/starch content. Other people need more protein and are highly sensitive to even small amounts of carbohydrates—starchy or nonstarchy.

Everyone is different, which means that the specific proportion of proteins, carbohydrates, and fats that might work well for you is not necessarily the same identical proportion of macronutrients that would work well for other people in your metabolic category.

Think of your Protein Type category as a sliding scale, or a continuum, or a spectrum of variable macronutrient requirements.

PROTEIN TYPES

Higher Protein: Lower Carb	Moderate Protein: Moderate Carb	Lower Protein: Higher Carb

What you need to do is to pinpoint your own highly individualized macronutrient ratio. In other words, you need to refine or tailor the general macronutrient ratio for Protein Types to your own particular needs. You need to identify what I call your "personal fuel mix."

Once you discover your personal fuel mix, you'll know how to combine your foods—proteins, carbohydrates, and fats—in proportions that are just right for you. This will make a huge difference in the way you feel following meals and snacks.

You'll know when you've hit your personal fuel mix because you will immediately have strong and lasting physical energy and mental clarity, a solid sense of well-being, and a sense of fullness and satisfaction, as opposed to persistent hunger and sweet cravings.

How do you find your personal fuel mix? It's really very simple. All you need to do is experiment a little by consuming varying amounts of carbohydrates.

Remember, as a Protein Type, excess amounts of carbohydrates—especially the starchy, sugary kind—are your downfall, since they produce lowered energy, mood swings, blood sugar problems, and food cravings.

As a first step, you'll need to restrict your carbohydrate intake for a few days. Once you know what it feels like to be almost entirely off carbohydrates, you can start adding them in again, a little at a time, until you hit your personal fuel mix.

If you go beyond your personal fuel mix, by eating excessive carbohydrates, you'll know it. Why? Because you'll lose your energy, sense of well-being, and feelings of satisfaction very quickly after eating. On the other hand, if you fail to reach your personal fuel mix by eating too few carbohydrates—you'll experience the very same kind of negative symptoms.

To find your personal fuel mix, all you need to do is follow the simple steps below.

Twelve Simple Steps for Finding Your Personal Fuel Mix

1. For the first five to seven days, eliminate all "caution carbs"—grains, cereals, breads, desserts, fruits, starchy vegetables—as well as milk products.
2. Eat freely of any of your allowable proteins and fats: meat, poultry, seafood, eggs, nuts, seeds, butter, and vegetable oils.
3. During these few days, limit your vegetable intake to the following nonstarchy varieties: asparagus, celery, green beans, cauliflower, spinach, and mushrooms. Start out with only a small portion of veg-

etables as compared to your protein amount. This is your baseline.

4. Eat until you are full but not to the point of feeling stuffed.

5. Have snacks between meals if you like, using the same food choices.

6. Most Protein Types will feel better almost immediately. They will be able to go longer between meals without eating, will lose their sweet cravings, and will feel a distinct energy boost. Some Protein Types can experience withdrawal from high-starch and sugary foods. This usually does not last for more than forty-eight hours. It might involve any number of symptoms such as headache, flulike sensations, or extreme sweet cravings. If this should happen to you, just hang in there for two to three days and you should start to experience some of the positive feelings listed above.

7. Typically, Protein Types will feel better for five to seven days after eliminating all the "caution carbs." Sometime thereafter they generally begin to feel irritable, short-tempered, and tired, and then crave sweets and feel hungry or unsatisfied after eating. When you reach this point, increase the amount of nonstarchy vegetables (eat only those on your Allowable Foods Chart) as compared to your quantity of protein, until you once again begin to feel well.

8. If you still do not feel well even after increasing your nonstarchy vegetables, begin to add a little starch to your meals, starting with only one tablespoon of a starchy vegetable from your Allowable Food Chart, such as artichoke, corn, peas, potato, or winter squash with dinner.

9. If you still feel well or even better by eating a little starchy vegetable with dinner, add one tablespoon of a starchy vegetable at lunch, and then one tablespoon at breakfast.

10. If all goes well, raise your starchy vegetable intake to two tablespoons per meal.

11. Then, if all is still fine, substitute some whole grain in place of starchy vegetables.

12. In this manner, you can continue to slowly increase your carbohydrate intake. At some point, you'll move beyond your personal fuel mix and begin to notice a reappearance of your "old" symptoms— fatigue, depression, mood swings, sweet cravings, digestive problems, and so on. When that happens, you'll know you need to start decreasing your carbohydrates gradually until you start feeling well

again. At this stage, if you have any degree of uncertainty, you can always return to your baseline and start over.

Remember, too many or too few carbohydrates in relation to protein will produce similar symptoms.

Once you've come this far, you'll know how to manage your meals with great precision. But there are more techniques you can use to customize and fine-tune your diet even further. Look for the fine-tuning guidelines in Chapter 9.

Characteristics of Your Metabolic Type

Many Carbo Types share similar characteristics. However, if you're a Carbo Type, that doesn't mean you're just like everyone else in your metabolic category in the way you react to foods, your strengths and weaknesses, your energy level, the strength of your appetite, and so on. After all, you're unique on a metabolic level!

Nonetheless, here are some typical tendencies you may have in common with other Carbo Types:

Relatively Weak Appetite

For Carbo Types, a little food tends to go a long way. You may eat three meals a day, but often the meals won't be large. Or you may be satisfied with one or two meals and several smaller snacks. Whatever your routine, chances are that food does not play a prominent role in your conscious daily awareness.

High Tolerance for Sweets

Unless they have hypoglycemia (low blood sugar), people with your style of metabolism usually handle sweets pretty well. This can be both a blessing *and* a curse, for although you can handle sweets, they can also be your downfall. Your tendency might be to reach for them whenever you're hungry or need an energy boost. So your tendency could easily be to overdo sweets, which could eventually lead to problems like hypoglycemia, insulin resistance, and diabetes.

Problems with Weight Management

People with your kind of metabolism are often lean, or at least start off that way. Yet the tendency for sweet-snacking often leads to problems with obesity. Your small appetite tends to complicate the issue. By eating very little, snacking on sweets, or by waiting long periods between eating, you have a tendency to lower your metabolic rate, thereby throwing your system into "starvation mode," a self-preservation mechanism in which the body thinks it's starving and therefore slows down its metabolism in order to conserve energy.

Type-A Personalities

Some Carbo Types—the sympathetic dominants—have classic Type-A personalities. They tend to be aggressive, goal-oriented, highly motivated workaholics. They can be abrupt, appear cool and aloof, and quick to anger. Their energy tends to come in spurts, so their physical stamina is relatively limited, yet their concentration tends to be excellent. Aside from the fact that they don't have large appetites, they often think they don't have time to eat—a quality that both horrifies and mystifies many people in the opposite metabolic category, the Protein Type.

Variable Energy Patterns

Another segment of the Carbo Type population—the slow oxidizers—tend to have very different personality and energy patterns from sympathetic dominants, even though they share the same general dietary characteristics. Slow oxidizers tend to have lower though steadier energy without the peaks and valleys that sympathetics experience.

Caffeine Dependency

Both sympathetic dominants and slow oxidizers frequently depend on caffeine to get them through the day. Sympathetics use caffeine to "jump-start" their adrenals, which tend to be strong anyway. Caffeine gives them a hormonal kick and an energy surge, but overuse can lead to a weakened appetite, a worsening of already poor dietary habits, adrenal exhaustion, or an actual shift in their metabolic type due to a loss of sympathetic strength. Caffeine can make slow oxidizers feel "half alive" again, and they may feel quite unable to function without it. But, unlike sympathetic dominants, slow oxidizers generally start out with weak adrenals that need to be rebuilt through a balanced nutritional regime. Caffeine only exacerbates the fundamental metabolic imbalances of slow oxidizers.

If any of these situations describes you, it's a clear indication that you're pumping the wrong kind of "body fuel" into your "engines of metabolism."

Dietary Emphasis for Carbo Types

As a Carbo Type, what you need is a diet comprised of relatively small amounts of proteins and fats compared to carbohydrates.

But all proteins are not created equal. You need to avoid the heavier, high-purine proteins and focus instead on lighter proteins that are low in fat and low in purines.

More than any other type, you have the freedom to eat a wide selection of carbohydrates—vegetables, grains, and fruits—of both starchy and nonstarchy varieties. Because your system converts carbohydrates into energy slowly, you can handle starchy or sugary foods better than other types, though you still have to be careful not to overdo it.

Your tendency to metabolize your food slowly is the very reason you need to avoid larger amounts of proteins and fats, especially the heavier proteins. These foods will slow down your energy production even more.

If you happen to be a Carbo Type, you definitely need a low-protein, low fat diet in order to lose weight, feel energized both physically and mentally, and stay on an even keel emotionally. Excess protein and fat will leave you feeling drained and sluggish—or even hyper, wired, quick to anger, and irritable.

Over the long haul, this type of diet, if properly followed and tailored to your metabolic individuality, can prevent you from developing all kinds of serious degenerative diseases (cardiovascular problems, immune deficiency, blood sugar abnormalities, osteoporosis, arthritis, digestive disorders, and many other chronic illnesses), all of which are rooted in metabolic imbalance.

THE CARBO TYPE DIET ALLOWABLE FOODS CHART

PROTEINS			CARBOHYDRATES				OILS / FATS	
MEAT/FOWL	SEAFOOD	DAIRY	GRAIN	VEGETABLE		FRUIT	NUT/SEED	OIL/FAT
light meats	light fish	non/low-fat	whole grains only	high starch	low starch	all are okay	use sparingly	use sparingly
chicken breast	catfish	cheese		potato	beet green	apple	walnut	butter
Cornish game hen	cod	cottage cheese	high starch	pumpkin	broccoli	apricot	pumpkin	cream
turkey breast	flounder	kefir	amaranth	rutabaga	Brussels sprout	cherry	peanut	ghee
pork, lean	haddock	milk	barley	sweet potato	cabbage	citrus	sunflower	oils:
ham	halibut	yogurt	brown rice	yam	chard	grape	sesame	almond
Only occasional	perch	eggs	buckwheat	moderate starch	collard	melon	almond	coconut
lean red meat or	scrod	LEGUMES	corn	beet	cucumber	peach	cashew	flax
restrict entirely	sole	use sparingly	couscous	corn	garlic	pear	Brazil	olive
	trout	high starch	kamut	eggplant	kale	pineapple	filbert	peanut
	tuna, white	dried beans	kasha	jicama	leafy greens	plum	pecan	sesame
	turbot	lentils	millet	okra	onion	tomato	chestnut	sunflower
		low starch	oat	parsnip	parsley	tropical	pistachio	walnut
		tempeh	quinoa	radish	peppers	LEGUMES	coconut	
		tofu	rice	spaghetti squash	scallion	high starch	hickory	
		NUTS	rye	summer squash	sprouts	dried beans	macadamia	
		sparingly	spelt	yellow squash	tomato	dried peas		
			triticale	turnip	watercress	lentils		
			wheat	zucchini				

Important Tips on Your Allowable Foods

Emphasize Low-Fat, Low-Purine Proteins.

Your metabolic type does very well on low-fat proteins. You should avoid high-fat proteins because they interfere with your body's ability to produce energy in an efficient manner. Likewise, you should avoid proteins high in purines—a special category of proteins that play an important role in the energy-producing processes in body tissues. High-fat, high-purine proteins are likely to make you feel lethargic, depressed, and fatigued. Any meat, fowl, or seafood that is *not* included in your Allowable Foods Chart tends to be too high in fat and purine for your type and should be avoided or at least greatly minimized to only occasional intake.

PROTEINS		
MEAT/FOWL	SEAFOOD	DAIRY
light meats	light fish	non/low fat
chicken breast	catfish	cheese
Cornish game hen	cod	cottage cheese
turkey breast	flounder	kefir
pork, lean	haddock	milk
ham	halibut	yogurt
Only occasional	perch	eggs
lean red meat or	scrod	LEGUMES
restrict entirely	sole	use sparingly
	trout	high starch
	tuna, white	dried beans
	turbot	lentils
		low starch
		tempeh
		tofu
		NUTS
		sparingly

Eat Protein at Most Meals.

Try to eat protein with most of your meals. Although your metabolism does best with a relatively higher percentage of carbohydrates in your diet, protein is still important for you and must not be ignored. Many people make the mistake of habitually eating carbohydrate alone for meals. Over time this can lead to severe disruptions in energy metabolism and blood sugar problems. As long as you get adequate protein with your meals, it will likely be okay to eat just a carbohydrate food (like fruit) for a snack. However, if you suffer with hypoglycemia or you find that eating fruit alone for a snack makes you more hungry or causes you to crave sugar, you'll need to include some protein with *every* intake of food, even your snacks.

Carefully Consider Dairy.

Dairy foods are a "mixed bag" for your type. On the one hand, your type needs the lighter, lower-fat, lower-purine proteins. Low-fat dairy products, like yogurt or cottage cheese, fit this bill nicely. However, your type also tends to do best by minimizing calcium intake, so in this regard dairy is not ideal for you. In general, the best thing to do is monitor your reactions to dairy products. If you feel a drop in energy or an adverse shift in your mood after eating dairy, you may need to restrict it from your diet.

Balance Your Carbohydrate Intake.

CARBOHYDRATES			
GRAIN	VEGETABLE		FRUIT
whole grains	high starch	low starch	all are okay
only	potato	beet green	apple
high starch	pumpkin	broccoli	apricot
amaranth	rutabaga	Brussels sprout	berry
barley	sweet potato	cabbage	cherry
brown rice	yam	chard	citrus
buckwheat	moderate starch	collard	grape
corn	beet	cucumber	melon
couscous	corn	garlic	peach
kamut	eggplant	kale	pear
kasha	jicama	leafy greens	pineapple
millet	okra	onion	plum
oat	parsnip	parsley	tomato
quinoa	radish	peppers	tropical
rice	spaghetti squash	scallion	LEGUMES
rye	summer squash	sprouts	high starch
spelt	yellow squash	tomato	dried beans
triticale	turnip	watercress	dried peas
wheat	zucchini		lentils

All plant-based foods—grains, vegetables, or fruits—are carbohydrates. But there are different kinds of carbohydrates and they don't all affect your metabolism in the same way. For example, some carbohydrates are higher in starch and some are lower in starch. Starchy carbohydrates break down easily into sugar, which means they hit your bloodstream quickly. This can cause a strong insulin response from your pancreas, which typically leads to increased fat storage and blood sugar problems like hypoglycemia. For this reason, grains, starchy vegetables, and fruits are "caution carbs." Over time, excess insulin secretion can contribute to more severe disorders such as allergies, asthma, alcoholism, atherosclerosis, cancer, carbohydrate addiction, heart disease, chronic fatigue, depression, diabetes, insulin resistance, glucose intolerance, hypertension, obesity, and peptic ulcers. Although your metabolic type handles starches better than other types, you still must take care to get a mixture of starchy and nonstarchy carbohydrates. This is particularly important if you have concerns about weight. So, eat all the nonstarchy vegetables you want, but limit the moderate and high starch carbohydrates to no more than one moderate-starch and one high-starch food per meal. If you eat a starchy vegetable, don't eat a grain product at the same meal. For example, if you eat a potato, don't eat bread at the same meal.

Go Ahead with Grains.

In general, grains are very good for your metabolic type. But remember, grains are starchy carbohydrates, so you shouldn't overdo them. Here's the way to tell if you're eating too many: Say you ate a chicken breast, small salad, and a large serving of rice for lunch. But afterward you were still hungry, felt sleepy, or had a strong desire for sweets. Chances are you ate too much starch (rice) relative to protein. So next time around, what you need to do is to increase the protein and decrease the starch, i.e., eat more chicken and less rice. As I'll show you in subsequent sections, your body will tell you when you achieve the right mix of carbohydrates and protein. When you use grains, remember to use only whole-grain products. Do not consume any refined grain products made with white flour or enriched flour. Any baked foods you consume should contain only whole-grain flours. Keep in mind, though, that all grains are starches, which means they readily break down into sugar, so they should be used wisely.

Enjoy Selected Juices.

Vegetable juices, as long as they're freshly made, are particularly good for your metabolic type and can be used freely. However, juices should be made only from vegetables that appear on your Allowable Foods Chart. The only exception is carrot juice. You can have a little from time to time even though carrots are not among your allowed vegetables. Avoid all canned juices. In general, it's best not to consume fruit juices, since they're very high in sugar. Eating fruit is fine and even encouraged for your type, but fresh fruit juices should be used only periodically for therapeutic reasons and not as a matter of routine or for quenching thirst. In place of fruit juice, make smoothies by blending the whole fruit. If you're thirsty, drink water—not juice, tea, or milk.

Limit Legumes.

Legumes—dried beans, peas, lentils—like dairy, have conflicting influences on your metabolism. They're an excellent source of carbohydrate and vegetable protein. However, they are also a source of purines, a category of protein that is not appropriate for your metabolic type. Legumes do not contain the same amount of purines as, say, steak or salmon, so you can have them from time to time, especially if you're eating a vegetarian meal. Just be careful not to eat too many or have them too often.

Minimize Fats and Oils.

The subject of fats and oils and their effects on human metabolism has been extensively researched and documented. An in-depth discussion of them is beyond the scope of this book (for a complete discussion, see *Fats and Oils*, an excellent book by Udo Erasmus).

Although fats and oils should be minimized in your diet, this does not mean a no-fat diet. It is important to consume some good, natural oils. They're critical to membrane structure, hormone production, immune function, and a whole host of important metabolic processes. Use only natural cold-pressed oils and unsalted butter. Recommended brands are Omega, Flora, or Bio-San, available in health food stores. Never consume margarine, hydrogenated oils, or fat substitutes. If you must

OILS / FATS	
NUT/SEED	OIL/FAT
use sparingly	use sparingly
walnut	butter
pumpkin	cream
peanut	ghee
sunflower	oils:
sesame	almond
almond	coconut
cashew	flax
Brazil	olive
filbert	peanut
pecan	sesame
chestnut	sunflower
pistachio	walnut
coconut	
hickory	
macadamia	

buy packaged foods, read the labels to make sure you do not consume these substances.

Go Easy with Nuts and Seeds.

Nuts are a source of nonpurine protein but are also very high in oils. So they're a double-edged sword for your metabolic type. They contain protein, but because of their high-fat content, their use must be limited. For example, if you find that a piece of fruit (pure carbohydrate) does not satisfy you as a snack and you need some protein to go with it, some nuts or nut butters may work perfectly. On the other hand, you must take care not to eat large quantities, especially if you are also eating animal proteins on that day.

Snack as Needed.

Of all the metabolic types, Carbo Types are the least dependent on snacks. If you want to eat them, that's fine. Just be careful not to overdose on carbohydrates. If you start craving sweets, you probably ate too many carbohydrates and didn't get enough protein in the meal or snack just prior to the sweet craving.

Get a Loaf.

Breads are okay for your metabolic type. But make sure to eat only breads made from whole-grain flours. Avoid the white breads made with refined, enriched flours. Fats and oils are limited in your diet, so go easy on the butter. Sprouted-grain breads like Ezekiel and Manna brands are best because sprouting increases the level of vitamin C and B vitamins, and destroys the enzyme inhibitors found in grains.

Be Conscious of Glycemic Values.

All carbohydrates—fruits, vegetables, grains—are converted to glucose in the body. Carbohydrates are categorized according to the rate or speed at which they hit the bloodstream as glucose, and ranked accordingly in what is known as the glycemic index (GI). High-glycemic foods such as grains and starchy vegetables hit your blood-stream much more rapidly than low-glycemic foods like proteins and fats. Although your metabolic type can handle high-glycemic foods better than other types, you still don't want to overdo them. You don't want to burden your system with too many foods that rapidly convert to glucose in your bloodstream. You need to place more emphasis on those foods that are lower on the GI. Whenever you do eat high-glycemic foods, it's a good idea to include some protein at the same time, since protein will help slow down the rate at which high-glycemic foods are converted to sugar. (Note: Check Chapter 9 for the complete glycemic index. It's very important for all metabolic types to become familiar with the GI.)

Foods to Avoid

Certain foods really aggravate your metabolic imbalances and should be avoided. You may have strong adverse reactions to these foods, or, if your metabolism is less sensitive, the reactions may be slight or even nonexistent. Or your reactions to these problem foods could vary from time to time. All these possibilities are common and reflect yet another facet of metabolic individuality

Keep in mind that *the effects of nutrition are cumulative*. The more you ingest a food, the stronger the effect becomes. So even if you don't display any noticeable adverse reactions, it's still best to minimize your intake of the following foods whenever possible.

In short, stick to your allowable foods. But if you simply must eat something not on that list, be aware that the following foods are particularly undesirable for your metabolism.

Alcohol.

Alcohol, plain and simple, is a poison to your body. Your body must detoxify it and neutralize its adverse effects. From this perspective, it isn't really good for anyone. However, of the three metabolic categories, your metabolic type is best-suited to handle alcohol. But don't get me wrong—it's still a simple sugar, so it can wreak havoc with your metabolism. It triggers excessive insulin secretion, which leads to blood sugar imbalances, increased fat storage, and the development of chronic degenerative processes. Thus, moderation with alcohol is strongly recommended.

Allergenic or Reactive Foods.

Your Allowable Foods Chart provides recommendations for foods that will specifically support your metabolic type. This means that they contain the right balance of nutrients for your type. Whether or not you are currently reactive or allergic to any of these foods is a completely different issue. If you have known reactions to any recommended foods, leave them out of your diet temporarily, but try them from time to time. As your chemistry changes, so too may your food reactivities. This is the experience of many individuals who have properly customized their diets to match their metabolisms.

Caffeine.

Avoid caffeine products as much as possible, including coffee, black teas, caffeine-containing herbs, and soft drinks. Because your metabolic type can tolerate caffeine better than other types can, it's easy for you to abuse it. If you do insist on drinking coffee, make sure it's organic and limit it to no more than one to two weak cups per day. Also, make sure to eat some protein, as this will help counter to a degree its adverse effects on your type. Bottom line: Caffeine is counterproductive for your type, whether you're a slow oxidizer or a sympathetic dominant. If you're a slow oxidizer, you may be so exhausted that you feel you need caffeine to get through the day. But too much caffeine will only exhaust your system further, like a whip applied to a tired horse. Short-term, the stimulation is pleasurable, but over the long term, caffeine can worsen your fatigue by further exhausting your adrenals. If you're sympathetic dominant, excess caffeine will worsen your existing imbalance.

Sugar.

In significant quantities, sugar is not good for anyone. However, unless you suffer from hypoglycemia or diabetes, your metabolic type typically handles sugar better than other types. This is the good news and the bad news, for it is generally easy for Carbo Types to overeat sugar-containing foods. When you start craving sugar foods, it's a signal that you're getting too much carbohydrate and not enough protein in your diet. For your metabolic type, sugar can be stimulating, and, if you're not watchful, addictive. You may find yourself reaching for sugar more and more to give you an energy boost. But sugar is empty calories and empty energy. It doesn't provide good nutrition or the right kind of energy for your body. A sugar habit now can lead to problems with sugar metabolism down the road. When you need energy, you're better off trying some protein first instead of sugar. Be especially watchful for hidden sugars in processed, packaged foods. Sugar is added to a great many commercial foods and can really add up if you're not careful, secretly sabotaging your best intentions to follow your dietary recommendations.

Foods High in Fat.

Make no mistake, a diet too low in natural fats and oils containing essential fatty acids is dangerous and can have serious health consequences. However, of the three metabolic types, your type requires the least amount of fat. So, relatively speaking, you belong on a low-fat diet. But this does *not* mean *no fat*. That's why you can have small amounts of butter and cold-pressed oils as a supplement to the fatty acids naturally occurring in your diet. If you don't get enough fatty acids in your diet, you're likely to experience sudden changes such as increased fatigue, diminished performance, hunger soon after eating, decreased fingernail strength, decreased hair quality, overly dense stool, constipation, increased need for sleep, grogginess upon awakening, decreased well-being, diminished concentration, and dry skin. Ironically, however, these same symptoms can be produced by either an excess *or* a deficiency of fatty acids. So try keeping your intake of fatty foods to a minimum. But if you feel poorly at this low level, slowly increase your fats until your symptoms diminish.

Foods High in Purines.

Essentially, all the animal proteins *not* listed in your Allowable Foods Chart tend to be high in purines. These are a special class of proteins that are particularly beneficial for some types, but they're an undesirable fuel for your kind of metabolism. Purines tend to oxidize too slowly, thereby slowing down even further the metabolisms of slow oxidizers. They also worsen the imbalances of sympathetic dominants. Therefore, eat purines only occasionally, if at all.

Thyroid-suppressing Foods.

Certain foods contain a chemical known as thiocyanate, which causes thyroid dysfunction. Thiocyanate belongs to a class of substances known as goitrogens. These substances block the production of thyroid hormone, a hormone that plays an integral role in the regulation of all your metabolic activities. Goitrogens are found in raw broccoli, Brussels sprouts, cabbage, cauliflower, kale, mustard, rutabaga, and watercress. If you eat these foods frequently, it's a good idea to supplement your diet with extra iodine in the form of kelp, since goitrogens work by blocking iodine absorption by the thyroid gland. Kelp can be ground and used in a salt shaker as a condiment. Also note that cooking will partially inactivate the thyroid-suppressing chemical found in these foods. So you'll want to use kelp, take care to cook these foods, and use them conservatively, especially if you've been diagnosed with hypothyroidism (slow thyroid).

Your Macronutrient Ratio

This diet is easy! There are only two things you need to remember:

1. Eat the right kinds of foods for your type and avoid the wrong foods for your type—in other words, stick to your allowable foods.
2. Eat the right proportions of macronutrients (proteins, fats, carbohydrates) at each meal.

If you think of your food as fuel, then the proportions of proteins, carbohydrates, and fats can be viewed as your fuel mixture. If you get the right fuel for your type and the right fuel mixture, you'll have a powerful force at work. Your food will be efficiently converted to energy rather than stored as fat.

Here's your general macronutrient ratio:

PROTEINS	&	OILS/FATS	CARBOHYDRATES
40%			**60%**
(approx. 25% proteins)		(approx. 15% fats)	
Lower Amounts of Proteins and Fats and Oils			*Higher Amounts of Carbos*
light meat fowl, seafood, low-fat dairy, some legumes, some nuts		limited vegetable oils, butter	fruits, vegetables, grains

Stick to your forty percent/sixty percent food ratio whenever you eat, getting approximately sixty percent of your calories from carbohydrates, and about forty percent of your calories from proteins and fats. Note that more of your calories should come from protein than from fat.

It's not necessary to be perfectly precise in terms of your percent-

ages. When combining your food, just try to approximate as best you can.

It's unnecessary to measure out by weight everything you eat, or to calculate the number of calories in a meal. When you get the right balance for your metabolism, your appetite will naturally be satisfied, and the calorie issue will eventually take care of itself. So it doesn't matter whether you eat a small meal or a large meal or something in between. What is important is eating the right foods for your type and in the right proportions for your type every time you eat.

If you happen to be especially concerned with weight loss, or if you need to lose a significant amount of weight, I will explain issues regarding calories and food quantities later on in the chapter on weight management. However, it's very important to realize that:

Your weight will begin to normalize just by eating the right foods in the right combinations. When you balance your macronutrients properly, you'll lose weight if you're overweight and gain weight if you're underweight.

Try to eat at regular intervals and stick to the same mealtimes every day if at all possible. It's also important to eat when you're hungry—preferably *before* you get hungry. This will keep you from overeating and will keep your blood sugar on an even keel.

A helpful way to think about your macronutrient percentages is in terms of a plate of food. The majority of food on your plate should be carbohydrate (primarily nonstarchy) and the rest should be protein with minimal fat.

A lot of people are very confused about how to eat a meal that contains fifteen percent fat. The Carbo Type diet is a low-fat diet, relatively speaking. However, you don't need to do anything special to get the right fat intake. Simply stick closely to your allowable foods and when you need some additional fat like butter or oil, just use a minimal amount.

Plate of food

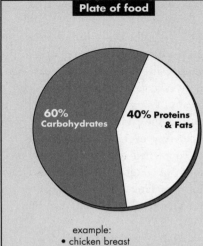

60% Carbohydrates

40% Proteins & Fats

Each time you eat, the majority of your food should be carbohydrate (primarily non-starchy), and the rest should be low fat proteins. To avoid disruptions in your blood sugar balance, try to eat protein with most of your meals and snacks. Note that many of your protein foods are also sources of natural fats and oils. This means your requirement for fats can be met just by eating your allowable proteins, and supplementing with small amounts of butter and oil.

example:
- chicken breast
- baked potato with low-fat yogurt
- steamed broccoli + beets
- green salad w olive oil + vinegar

Note that the 60%/40% ratio is just a general guideline for carbo types. So you will need to follow the twelve steps on page 208 to identify the specific macronutrient ratio or personal fuel mix that meets your highly individualized needs.

Sample Menus

The following are *suggestions only* for possible meal plans. Feel free to create your own menus, combining your allowable foods in any manner that suits your taste at any given meal. *Bon appétit!*

MEAL	DAY ONE	DAY TWO
BREAKFAST	soft-boiled egg(s), whole wheat toast, teaspoon butter, apple	hot whole-grain cereal, low-fat milk, grapes
LUNCH	sandwich made with white tuna on whole-grain bread with tomato, sprouts, celery, onions, and mayonnaise, small bowl of vegetable soup	soup made with chicken, broccoli, cabbage, potato, onion rice
SNACK	pineapple and low-fat cottage cheese, Manna bread	apple and almonds
DINNER	chicken breast, baked potato with low fat yogurt steamed broccoli and beets, green salad with olive oil and vinegar	baked cod, romaine lettuce, tomato, parsley, onion, with fresh lemon juice and olive oil dressing, millet, steamed zucchini with teaspoon butter

MEAL	DAY THREE	DAY FOUR
BREAKFAST	protein shake (whey or egg white protein) in low-fat milk with fresh or frozen fruit, whole grain toast, teaspoon butter	poached egg(s) hot, whole-grain cereal with low-fat milk, fruit
LUNCH	tossed green salad with lettuce, tomato, onion, radish, peppers, olive oil, and lemon juice with choice of grilled chicken, turkey, or ham, whole-grain bread and small amount of butter	ham sandwich on whole-grain bread with tomato, sprouts, onions, and mayonnaise or mustard, small bowl of vegetable soup
SNACK	plain, low-fat yogurt with fresh fruit	low-fat Swiss or mozzarella cheese on Ry-Krisp crackers
DINNER	broiled pork chops with rice, corn on the cob, green, leafy salad with green peppers, cucumbers, and scallions with vinaigrette dressing	broiled trout with lemon, steamed broccoli, baked yam with teaspoon butter, sliced cucumber with chopped onion and vinegar

MEAL	DAY FIVE
BREAKFAST	low-fat cottage cheese or plain, low-fat yogurt with fruit, whole-grain toast, teaspoon butter
LUNCH	vegetable soup made with turkey and barley
SNACK	wheat thins with cashew butter (1–2 teaspoons only)
DINNER	baked Cornish game hen with stuffing, Brussels sprouts, cole slaw with chopped scallion and green pepper, vinaigrette dressing

Finding Your Personal Fuel Mix

It's important to keep in mind that the forty percent/sixty percent macronutrient ratio is a general guideline for Carbo Types. Think of it as a starting point or a first step. It provides you with the *general parameters* you need to follow in order to be at your best. Due to metabolic individuality, however, different people within the Carbo Type category have different macronutrient requirements.

As an example, some Carbo Types can get by on less carbohydrate and tolerate larger amounts of protein, even those with a higher fat and purine content. Other people need more carbohydrate and are highly sensitive to even small amounts of additional protein.

Everyone is different, which means that the specific proportion of proteins, carbohydrates, and fats that might work well for you is not necessarily the same identical proportion of macronutrients that would work well for other people in your metabolic category.

Think of your Carbo Type category as a sliding scale, or a continuum, or a spectrum of variable macronutrient requirements.

CARBO TYPES

Lower Protein: Higher Carb	Moderate Protein: Moderate Carb	Lower Carb: Higher Protein

⟵———————————————————⟶

What you need to do is to pinpoint your own highly individualized macronutrient ratio. In other words, you need to refine or tailor the general macronutrient ratio for Carbo Types to your own particular needs. You need to identify what I call your personal fuel mix.

Once you discover your personal fuel mix, you'll know how to combine your foods—proteins, carbohydrates, and fats—in proportions that are just right for you. This will make a huge difference in the way you feel following meals and snacks.

You'll know when you've hit your personal fuel mix because you will immediately have strong and lasting physical energy and mental clarity, a solid sense of well-being, and a sense of fullness and satisfaction—as opposed to persistent hunger and sweet cravings.

How do you find your personal fuel mix? It's really very simple. All you need to do is experiment a little by consuming varying amounts of carbohydrates.

Remember, as a Carbo Type, excess amounts of carbohydrates—especially the starchy, sugary kind—can be your downfall, producing lowered energy, mood swings, blood sugar problems, and food cravings.

As a first step, you'll need to restrict your carbohydrate intake for a few days. Once you know what it feels like to be almost entirely off carbohydrates, you can start adding them in again—a little at a time—until you hit your personal fuel mix.

If you go beyond your personal fuel mix by eating excessive carbohydrates, you'll know it. Why? Because you'll lose your energy, sense of well-being, and feelings of satisfaction very quickly after eating. On the other hand, if you fail to reach your personal fuel mix by eating too few carbohydrates—you'll experience the very same kind of negative symptoms.

To find your personal fuel mix, all you need to do is follow the simple steps below.

Twelve Simple Steps for Finding Your Personal Fuel Mix

1. For the first two to seven days, eliminate all "caution carbs"—grains, cereals, breads, desserts, fruits, starchy vegetables—as well as milk products.
2. Eat freely of any of your allowable proteins and fats: meat, poultry, seafood, eggs, nuts, seeds, butter, and vegetable oils.
3. During these few days, limit your vegetable intake to the non-starchy varieties listed in your Allowable Foods Chart. Start out with only a small portion of vegetables as compared to your protein amount. This is your baseline.

4. Eat until you are full but not to the point of feeling stuffed.

5. Have snacks between meals if you like, using the same food choices.

6. Some Carbo Types, particularly those with blood sugar problems, will feel better almost immediately. They will be able to go longer between meals without eating, lose their sweet cravings and will feel a distinct energy boost. But other Carbo Types will not feel well. They may experience symptons of withdrawal from high-starch and sugary foods. This usually does not last for more than two to three days. It might involve any number of symptoms such as headache, flulike sensations, or extreme sweet cravings. If this should happen to you, just hang in there and you should start to experience some of the positive feelings listed above.

7. True Carbo Types who are already eating correctly will not feel well by cutting back on their carbohydrate intake this way. However, a majority of Carbo Types, will actually feel better for a few days by eliminating the "caution carbs." But shortly thereafter they will begin to feel irritable, short-tempered, and tired, and then crave sweets, feel hungry or unsatisfied after eating. Whenever you reach this point, increase the amount of nonstarchy vegetables (eat only those on your Allowable Foods Chart) as compared to your quantity of protein, until you once again begin to feel well.

8. If you still do not feel well even after increasing your nonstarchy vegetables, begin to add a little starch to your meals, starting with only 1 tablespoon of a starchy vegetable such as potato, rutabaga, sweet potato, or yam with dinner.

9. If you still feel well or even better by eating a little starchy vegetable with dinner, add one tablespoon of a starchy vegetable at lunch, and then one tablespoon at breakfast.

10. If all goes well, raise your starchy vegetable intake to two tablespoons per meal.

11. Then, if all is still fine, substitute some whole grain in place of the starchy vegetables.

12. In this manner, you can continue to slowly increase your carbohydrate intake. At some point, you'll move beyond your personal fuel mix and begin to notice a reappearance of your "old" symptoms— fatigue, depression, mood swings, sweet cravings, digestive problems, and so on. When that happens, you'll know you need to start

decreasing your carbohydrates gradually until you start feeling well again. At this stage, if you have any degree of uncertainty, you can always return to your baseline and start over.

Remember, too many or too few carbohydrates in relation to protein will produce similar symptoms.

Once you've come this far, you'll know how to manage your meals with great precision. But there are more techniques you can use to customize and fine-tune your diet even further. Look for the fine-tuning guidelines in Chapter 9.

Characteristics of Your Metabolic Type

Mixed types fall somewhere on the metabolic type scale between the Protein Types and Carbo Types. In this sense, they're a blend or mixture of the two.

There are two categories of Mixed Types—which one you fall into has a lot to do with the kinds of characteristics you manifest. The first category of Mixed Type can be referred to as the A-Mixed Type. The A stands for Actual. This means that most of your characteristics do not display either a Protein Type or a Carbo Type predominance, but are truly in the middle.

The second category of Mixed Type is the R-Mixed Type. Here the R stands for Relative. This signifies a relatively equal number of Protein Type traits and Carbo Type traits that offset each other—like a teeter-totter with an equal weight on either end. Instead of middle-of-the-road traits predominating, the R-Mixed Type has strong traits from both sides of the metabolic fence, with neither side dominating the other.

Many Mixed Types share similar kinds of characteristics. However, if you're a Mixed Type, that doesn't mean you're just like everyone else in your metabolic category in the way you react to foods, your strengths and weaknesses, your energy level, the strength of your appetite, and so on. After all, you're unique on a metabolic level!

Nonetheless, here are some *typical tendencies* that you may have in common with other Mixed Types:

Variable Appetite

A-Mixed Types tend to have average appetites. They tend to feel hungry at mealtimes but typically do not get hungry at other times.

R-Mixed Types tend to vacillate—sometimes feeling ravenous, while at other times they are not hungry to the point of skipping meals.

Cravings for Sweets and Carbohydrates

Typically, Mixed Types don't get cravings. However, if they don't carefully manage their diet by making sure they get a good balance of foods, they could shift into a Protein Type or a Carbo Type pattern and develop sweet cravings—or any other kind of craving, for that matter.

Weight Control

Mixed types have the capacity to do well on the widest range of foods, and for this reason they're less likely to have a problem with weight. But the freedom to eat a wide range of foods is not the unrestricted free-for-all it may seem at first glance—it's also a requirement. When Mixed Types slip into eating a restricted, or one-sided, diet (metabolically speaking), they can develop weight problems.

Fatigue, Anxiety, Nervousness

In one sense, it's great to be a Mixed Type because Mixed Types tend to have access to all the good traits of both Protein Types and Carbo Types. However, this equal access also means that Mixed Types can develop problems from both sides as well. Depending on the type of imbalance that develops, Mixed Types can develop fatigue, lethargy, or depression just as readily as hyperactivity, nervousness, and anxiety. Although Mixed Types have the potential to develop more problems than other types, they're also less likely to do so.

Dietary Emphasis for Mixed Types

In some ways, the diet for the Mixed Type is the most liberal of the three, since it's a mixture of the diets for Protein Types and for Carbo Types. This means that you *need* to get a good balance of high-purine, high-fat proteins *and* low-purine, low-fat proteins. Likewise, you need to make sure you get a good mix of vegetables and fruits that are good for *both* Protein Types and Carbo Types.

In other words, Mixed Types must take care not to get into the habit of eating too many Protein Type foods or too many Carbo Type foods on any given day. Each day your meals need to include foods from both groups. For this reason, you'll need to become familiar with the Allowable Foods Charts for both Protein Types (page 167) and Carbo Types (page 191).

The first thing to understand is that all proteins are not created equal. There are different kinds of proteins. There are those that are high in fat and high in purines. And there are those that are low in fat and low in purines.

More than any other kinds of foods, the high-fat, high-purine proteins provide the best fuel for Protein Types, but are inappropriate for Carbo Types. On the other hand, low-fat, low-purine proteins are perfect for Carbo Types but inadequate for Protein Types. So you must be sure to get a good balance of both types of proteins.

At the opposite end of the spectrum from proteins are carbohydrates. Because of their mineral balance, protein and fat content, and purine or non-purine status, certain vegetables contribute to balancing the body chemistry of Protein Types, while other vegetables do the same for Carbo Types. In addition, Carbo Types tend to handle starchy foods quite well, whereas starches can pose major problems for Protein Types. For these reasons, Mixed Types do best when they get a balance of both types of vegetables.

Overall, Protein Types *need* to focus on obtaining *larger amounts* of protein and fat in their diet, and *minimizing* their carbohydrate intake. As a rule, Carbo Types need to do just the opposite—eat less protein and fat and increase their intake of carbohydrates.

But, if you're a Mixed Type, you will do best on a good *balance* of proteins, fats, and carbohydrates—the typical "balanced meal." In the next few pages, I'll show you simple techniques for identifying the balance of macronutrients that is just right for your type.

Finding the right balance among protein, fat, and carbohydrate is your key to losing weight, feeling energized both physically and mentally, and staying on an even keel emotionally. Over the longer term, such a diet, if properly followed and tailored to your metabolic individuality, can prevent you from developing all kinds of serious degenerative diseases—cardiovascular problems, immune deficiency, blood sugar abnormalities, osteoporosis, arthritis, digestive disorders, and many other chronic illnesses—all of which are rooted in metabolic imbalance.

THE MIXED TYPE DIET ALLOWABLE FOODS CHART

PROTEINS			CARBOHYDRATES			OILS/FATS	
MEAT/FOWL	SEAFOOD	DAIRY	GRAIN	VEGETABLE	FRUIT	NUT/SEED	OIL/FAT

As a *Mixed Type*, you need to eat foods from *both* the Protein Type Diet and the Carbo Type Diet each day, and *not* get in the habit of eating foods from just one group or the other.

For this reason, you need to become familiar with the allowable foods charts of *both* the Protein Type Diet (page 167) *and* the Carbo Type Diet (page 191).

In addition, you may find it helpful to read the sections entitled "Important Tips on Your Allowable Foods" and "Foods to Avoid" in *both* the protein and carbo diets.

Important Tips on Your Allowable Foods

Eat Protein at Every Meal.

Eating sufficient protein at every meal will maximize your energy, trim your waistline, and assure peak performance. Failure to do this can lead to chronic fatigue, diminished well-being, and emotional imbalances such as depression, anxiety, and melancholy. Many people make the mistake of eating carbohydrate alone at a meal or snack. This is a mistake, as it can trigger excess insulin output from the pancreas, leading to food cravings, particularly for sugar or

PROTEIN TYPE PROTEINS[1]		
MEAT/FOWL	SEAFOOD	DAIRY
high purine	high purine	whole fat
organ meats	anchovy	low purine
pâté	caviar	cheese
beef liver	herring	cottage cheese
chicken liver	mussel	cream
medium purine	sardine	eggs
beef	medium purine	kefir
bacon	abalone	milk
chicken[2]	clam	yogurt
duck	crab	LEGUMES
fowl	crayfish	low purine
goose	lobster	tempeh
kidney	mackerel	tofu
lamb	octopus	medium purine
pork chop	oyster	beans, dried
spare rib	salmon	lentils
turkey[2]	scallop	NUTS
veal	shrimp	all are okay
wild game	snail	
	squid	
	tuna, dark	

1. Every meal should contain a protein from these sources, but dairy, legumes, or nuts are not a substitute for meats at main meals.
2. Dark meat is best.

other sweets, blood sugar regulation problems, increased fat storage, and a whole host of degenerative processes. It can also potentially shift you into a new imbalance—a Protein Type metabolic pattern.

Get a Good Mix of Protein Type and
Carbo Type Proteins Each Day.

Purines are special protein substances derived from a class of proteins called nucleoproteins, which play an important part in your body's energy-producing processes. They have particular benefit for Protein Types and directly contribute to balancing their body chemistry.

Carbo Types fare better on the lower-fat, lower-purine proteins. As a Mixed Type, *any* protein is permissible in your diet. But because of the special needs of your metabolic type, you fare better on a daily mixture of high-fat, high-purine proteins *and* low-fat, low-purine proteins. Too much or not enough of one or the other will result in disturbances in your energy, mood, and well-being.

CARBO TYPE PROTEINS		
MEAT/FOWL	*SEAFOOD*	*DAIRY*
light meats	light fish	non/low fat
chicken breast	catfish	cheese
Cornish game hen	cod	cottage cheese
turkey breast	flounder	kefir
pork, lean	haddock	milk
ham	halibut	yogurt
Only occasional	perch	eggs
lean red meat or	scrod	*LEGUMES*
restrict entirely	sole	use sparingly
	trout	high starch
	tuna, white	dried beans
	turbot	lentils
		low starch
		tempeh
		tofu
		NUTS
		sparingly

Snack as Needed.

Typically, Mixed Types don't often feel the need for snacks. But if you want to eat snacks, it's okay to do so. Generally speaking, it's best to eat a little protein when you snack so as not to over-stimulate insulin production. However, eating just carbohydrate (like fruit) alone from time to time is okay as well. As a Mixed Type, any snack will work for you, theoretically. But it's important to find what works *best*. Just keep in mind that whatever you eat should result in improved energy and well-being, should satisfy your appetite, and should not cause a desire for sweets. With these ideas as guidelines, learn to listen to your body!

Carefully Consider Dairy.

Dairy foods are optional for your type. As long as you don't react badly to dairy, it's fine for you. Generally speaking, dairy is not a good source of protein for Protein Types, but often works well for Carbo Types. So if your appetite is very strong, dairy is not likely to be the best protein choice. At such times, the heavier proteins are usually required to provide the right fuel for your metabolism. But when your appetite is less acute, dairy might be just the right protein for the occasion.

Consider Carbohydrates Carefully.

Any plant-based foods—grains, vegetables or fruits—are carbohydrates. But there are different kinds of carbohydrates and they don't all affect your metabolism the same way. For example, some carbohydrates are higher in starch and some carbohydrates are lower in starch. Starchy carbohydrates break down easily into sugar, which means they hit your bloodstream quickly.

PROTEIN TYPE CARBOS		
GRAIN	*VEGETABLE*	*FRUIT*
whole grains only	nonstarchy	avocado
	asparagus	olive
high starch	beans, fresh	not fully ripe—
amaranth	cauliflower	apple (some)
barley	celery	pear (some)
brown rice	mushroom	high starch
buckwheat	spinach	banana
corn	high starch	
couscous	artichoke	
kamut	carrot	
kasha	pea	
millet	potatoes, fried in butter, only	
oat		
quinoa	squash, winter	
rye	*LEGUMES*	
spelt	nonstarchy	
triticale	tempeh	
sprouted-grain bread is the only bread allowed[1]	tofu	1. Sprouted-grain brands such as Ezekiel or Manna breads
	high starch	
	beans, dried	
	peas, dried	
	lentils	

This can cause a strong insulin response from the pancreas, which typically leads to increased fat storage and blood sugar problems such as hypoglycemia. Over time, excess insulin secretion can contribute to more severe disorders such as allergies, asthma, alcoholism, atherosclerosis, cancer, carbohydrate addiction, heart disease, chronic fatigue, depression, diabetes, insulin resistance, glucose intolerance, hypertension, obesity, and peptic ulcers. Thus, grains, starchy vegetables, and starchy fruits are "caution carbs." For this reason, Protein Types need to emphasize *nonstarchy vegetables* as their *primary source* of carbohydrates. Although Carbo Types handle starches better than Protein Types, they can still run into trouble by overeating starches. So as a Mixed Type, you need to get a good mixture of vegetables from the Protein Type group *and* the Carbo Type group.

Use Grains in Moderation.

Use only whole-grain products. Do not consume any refined grain products made with white flour or enriched flour. All baked foods should contain only whole-grain flours. If you are carbohydrate sensitive or have blood sugar problems, avoid wheat and wheat products as much as possible, since wheat breaks down into sugar faster than any other grain and, therefore, has a disruptive influence on insulin metabolism. Here's a tip: Try using spelt instead of wheat, since spelt shares many of wheat's desirable attributes for baking but not wheat's influences on insulin. Keep in mind, though, that all grains are starches, which means they readily break down into sugar, so they should be used sparingly. For this reason, cooked whole grains are preferable to products like breads and crackers. The *worst* offenders for your metabolism are refined grains of all kinds. If you start craving sweets after a meal with grains, you probably ate too many grains and need to increase your proportion of protein next time around.

Don't Overdo Bread.

Avoid white breads made with refined, enriched flours. Instead, opt for sprouted-grain breads such as Ezekiel or Manna brands. Unlike regular breads, sprouted-grain breads won't inhibit calcium absorption. In addition, sprouted bread has enhanced quantities of vitamins B and C and does not contain the enzyme inhibitors typically found in grains. When you do eat bread, always use butter, which will minimize any potential adverse blood sugar fluctuations. Note that the process of making bread refines grains to some degree, which only increases the starchlike qualities of the grains, further increasing the insulin response. So if you have problems with carbohydrates or blood sugar problems, minimize your intake of bread.

Closely Monitor Fruits.

Because Protein Types tend to be fast oxidizers or parasympathetic dominants, they are predisposed to low blood sugar problems. Due to the high sugar and potassium content of

CARBO TYPE CARBOHYDRATES			
GRAIN	VEGETABLE		FRUIT
whole grains only	high starch	low starch	all are okay
	potato	beet green	apple
high starch	pumpkin	broccoli	apricot
amaranth	rutabaga	Brussels sprout	berry
barley	sweet potato	cabbage	cherry
brown rice	yam	chard	citrus
buckwheat	moderate starch	collard	grape
corn	beet	cucumber	melon
couscous	corn	garlic	peach
kamut	eggplant	kale	pear
kasha	jicama	leafy greens	pineapple
millet	okra	onion	plum
oat	parsnip	parsley	tomato
quinoa	radish	peppers	tropical
rice	spaghetti squash	scallion	LEGUMES
rye	summer squash	sprouts	high starch
spelt	yellow squash	tomato	dried beans
triticale	turnip	watercress	dried peas
wheat	zucchini		lentils

fruit, Protein Types need to limit their fruit intake. On the other hand, Carbo Types, as slow oxidizers or sympathetic dominants, typically do well with a higher potassium intake, so they usually handle fruit just fine. Mixed Types fall somewhere in between these two extremes. Normally, fruit is not a problem, but overeating fruit can shift a Mixed Type's metabolism to that of a Protein Type, potentially causing insulin regulation problems, sweet cravings, or weight gain. When very hungry, Mixed Types would do well to eat some protein instead of fruit. If you develop a sweet craving after eating fruit, it's almost a certain indication that you've had too much carbohydrate and not enough protein.

Use Juices Judiciously.

Avoid canned juices of any kind. Vegetable juices, as long as they're freshly made, are allowed in moderation. It's best to use a combination of starchy and nonstarchy vegetables such as carrot, celery, and spinach, and not overdo juices made from purely starchy vegetables. However, it's best to avoid fruit juices completely. Fruit juices, or even excessive amounts of vegetable juice, can potentially imbalance your metabolic type and lead to weight gain, food cravings, blood sugar fluctuations, and a desire for sugar. Eating fruit is permissible, but fresh fruit juices should be used only periodically for therapeutic reasons and not as a matter of routine or for quenching thirst. In place of fruit juice, make smoothies by blending whole fruits. If you're thirsty, drink water—not juice, tea, or milk.

Freely Use Fats and Oils.

The subject of fats and oils and their effects on human metabolism has been extensively researched and documented. An in-depth discussion of them is beyond the scope of this book (for a complete discussion, see *Fats and Oils*, an excellent book by Udo Erasmus). In general, what you need to know is that fats and oils in their natural state are not bad for you and eating them will not produce high cholesterol or heart disease any more than eating any other natural food. Fats contain fatty acids that are essential for good health, efficient immune function, normal hormonal production, cellular respiration (energy production), proper cell membrane permeability —in short, for life itself. Whether a food is good or bad depends on the quality of the food and the metabolic type of the person consuming the food. Fats are no exception. Protein Types need to support their metabolisms by consuming liberal amounts of natural oils and fats. Carbo Types do best limiting fat intake. Mixed Types should neither eat excessive amounts of fat nor restrict fat unnecessarily. Simply by including the higher fat-containing proteins in your diet

OILS / FATS	
NUT/SEED[1]	OIL/FAT
all are okay	all are okay
walnut	butter
pumpkin	cream
peanut	ghee
sunflower	oils:
sesame	almond
almond	flax
cashew	olive
Brazil	peanut
filbert	sesame
pecan	sunflower
chestnut	walnut
pistachio	
coconut	
hickory	
macadamia	

1. Nuts are listed from highest to lowest protein content. Higher protein is preferable.

and by using butter and vegetable oils, particularly olive oil, where appropriate according to your taste, you'll easily obtain sufficient fatty acids to meet your requirement. But never consume margarine, hydrogenated oils, or fat substitutes, as research is uncovering the fact that these substances can have a serious negative impact on your health! If you must buy packaged foods, read the labels to make sure they do not contain these substances. Use only real butter (organic if possible) and natural cold-pressed oils that have been properly manufactured. Recommended brands are Omega, Flora, and Bio-San, widely available in health food stores.

Be Conscious of Glycemic Values.

All carbohydrates—fruits, vegetables, grains—are converted to glucose in the body. Carbohydrates are categorized according to the rate or speed at which they hit the bloodstream as glucose, and are ranked accordingly in what is known as the glycemic index (GI). High-glycemic foods, such as grains and starchy vegetables, hit your bloodstream much more rapidly than low-glycemic foods such as proteins and fats. Protein types need to carefully regulate high-glycemic foods. On the other hand, Carbo Types can handle high-glycemic foods fairly well, although they still must be careful not to overdo them. As a Mixed Type, it's a good idea for you to carefully regulate high-glycemic foods like grains and starchy vegetables and to place much more focus on those foods lower on the glycemic index. Here's a tip: By including some protein whenever you do eat high-glycemic foods, you'll help slow down the rate at which the high-glycemic foods are converted to sugar. (Note: Check Chapter 9 for the complete glycemic index. It's very important for all metabolic types to become familiar with the GI.)

Foods to Avoid

Certain foods aggravate your metabolic imbalances and should therefore be avoided. You may have strong adverse reactions to these foods, or, if your metabolism is less sensitive, the reactions may be slight or even nonexistent. Or your reactions to these problem foods could vary from time to time. All these possibilities are common and reflect yet another facet of metabolic individuality.

Keep in mind that the effects of nutrition are cumulative. The more you ingest a food, the stronger the effect becomes. So even if you don't display any noticeable adverse reactions, it's still best to minimize your intake of the following foods whenever possible.

In short, stick to your allowable foods. But if you simply must eat something not on that list, be aware that the following foods are particularly undesirable for your metabolism.

Alcohol.

Alcohol, plain and simple, is a poison to your body. Your body must detoxify it and neutralize its adverse effects. From this perspective, it isn't good for anyone. Being a simple sugar, it can wreak havoc with your metabolism. It triggers excessive insulin secretion, which leads to blood sugar imbalances, increased fat storage, and the development of chronic degenerative processes. Thus, moderation with alcohol is strongly recommended.

Allergenic or Reactive Foods.

Your Allowable Foods Chart provides recommendations for foods that will specifically support your metabolic type. This means that they contain the right balance of nutrients. Whether or not you are currently reactive or allergic to any of these foods is a completely different issue. If you have known reactions to any recommended foods, leave them out of your diet temporarily, but try them from time to time. As your chemistry changes, so too may your food reactivities. This is the experience of many individuals who have properly customized their diet to match their metabolism.

Caffeine.

Avoid caffeine products as much as possible, including coffee, black teas, caffeine-containing herbs, and soft drinks. If you do insist on drinking coffee, make sure it's organic and limit it to no more than one to two weak cups per day. Also, when drinking caffeinated beverages, it's a good idea to eat some protein, as protein will help combat to a degree caffeine's adverse effects on your type. Bottom line: Caffeine is counterproductive for all metabolic types. Although some of the specific reasons differ for each type, coffee has a universally stimulating effect on the body's energy-producing glands. Those people who feel they need coffee have weak or exhausted energy glands. The stimulation of those glands by coffee is akin to whipping a tired horse. Short-term, this stimulation is pleasurable, but long-term it only worsens the problem by further exhausting the energy glands.

Fruit Juices.

Fruit juices are best avoided, as they are too high in sugar. Devoid of fiber, the concentrated fruit sugar has a particularly powerful negative impact on insulin and blood sugar control. Sugar flooding into your bloodstream causes a strong insulin surge that rapidly lowers blood sugar and increases fat storage.

Sugar.

In significant quantities, sugar is not good for anyone, so avoid or minimize it as much as you can. Be especially watchful for hidden sugars in processed packaged foods. Sugar is added to a great many commercial foods, and it can really add up if you're not careful, secretly sabotaging your best intentions to follow your dietary recommendations. By the way, by sugar I mean *all* forms of sugar—processed and natural—including beet sugar, cane sugar, brown sugar, molasses, honey, fructose, maltose, dextrose, corn syrup, maple syrup, etc.

Foods High in Oxalic Acids.

Oxalic acid is a naturally-occurring acid in some foods that interferes with the absorption of calcium. For this reason, Protein Types have to be especially careful to avoid or limit foods high in oxalic acid. Mixed types have more freedom with these foods, but you still must be careful not to overeat foods high in oxalic acid, such as apples, asparagus, black tea, blackberries, beets, beet greens, chard, chocolate, cocoa, cranberries, currants (red), endive, gooseberries, grapes, green peppers, plums, raspberries, rhubarb, spinach, strawberries, and tomatoes. The good news is that cooking destroys the oxalic acid, so items such as asparagus, beets, beet greens, chard, cranberries, green peppers, rhubarb, and spinach are all best eaten cooked.

Foods High in Phytates.

As Sally Fallon and Mary Enig point out in their wonderful book *Nourishing Traditions* (1-877-707-1776 or www.newtrendspublishing.com), in every traditional culture in the world, for thousands of years, whole grains have been prepared by soaking or fermenting them prior to cooking. Modern science has revealed the wisdom of these traditions by discovering that all grains and legumes contain substances called phytates. Phytic acid is a chemical found in the bran portion of grains and the skins of legumes. It binds with calcium (and iron, magnesium, phosphorous, and zinc) in the intestinal tract, thereby preventing absorption. When consumed excessively, phytates can cause serious mineral deficiencies, allergies, intestinal distress, and bone loss. All grains contain phytates, but wheat, oats, soy, and soy milk have the highest concentration. What to do? Simply soak any grains (such as oats, millet, rye, barley, quinoa) overnight before you cook them. You can also liberally use miso, soy sauce, and tempeh, since these are fermented products, and fermentation destroys phytates. However, tofu, soy milk, and soy protein powders are not fermented and do contain phytates, so you should limit consumption of these food items. Sprouted-grain breads, and sourdough bread with its long fermentation process, are also almost entirely free of phytates. All other breads are full of phytates and should be limited or avoided.

Foods High in Gluten and Enzyme Inhibitors.

Grains contain hard-to-digest proteins like gluten. Insufficient digestion of such proteins has been linked to problems such as allergies, celiac disease (sprue), mental illness, indigestion, and yeast overgrowth (candida albicans). But here again, soaking and fermentation renders such proteins more digestible and their nutrients more readily available. So, sourdough breads and sprouted breads are preferable to other varieties. Soybeans also contain potent enzyme inhibitors that need to be neutralized through fermentation or soaking.

Thyroid-Suppressing Foods.

Certain foods contain a chemical known as thiocyanate, which causes thyroid dysfunction. Thiocyanate belongs to a class of substances known as goitrogens. These substances block the production of thyroid hormone—a hormone that plays an integral role in the regulation of all your metabolic activities. Goitrogens are found in raw broccoli, Brussels sprouts, cabbage, cauliflower, kale, mustard, rutabaga, and watercress. If you eat these foods frequently, it's a good idea to supplement your diet with extra iodine in the form of kelp, since goitrogens work by blocking iodine absorption by the thyroid gland. Kelp can be ground and used in a salt shaker as a condiment. Also note that cooking will partially inactivate the thyroid-suppressing chemical found in these foods. So you'll want to use kelp, take care to cook these foods, and use them conservatively, especially if you've been diagnosed with hypothyroidism.

Your Macronutrient Ratio

This diet is easy! There are only two things you need to remember:

1. Eat the right kinds of foods for your type, and avoid the wrong foods for your type—in other words, stick to your allowable foods.
2. Eat the right proportions of macronutrients (proteins, fats, carbohydrates) at each meal.

If you think of your food as fuel, then the proportions of proteins, carbohydrates, and fats can be viewed as your fuel mixture. If you get the right fuel for your type *and* the right fuel mixture, you'll have a powerful force at work. Your food will be efficiently converted to energy, rather than stored as fat.

Here's your general macronutrient ratio:

PROTEINS	&	FATS	CARBOHYDRATES
50%			50%
(approx. 30% proteins)		(approx. 20% fats)	
Equal Amounts of Proteins and Fats			*Equal Amounts of Carbos*
red meats, fowl, seafood, dairy, legumes, nuts		fatty meats, fowl and seafood, dairy, nuts, seeds, oils, butter	fruits, vegetables, grains

Stick to your 50 percent/50 percent food ratio whenever you eat, getting approximately 50 percent of your calories from carbohydrates, and 50 percent from proteins and fats. Note that more of your calories should come from protein than from fat.

It's not necessary to be perfectly precise in terms of your percent-

ages. When combining your food, just try to approximate as best you can.

It's unnecessary to measure out by weight everything you eat, or to calculate the number of calories in a meal. When you get the right balance for your metabolism, your appetite will naturally be satisfied, and the calorie issue will eventually take care of itself. So it doesn't matter whether you eat a small meal or a large meal or something in between. What is important is eating the right foods for your type and in the right proportions for your type, every time you eat.

If you happen to be especially concerned with weight loss, or you need to lose a significant amount of weight, I'll explain issues regarding calories and food quantities later on, in Chapter 10. However, it's very important to realize that:

Your weight will begin to normalize just by eating the right foods in the right combinations. When you balance your macronutrients properly, you'll lose weight if you're overweight and gain weight if you're underweight.

Try to eat at regular intervals and stick to the same mealtimes every day if at all possible. It's also important to eat when you're hungry, preferably before you get hungry, so snack if you need to. This will keep you from overeating and keep your blood sugar on an even keel.

A helpful way to think about your macronutrient percentages is in terms of a plate of food. Almost half the food on your plate should be carbohydrate (primarily nonstarchy) and the rest should be protein and fat-containing foods.

A lot of people are very confused about how to eat a meal comprised of twenty percent fat. But your requirement for fats can easily be met by just eating your protein foods that are also sources of natural fats and by making use of butter and oils on your foods according to your taste.

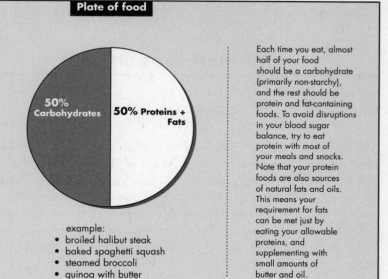

Plate of food

50% Carbohydrates

50% Proteins + Fats

Each time you eat, almost half of your food should be a carbohydrate (primarily non-starchy), and the rest should be protein and fat-containing foods. To avoid disruptions in your blood sugar balance, try to eat protein with most of your meals and snacks. Note that your protein foods are also sources of natural fats and oils. This means your requirement for fats can be met just by eating your allowable proteins, and supplementing with small amounts of butter and oil.

example:
- broiled halibut steak
- baked spaghetti squash
- steamed broccoli
- quinoa with butter

Note that the 50%/50% ratio is just a general guideline for Mixed Types. So you will need to follow the twelve steps on page 233 to identify the specific macronutrient ratio or the personal fuel mix that meets your highly individualized needs.

Sample Menus

The following are suggestions only for possible meal plans. These are not intended as receipes, but are provided as ideas for good ways to use your allowable foods. Feel free to create your own menus, combining your allowable foods in any manner that suits your taste at any given meal. Your metabolic type needs to make sure that you get protein every time that you eat. Refrain from eating carbohydrate all by itself. Note that most snacks should always contain proteins. *Bon appétit!*

MEAL	DAY ONE	DAY TWO
BREAKFAST	hot whole grain cereal with whole milk and berries (optional: eggs or cottage cheese)	oatmeal with half and half, banana, protein shake with whey or egg-white protein powder, fruit
LUNCH	cheese sandwich comprised of 1 or 2 pieces of whole-grain bread and tomato, lettuce, onion, pickle, and mayonnaise, coleslaw	dark or light tuna salad made with tomato, artichoke hearts, celery, scallions, lettuce, olive oil, and lemon juice, toasted spelt bread
SNACK	cottage cheese with olives and rye cracker	nuts and raisins
DINNER	roast beef, steamed beets with butter, spinach salad with onions, croutons, olive oil, and vinegar	Cornish game hen with wild rice, steamed asparagus and butter, lettuce, tomato, radish and onion salad with olive oil and vinegar

MEAL	DAY THREE	
BREAKFAST	bacon and eggs, wheat toast with butter, ½ grapefruit or apple	
LUNCH	turkey sandwich on 1 or 2 pieces of whole-grain bread, salad with vinaigrette dressing	chicken salad san (light and/or dark mayonnaise, chopped t onion, celery, and sprout
SNACK	fruit salad and whole milk yogurt	whole-wheat toast or apple with almond butter
DINNER	broiled pork chops, steamed zucchini, sweet potato with butter	leg of lamb with roast potatoes, broccoli, mixed green salad

MEAL	DAY FIVE
BREAKFAST	vegetable omelette with potatoes fried in butter (optional: 1 piece of sprouted toast)
LUNCH	hamburger on sprouted-grain bun, coleslaw with pickle
SNACK	leftover chicken with carrot and celery sticks
DINNER	broiled halibut steak, baked spaghetti squash, steamed Swiss chard

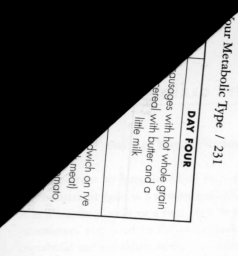

IET

Fuel Mix

...fty percent/fifty percent
...or Mixed Types. Think of
...ides you with the general
...be at your best. Due to
...people within the Mixed
...requirements.

As an example, some Mixed Types can get by on less protein and tolerate larger amounts of carbohydrates, even those with a higher sugar and starch content. Other people need more protein and are highly sensitive to even small amounts of carbohydrates—starchy or nonstarchy.

Everyone is different, which means that the specific proportion of proteins, carbohydrates, and fats that might work well for you is not necessarily the same proportion of macronutrients that would work well for other people in your metabolic category.

Think of your Mixed Type category as a sliding scale, or a continuum, or a spectrum of variable macronutrient requirements.

MIXED TYPES

Higher Protein: Lower Carb   Moderate Protein: Moderate Carb   Lower Protein: Higher Carb

What you need to do is pinpoint your own highly individualized macronutrient ratio. In other words, you need to refine or tailor the general macronutrient ratio for Mixed Types to your own particular needs. You need to identify what I call your personal fuel mix.

Once you discover your personal fuel mix, you'll know how to combine your foods—proteins, carbohydrates, and fats—in proportions that are just right for you. This will make a huge difference in the way you feel following meals and snacks.

You'll know when you've hit your personal fuel mix because you will immediately have strong and lasting physical energy and mental clarity, a solid sense of well-being, and a sense of fullness and satisfaction—as opposed to persistent hunger and sweet cravings.

Remember, as a Mixed Type, excess amounts of carbohydrates (especially the starchy, sugary kind) *or* excess proteins are your downfall, and an imbalance between the two can produce decreased energy, mood swings, blood sugar problems, and food cravings.

How do you find your personal fuel mix? It's really very simple. All you need to do is experiment a little by consuming varying amounts of carbohydrates.

As a first step, you'll need to restrict your carbohydrate intake for a few days. Once you know what it feels like to be almost entirely off carbohydrates, you can start adding them in again, a little at a time, until you hit your personal fuel mix.

If you go beyond your personal fuel mix by eating excessive carbohydrates, you'll know it. Why? Because you'll lose your energy, sense of well-being, and feelings of satisfaction very quickly after eating. On the other hand, if you fail to reach your personal fuel mix by eating too few carbohydrates, you'll experience the very same kind of negative symptoms.

To find your personal fuel mix, all you need to do is follow the simple steps below.

Twelve Simple Steps for Finding Your Personal Fuel Mix

1. For the first five to seven days, eliminate all "caution carbs"—grains, cereals, breads, desserts, fruits, and starchy vegetables—as well as milk products.
2. Eat freely of any of your allowable proteins and fats: meat, poultry, seafood, eggs, nuts, seeds, butter, and vegetable oils.
3. During these few days, limit your vegetable intake to the non-

starchy carbohydrates. Start out with only a small portion of non-starchy vegetables as compared to the amount of protein you eat. This is your baseline.

4. Eat until you are full but not to the point of feeling stuffed.

5. Have snacks between meals if you like, using the same food choices.

6. Many Mixed Types will feel better almost immediately. They will be able to go longer between meals without eating, will lose their sweet cravings, and will feel a distinct energy boost. But some Mixed Types can experience withdrawal from high-starch and sugary foods. This usually does not last for more than forty-eight hours. It might involve any number of symptoms such as headache, flulike sensations, or extreme sweet cravings. If this should happen to you, just hang in there for two to three days and you should start to experience some of the positive feelings mentioned earlier.

7. Typically, Mixed Types will feel better for five to seven days after eliminating all the "caution carbs." But shortly thereafter they generally begin to feel irritable, short-tempered, and tired, then crave sweets, and feel hungry or unsatisfied after eating. When you reach this point, increase the amount of nonstarchy vegetables as compared to your quantity of protein, until you once again begin to feel well.

8. If you still do not feel well even after increasing your nonstarchy vegetables, begin to add a little starch to your meals, starting with only one tablespoon of a starchy vegetable like artichokes, corn, peas, potato, sweet potato, yam, or winter squash with dinner.

9. If you still feel well or even better by eating a little starchy vegetable with dinner, add one tablespoon of a starchy vegetable at lunch and then one tablespoon at breakfast.

10. If all goes well, raise your starchy vegetable intake to two tablespoons per meal.

11. Then, if all is still fine, substitute some whole grain in place of the starchy vegetables.

12. In this manner, you can continue to slowly increase your carbohydrate intake. At some point, you'll move beyond your personal fuel mix and begin to notice a reappearance of your "old" symptoms—fatigue, depression, mood swings, sweet cravings, digestive problems, and so on. When that happens, you'll know you need to start

decreasing your carbohydrates gradually until you start feeling well again. At this stage, if you have any degree of uncertainty, you can always return to your baseline and start over.

Remember, too many or too few carbohydrates in relation to protein will produce similar symptoms.

Once you've come this far, you'll know how to manage your meals with great precision. But there are more techniques you can use to customize and fine-tune your diet even further. Look for the fine-tuning guidelines in Chapter 9.

Chapter 8

FREQUENTLY ASKED QUESTIONS

Quick and Easy Steps to Success

Once you've taken the self-test and carefully reviewed the diet section that applies to you, you might want to just go ahead and plunge right in and start eating according to the food lists and dietary instructions provided there.

Keep in mind that your metabolic type diet is the key to your success. So you'll want to focus on your *own dietary section* very closely. Even if you skim the rest of this book, be sure to spend plenty of time reading and reviewing your diet section as often as necessary, until you're extremely familiar with it, and know it almost by heart!

It won't take a lot of time and it will be easy to do! Each individual diet section is not very long, and you'll find that your dietary tips and guidelines are presented in a very clear, easy-to-read, and digestible format.

Of course, if you can spare the time, it's always a good idea to review and familiarize yourself with the *other two* diet sections as well—in other words, even the metabolic type diets that *don't* apply to you.

This will simply broaden your perspective and give you a more in-depth understanding of your own nutritional needs. And your dietary needs may shift over time. So the more you know now about the full spectrum of metabolic requirements, the easier it will be to adjust your own diet if the need arises.

Then again, you may simply be the chief cook in your household, and your family members may have dietary needs distinctly different from your own. If that's the case, you'll definitely need to become closely familiar with whatever diet section in Chapter 7 applies to anyone for whom you prepare meals.

If you feel a little overwhelmed by all the information, never fear. It's really much simpler than it might first appear!

When pursuing any new dietary direction, it's not unusual for people to feel a little challenged at first. New approaches of any kind can seem challenging, especially to those of us with busy, stress-filled lives who have little time to focus on meal planning and food preparation.

The two biggest concerns people typically have are:

1. uncertainty about what to do first or how to get started
2. confusion about "putting it all together," or how to juggle the multiple aspects of a new regime all at once

If these are your concerns, don't worry, because in Chapter 12, "Indispensable Tips for Savvy Consumers," you'll find practical tips that will make your new metabolic diet very easy to implement and follow.

So if you've read and reviewed your diet section and you're all ready to go but would like *practical hints* about getting started—how to get organized, how and where to food-shop, how to prepare meals, what to focus on first, how to integrate your diet into your life with ease and efficiency—just flip directly to Chapter 12.

You can always come back to this chapter a little later on, once you're "up and running" with your new diet.

On the other hand, if you've read your dietary section and you have other kinds of questions and concerns—more fundamental issues about your health or your weight or symptoms you may have, or why certain foods are recommended for your metabolic type—*then you'll want to review this chapter now*, because the answers are all here in a convenient question-and-answer format.

Problem Solving

Rest assured that you are not about to embark on the latest new dietary fad! Remember, the science of metabolic typing has been evolving for a very long time, and nutritionists and health professionals all over the world have been using various forms of metabolic typing in their clinical practices for over two decades.

It's a dietary approach that thousands of people have used very successfully. Nonetheless, in the process of getting acclimated and learning about their metabolic type diets, many people have questions or problems from time to time.

Interestingly, the very same kinds of questions crop up again and again. Despite our biological diversity, those of us who live in industrialized societies all share remarkably similar dietary issues and dilemmas.

On the following pages you'll find several Q&A sections where I've gathered many of the questions that people most commonly ask, along with answers that I think you'll find useful.

For your convenience I've organized the questions and answers according to the three primary metabolic categories (Protein Types, Carbo Types, and Mixed Types). I've also added an introductory Q&A section to cover general questions that apply to everyone, regardless of their metabolic type.

Frequently Asked Questions for All Metabolic Types

I've tried many weight loss programs but have never been able to lose weight and keep it off. Why would your system be more successful than any other?

The reason most weight loss programs fail is that they address the symptoms rather than the causes of being overweight. Like chronic fatigue, headaches, or constipation, excess weight and obesity are expressions of underlying biochemical imbalances within the body's fundamental homeostatic controls. That's why it's so critical for you to identify your metabolic type. Eating accordingly will help to correct those underlying imbalances. This explains why some people lose weight on a high-protein diet and others lose weight on a high-carbohydrate diet—or anything in between. The best way to lose weight and keep it off is to address your genetic dietary requirements. This is why you don't find obese people in native cultures around the world. For more details on weight control, see Chapter 10.

I feel poorly all the time. I have a lot of nagging ailments and I'm terribly run down and fatigued. Can this program help me? If so, when can I expect to feel better?

Remember that your body is designed to be healthy. A blueprint for your own perfect health is present in each of your cells. But the only way you can fulfill this potential is by providing your body with the right raw materials and avoiding foods that are inappropriate for your metabolic type. When you cut yourself, your body "knows" how to heal itself. Similarly, your body knows how to generate ideal health. All you need to do is give it what it needs and then let it take over. It's difficult to say precisely when you can expect to feel better. Every person is unique and there are many factors that come into play in each individual case: age, stress, environment, exercise, toxicity, seriousness of the problem, length of time it has been present, and so on. However, some positive changes are bound to occur shortly after fully adopting a new metabolically correct diet. Use every such occurrence of positive change, no matter how small, as a stepping-stone to increase your faith in your body's ability to be healthy and you'll be richly rewarded. Realistically, though, if you've been eating improperly and following an unhealthy lifestyle for a long time, you can't always wave a magic wand and expect to feel great overnight. Remember, you have to build health from the ground up, so it can take time.

I took the Metabolic Type Self-Test but am not certain I answered the questions as well as I could have. So I'm not sure if I've identified my metabolic type correctly. What should I do?

It's not unusual for people to be concerned about this. But don't worry, there are several different ways to verify your results. First, you can retake the Metabolic Type Self-Test as often as you want. Second, ask someone close to you to review your answers to see if he or she agrees with your responses. Third, you can use the Troubleshooting Test in Appendix A as a powerful additional tool to verify the results of the self-test. Finally, remember that the "proof is in the pudding." In other words, once you begin your new diet, your body will send you signals to let you know if you're moving in the right direction. Use the Fine-Tuning Mini-Quiz in Chapter 9 to assist you in interpreting the signals your body will be sending you.

Why am I hungry all the time? And why do I crave bread, pastry, doughnuts, corn chips, and all the things that aren't good for me?

Generally speaking, cravings are an indication that your body is not getting the right fuel mix. The result is that your cells are unable to generate sufficient energy. When this happens, the message "We need energy!" is transmitted to your brain by a hundred trillion screaming body cells. This demand gets translated into a strong desire for food—most often for sugar and other forms of carbohydrate. But when you eat carbohydrate and do not get the right proportion of protein along with it, your fuel mixture is insufficient for maximum energy production. Instead of being fully converted to energy, a portion of your food gets stored as fat and you're soon hungry all over again. It becomes a vicious cycle. You can resolve your cravings by going back to your dietary section in Chapter 7 and reviewing your Allowable Foods Chart and the twelve simple steps for finding your personal fuel mix.

I don't like the foods recommended for my metabolic type. How long do I have to eat this way?

To start, eat any of the foods on your list that you do like. As your body chemistry balances, you'll be surprised by the way your tastes also change. You'll actually begin to enjoy more foods that are truly good for you, and, in a very natural way, you'll lose interest in foods that are bad for you. Human beings have the capacity to instinctively know which foods are good for them and which foods are not. But this ability has been lost or distorted by the excess use of sugar, alcohol, nicotine, and junk foods, by air and water pollution, by eating the wrong foods for one's type, and by the addition of over ten thousand chemicals to our food supply. Fortunately, however, our distorted appetites can be restored once we begin to eat according to our metabolic type. In addition, as your chemistry balances and your health improves, you'll be able to eat and enjoy a broader range of foods.

Should I feed my whole family the way I eat?

No, I do not recommend that you force your metabolic type diet on others if you don't know that it's right for their metabolism. Nutrition is very powerful. Just as you can correct imbalances with nutrition, you can also create imbalances if you use it improperly. When everyone in your family is meeting their individual nutrient requirements, you will all be healthier and happier and your home environment will be far more harmonious. Use the fine-tuning tool in Chapter 9 to learn how your body communicates the success or failure of a meal. Then use that information to judge the results of meals on family members. For example, if one child's energy picks up and his/her mood improves, while another child noticeably becomes lethargic or throws a tantrum while insisting on having a dessert, it's likely that the meal was good for one child and not the other. It's important to tailor your kids' diets to their highly individualized needs if you want them to be able to function well at home and in school.

I have three children between the ages of five and twelve and I have no idea how to go about determining their metabolic type. They're not old enough to do the Metabolic Type Self-Test. What can I do?

You might try filling out the Metabolic Type Self-Test for your children. Parents sometimes find this fairly easy to do, especially for older children. If that's not feasible, there are other ways to provide your child with a healthy, metabolically appropriate diet. To begin with, you and your spouse can both do the self-test and learn the signals that your bodies send when you're eating the wrong foods, combining them inappropriately, waiting too long between meals, and so on. Once you learn to interpret your own "body language," you'll be much better equipped to spot any diet-related problems your kids might have. Then just fill your house with good foods and see what happens. As long as kids are off junk food, they will tend to gravitate naturally toward the foods they need. For example, when meat is too rich for them, they will resist eating it. You can also try keeping a diary of meals and snacks so that you can more easily observe and recall what kinds of meals and snacks provoke negative symptoms in your children.

My eight-year-old son is hyperactive and has terrible problems in school. He can't concentrate or sit still and his teachers are pressuring me to put him on Ritalin. What should I do?

Since all children are in an "anabolic" or "growth" phase of life, they tend to need higher amounts of protein and fat regardless of their metabolic type. When they get adequate amounts of protein and the right balance of macronutrients, their behavioral problems often disappear. But failure to get the right balance of nutrients frequently causes children to become apathetic, anxious, depressed, irritable, hyperactive, withdrawn, lethargic, aggressive, combative, violent, and subject to low self-esteem, panic attacks, attention deficit disorder, and other psychological problems. So, what you need to do first is minimize starches and sugars and increase protein in your child's diet. Sugar is the absolute worst type of fuel for children's metabolisms. Try restricting all sugar—including all hidden sugars in processed and packaged foods. In addition, use only whole, natural foods and avoid any foods with artificial food coloring and dyes, as these chemicals can exacerbate behavioral problems. To keep your children's blood sugar stable, be sure to give them protein-based snacks between meals. In general, be aware that food exerts an extremely powerful influence on the personality as well as on the emotional and psychological status of all of us, adults and children alike. In fact the "biochemistry of behavior" is a complex, emerging area in itself. In short, from an emotional or psychological perspective, it's important for everyone to eat a metabolically appropriate diet.

I like to play tennis and basketball but I don't have enough physical endurance to enjoy these sports. I also like to exercise but feel wiped out afterward. What kinds of foods would give me more stamina?

Sports activities require two different types of cellular metabolism: aerobic and anaerobic. Aerobic metabolism comes into play during activities that require oxygen, such as jogging or biking. Anaerobic metabolism is required for activities such as weight lifting or sprinting, which do not require oxygen. All of the qualities necessary for excellence in athletics—speed, endurance, reaction time, strength— require that the body have ready access to both aerobic and anaerobic metabolism "on demand." This capacity is maximized when you balance your body chemistry. If you follow your metabolic type diet carefully, you will see your athletic performance soar. The best way to do this is to follow the twelve steps in Chapter 7 and use the related Fine-Tuning Mini-Quiz in Chapter 9. The important thing is to ignore everything you have read about what is supposed to be the next sports nutrition "miracle" and learn to listen to your body and understand what it needs as opposed to what works for somebody else. You'll be amazed at the results.

Should I eat the same diet all the time, regardless of what sporting event I'm participating in?

Not necessarily. Sometimes your macronutrient requirement (i.e., ratio) may vary somewhat, depending on the type of sport you're doing. At other times your macronutrient requirement will stay the same as it is on a daily basis. It's a function of whether your kind of metabolism matches the kind of metabolism required for the sport. For example, if you happen to have an anaerobic metabolism, you're already perfectly suited for weight lifting. On the other hand, if you're functioning in an anaerobic mode and planning to run a marathon, you'll most likely need to make significant adjustments to your macronutrient ratio. This aspect of sports nutrition is far too complex to address here, but the bottom line is that your macronutrient ratio can make an enormous difference in your sports performance, so you'll need to experiment to determine what macronutrient ratio works best for you for each specific sports activity.

I take a variety of medications. Would this dietary program interfere with their effects, and if so, should I stop my medications?

If you have a serious health problem, you should be working with a licensed health practitioner. Don't think you can simply stop your medication and quit seeing your doctor because you're changing your diet. Talk to your doctor about any changes you are now seeking to make in your diet. It's unlikely that he or she will object to the idea of your following a more sophisticated, metabolically appropriate dietary regime. But remember, even people with a serious chronic degenerative disorder can see substantive improvements in their condition by eating the right foods to help balance their body chemistry. This is very common even for people who pursue a beginner-level dietary approach like the one presented in this book. For this reason, you need to stay in close contact with your health practitioner to monitor your condition and decrease your medication if necessary.

I have a friend/relative with an advanced degenerative disease. Should I get this person on this program?

The dietary programs outlined in this book can be helpful to anyone who needs to make more informed choices about what foods to select on a day-to-day basis, but they're certainly not designed to be therapeutic protocols for people with serious chronic degenerative diseases. Rather, the introductory level approach to metabolic typing provided here is well suited for people who do not have full-blown diseases but who may suffer with a wide range of very common, midlevel symptoms (see the Chronic Degeneration Pathways chart on page 86) such as chronic fatigue, indigestion, obesity, aches and pains, low blood sugar, mood swings, and so on.

I seem to have poor resistance to colds and flu infections. I seem to "catch" every "bug" that goes around. Can this be avoided?

In one study where viruses were implanted in the mucous membranes of test subjects, some became ill while others did not! This demonstrates that whether or not you get sick depends more on you than on the virus. Like all living entities, viruses need a suitable environment in which to flourish. Typically, cold and flu viruses take hold when your body chemistry is too alkaline. Cold temperatures result in an alkaline shift in the body. And the most powerful alkalinizing substances are alcohol, sugar, salt, caffeine, and nicotine. Coincidentally, people tend to consume more of these substances during the Thanksgiving, Christmas, and New Year's holidays, the start of the typical cold and flu season. Science has also proven that the immune system is dependent on the proper biochemical balance to function efficiently. So if you follow your metabolic type diet, you'll be much more resistant to colds and flu infections, or, if you do get them, your symptoms will be much less severe and your recovery time much faster. Your best bet overall is to minimize your intake of alkalinizing foods during the flu season and boost your immune system by sticking to your metabolic type diet.

I'm a vegetarian and refuse to eat animal proteins. Can I still benefit from this approach?

If your body has a genetic need for intrinsic factors found only in animal protein, you may not get all the benefits you're hoping for. However, you can still adhere to the macronutrient ratio appropriate to your metabolic type and stick with your other allowable foods. Doing so can considerably help to balance your body chemistry.

I'm eating the foods from my list, but I'm still suffering from mood swings. I just feel angry and irritable a lot of the time and I'm prone to depression. What should I do?

Blood sugar imbalances are often responsible for these problems. You need to be sure that you eat at regular intervals each day and don't wait too long between meals. Many people also need to eat a snack between meals to keep their blood sugar on an even keel. In addition, be sure you're getting the right macronutrient ratio at all your meals. To do so, follow the twelve steps in Chapter 7, and the Fine-Tuning Mini-Quiz and Circadian Rhythm Indicator in Chapter 9. If your mood swings are still not relieved, use the Glycemic Index, also in Chapter 9. You may be inadvertently eating too many foods that are high on the glycemic index, preventing the proper regulation of your blood sugar levels. Finally, you may be severely reactive to a food you eat regularly. See the information on the ALCAT test in Chapter 11, "Key Considerations Beyond Diet."

I feel sleepy and hungry shortly after eating even small quantities of healthful foods such as whole-grain breads, crackers, or cereals, or healthful snack foods like rice cakes or granola. Yet I also get very fatigued if I go without these kinds of carbohydrates. What can I do?

Try substituting cooked whole-grain cereals such as rice, oatmeal, quinoa, or buckwheat for grain foods that have been baked—such as breads, dry cereals, or crackers. Any grains that have been ground into flour and baked (even whole-grain breads or crackers) break down into sugar faster than slow-burning whole-grain cereals that you cook yourself. That's why cooked whole grains like rice and oatmeal fill you up longer than bread and give you a longer, steadier supply of energy. In general, you'll want to be aware of the glycemic-index rating of all the grain products you typically consume, and focus on those with lower ratings, especially if you're a Protein Type or a Mixed Type. Be aware that even many high-quality packaged products found in health food stores—like rice cakes, popped cereals, and cornflakes—have very high GI ratings. Granola is another "healthful" food, but it's generally loaded with sugar and, therefore, often causes problems. When you do eat bread, note that some varieties, such as rye bread, have a much lower GI rating than others, such as whole-wheat bread.

Will my metabolic type ever change? How often should I take the Metabolic Type Self-Test?

Your body is a dynamic biological system characterized by change and flux and its own unique cycles and rhythms. And your dietary needs can change anytime, for any number of reasons—stress, illness, hormonal shifts, aging, and so on. If your nutrient requirements do shift, they're likely to do so in small incremental ways. But you can also experience a more dramatic change in your body chemistry and actually shift into another metabolic type category. For example, years of poor eating habits may have pushed you out of your real metabolic category (your "genetic type") into another category (your "functional type"). The important thing is to focus on meeting your dietary needs of the moment, whatever they may be. In that way, your body can repair and rebuild and balance itself. If your dietary needs change, your body will send you clear signals and you can make the necessary adjustments. The Fine-Tuning Mini-Quiz and Circadian Rhythm Indicator in Chapter 9 are indispensable tools that will help you detect subtle shifts in your body chemistry. If at some point you suspect that your metabolic type category has changed, you can retake the self-test in Chapter 6. Since everyone is different, there are no set rules for how often you should retest yourself.

Even though I am following my diet closely and taking digestive aids, I still have problems with indigestion, gas, bloating, and irritable bowel. Can you suggest something for me?

Although a metabolically correct diet is the most essential "building block" necessary to restore health, any chronic health disorder can be influenced by, or even caused by, a multiplicity of factors. So be sure to review Chapter 11, where you'll find a discussion of the key factors beyond diet that you should consider, whether you have digestive problems or any other kind of chronic ailment. For example, you might have a parasite or a candida infection, an imbalance in bowel flora, heavy metal toxicity, a structural problem such as TMJ stress (improper bite), or a spinal (vertebrae) misalignment that requires chiropractic care. Perhaps you need a more fiber-rich diet and plenty of water to assist normal peristaltic activity. Or perhaps you have food allergies. To test for allergies, consider using the ALCAT test described in Chapter 11. It's an effective way to identify any severely reactive foods that can play a direct role in digestive and eliminative disturbances of all kinds. I also recommend that you try the simple Food-Combining Assessment in Chapter 9. Food combining can relieve certain types of indigestion by reducing stress on the digestive organs and minimizing any toxicity resulting from insufficient digestion. You should also try eliminating any blood-type-specific foods that contain "lectins," substances that cause the red blood cells to agglutinate, or stick together. This effect can produce immune reactions and damage the intestinal mucosa. See page 279 in Chapter 9 for a list of foods to avoid for your blood type, and information on how to determine your blood type if you don't already know it.

Initially, I reacted very well to my metabolic type diet. But after about 2 weeks, I didn't feel that great. Then, for no apparent reason, I suddenly started feeling good again. I'm a thirty-seven-year-old female. Could this be related to my periods and other symptoms of PMS?

For some women, the monthly change in hormonal balance is strong enough to require a significant adjustment to their regular macronutrient ratio. More often than not, whatever imbalance a woman has tends to be more pronounced in the two weeks prior to her period. This means that if you're a Protein Type, for example, you might need to increase your protein even further for those two weeks and then return to your usual ratio the other two weeks. Or you may require just the opposite. Use the Fine-Tuning Mini-Quiz in Chapter 9 to help you adjust your diet to meet the changes in food requirements dictated by the monthly changes in your hormonal balance, and say good-bye to fluctuating energy levels and other undesirable symptoms of PMS.

Do you have any advice on a cancer prevention diet? Breast cancer and colon cancer are prevalent in my family. Should I stick to a low-fat diet to help prevent these diseases, as many medical experts advise?

How efficiently your immune system functions is greatly dependent on how successful you are in meeting your genetically based needs for nutrition. In our experience over the course of several decades, an excess of fat *or* a deficiency of fat in the diet can contribute to the development of cancer, or any other degenerative disease. A recent study published by the *Journal of the American Medical Association* found that, contrary to conventional wisdom, low-fat diets do *not* help to prevent breast cancer. There is also vast historical evidence to show that populations in remote (non-industrialized) regions of the world have virtually no incidence of cancer, heart disease, or other serious degenerative disorders. This includes cultures in which people have thrived for centuries on very high-fat, high-protein diets. Increasingly, physicians and nutritionists throughout the world are coming to understand the key role played by the homeostatic control mechanisms in the prevention and reversal of all forms of chronic disease. In turn, growing numbers of practitioners have realized that there are no "one-size-fits-all" nutrition-based therapeutic solutions for any given disease. They recognize that the successful prevention or management of chronic disease requires that diet/nutrition regimes be carefully tailored to the highly individualized needs of each patient.

Frequently Asked Questions for *Protein Types*

Isn't it dangerous to eat all this meat and fat? I'm concerned my cholesterol will go up.

Remember the old adage, "One man's food is another's poison." This is literally true. So, whether or not any food is "dangerous" for you is a question that can be answered only within the context of your metabolic type. Bear in mind that there is no scientific research to demonstrate that eating meat or fat actually raises cholesterol. Yet we've observed over and over again that Protein Types who consume high-protein, high-fat diets actually *lower* their cholesterol. What is even more striking is that high-carbohydrate, low-fat, low-protein diets actually *elevate* the cholesterol of Protein Types. If you track your cholesterol levels with regular blood tests, be aware that blood cholesterol levels can temporarily elevate while your body mobilizes cholesterol from sites of arteriosclerotic plaque.

I thought vegetables were good for you. Why do I have such a limited number of vegetables in my program?

Vegetables are good for everyone and, unfortunately, most people do not eat enough of them. However, different vegetables have different effects on different metabolic types. The various combinations of minerals, vitamins, phytonutrients, proteins, purines, fatty acids, carbohydrates, and other intrinsic factors produce varying effects on the body's biochemistry. For example, research has shown that the effect of certain vegetables on one metabolic type will be acidifying, while other vegetables will be alkalinizing. All vegetables listed as allowable foods for your diet have a similar, positive effect on the metabolism of Protein Types by working to balance body chemistry. Vegetables *not* listed on your chart will produce the opposite effect, essentially pushing your chemistry in the wrong direction—further out of balance. But the good news is, once your chemistry improves and your nagging health problems are resolved, you can add vegetables to your diet that are not on your list. In the event that your problems return, however, you will need to once again adhere closely to your original recommendations.

I have very persistent digestive problems. I just can't seem to digest most foods very well. I've tried everything, but nothing has helped. I don't think I'll be able to handle these foods you are recommending.

A chronic deficiency of the nutrients required by one's metabolic type leads to a lack of balance and efficiency in all the body's cells, tissues, organs, and systems. Where this degenerative process manifests itself in the body is believed to be related to one's genetic "weak link." Eating a diet that is right for your metabolic type can do much to reverse this trend. However, if you have weak digestion, you have a bit of a catch-22 problem. Since you can't digest food properly, you won't be able to make effective use of the nutrients it contains. Your digestive efficiency can be restored over time, but in the meantime you might find it very helpful to supplement your diet with digestive aids. The best product I've found for this purpose over the years is called Enzigest and is available from CX Research: (800) 690-1088. It's a potent, broad-spectrum, non-animal-based enzyme formulation. One can take anywhere from one to four capsules with meals and can even take them between meals or at bedtime to "police" any poorly digested food remnants. Your body will tell you if you take too many enzymes. In some people, too many enzymes will cause sleepiness or tiredness or some burning sensation in the stomach. If this occurs, simply decrease your enzyme intake to a level that does not produce these reactions. You also might try taking some HCL (hydrochloric acid) at the start of your meals, particularly if you feel that food stays in your stomach too long, or you have problems with belching or burping. Good quality HCL is available through CX Research.

Is it possible to overdose on high-purine proteins? Can I substitute the leaner, lighter proteins some of the time? I would like to be able to eat a broader range of meats, seafoods, poultry, etc.

Too much of anything—even a food that is good for you—can create problems. Remember, though, Protein Types *need* larger amounts of protein relative to carbohydrate and do best on the higher purine proteins. That's why most Protein Types find that their performance suffers when they try to substitute lower-purine proteins such as eggs, dairy, and lighter seafoods at main meals. However, not all Protein Types are the same. Some require heavier proteins with every meal, and others don't. You'll need to experiment and go by what your body tells you. In addition, some people are sensitive to arachidonic acid (AA), a substance found in high-purine foods, particularly organ meats and red meats. For these people, excess AA may produce dry, brittle, lifeless hair; skin dryness; fatigue; grogginess upon awakening; constipation; and sleep disturbances. If these problems suddenly appear, stop all red meat and organ meat intake for five days. If your symptoms noticeably improve, you may be sensitive to AA and will need to decrease your intake of red meat and organ meat. Stop these for one week, then gradually add back in.

What foods do I snack on? These foods all look like dinner foods to me.

Any of your allowable foods can be used as snacks, but as a Protein Type, it's important that your snacks contain protein. Leftovers (one day only) can be put to good use as snacks. Often the lighter proteins like hard-boiled eggs, cheese, yogurt, nuts, and seeds work well as snacks. Keep in mind that when you eat meals that are proper for your metabolic type, your need for snacks will greatly diminish. The important thing is to find what works best for you.

How can I possibly lose weight on all the high-fat foods recommended in my diet?

The short answer is that fat will make you fat only if it's the wrong type of fuel for your body's engines of metabolism. But so can protein or carbohydrate if they're eaten in the wrong proportion for your body's requirements. If fat is right for your type, eating fat can make you thin and *not* eating fat can make you fat. The key issue is whether or not the nutrients you consume—whether protein, carbohydrate, *or* fat—are fully converted to energy. If your food isn't converted to energy, your body has no recourse but to store what's left as fat. That's why you need to focus on balancing your macronutrient ratio in a manner that's compatible with your genetic requirements.

There are no dessert foods listed on this diet. That seems quite austere.

Your metabolic type diet is not intended to be a "restriction diet." It merely lists all the foods that specifically help to balance and support your kind of metabolism. This does *not* mean that you can't enjoy desserts, other sweet treats, or small amounts of your favorite fruits from time to time. If you eat correctly ninety-five percent of the time, you can "cheat" the other five percent of the time. This should pose no problem and can be your just reward for sticking to your metabolic type diet. Having said that, be aware that some Protein Types are much more reactive to sugar than others and will need to take special care to get adequate protein and fat around the times they indulge in sweet treats. Such problems, however, will lessen as your body chemistry balances over time from following a metabolic type diet.

I'm feeling much better on my Protein Type diet and find that I do best with just a small amount of carbohydrate. But I don't think I'm getting enough fiber, since my bowels seem more sluggish than before. Is there anything I can do?

Until your metabolic balance improves, you'll need to maintain minimal carbohydrate intake relative to protein. Later on, you'll be able to add more carbohydrate back into your diet and still maintain the good response you're getting now. In the meantime, try adding some fiber to your diet in the form of psyllium seed husk powder or freshly ground flaxseed. You'll need to experiment to see which one and how much work best for you. Try starting with one teaspoon of psyllium powder shaken in a jar with 6 ounces of water, followed by another glass of water. Or try stirring one to two tablespoons of freshly ground flaxseed into some yogurt or hot cereal. Whichever you use, be sure to drink enough fluids, *and don't use too much fiber* or you could end up lengthening transit time instead of shortening it.

Frequently Asked Questions for *Carbo Types*

Protein foods give me indigestion. How much protein do I have to eat?

Many Carbo Types, particularly sympathetic dominants, are not genetically designed to handle either large amounts of protein or heavier proteins—those higher in purines and fats. Also, remember that different people within any given metabolic category will have different requirements for protein. So you'll need to discover what amount of protein is right for you, and the best way to determine this is to follow the twelve steps provided in Chapter 7. You might find that you have trouble digesting the amount of protein that is right for you, even though it improves your energy and reduces your food cravings. This ironic predicament occurs when you fail over a prolonged period of time to acquire the foods and nutrients that are right for your metabolic type. This results in a lack of metabolic efficiency that weakens your digestion. In turn, the adverse effects of poor digestion cause you to drop from your diet the very foods that you *desperately need,* further exacerbating your digestive inefficiency. The result is a self-perpetuating downward spiral of degenerating digestive capacity. The only way to break this cycle is to start giving your body what it needs. Little by little, your metabolic efficiencies will be restored. In the meantime, take some digestive support in the form of enzymes and/or HCL (hydrochloric acid).

I am never hungry. When should I force myself to eat?

Typically, Carbo Types have diminished appetites. Often, when they do feel hungry, they'll eat something sweet, and because they handle carbohydrates well, sweets will appease their appetite. However, this is not a good practice and can lead to serious degenerative processes down the road. The body *must* obtain specific quantities of vitamins, minerals, enzymes, proteins, fats, and carbohydrates on a daily basis. Failure to provide these forces the body to cannibalize its own tissues, tearing down muscle for protein, bone for calcium, and so on, in order to survive. Obviously, this is not a good situation, because when the body's reserves are used up, degenerative disease is just around the corner. Paradoxically, it often happens that the more often Carbo Types skip meals, the less interested they become in food. Enzyme systems become deactivated and the metabolic rate slows down, both of which contribute to decreased interest in food. However, when someone with this problem begins to eat on a regular routine basis, the appetite returns to a more normal pattern. Since it's important for you to get sufficient quantities of macronutrients and micronutrients on a daily basis, you should establish a daily schedule for breakfast, lunch, and dinner, and routinely eat at those times even if you're not hungry. You don't have to eat large meals, but you should eat something, even if it's only a small quantity. Additionally, it's important for you to get protein, fat, and carbohydrate at all three meals. Not only will your appetite improve, so, too, will your overall health and well-being.

I feel fine on sweets and starchy foods. Why do I need to give up these foods?

It's important to remember that metabolic type diets are not restriction diets, and no one needs to give up sweets and starches entirely. In fact, there are six tastes found in foods: bitter, sour, salty, pungent, astringent, and sweet. The regular inclusion in the diet of foods that provide all six tastes actually helps to optimize everyone's health. The problem is not with sweets or starches per se, but with the *quantity* of starches that most people consume at the *expense* of other foods. As a Carbo Type, you have the ability to tolerate larger quantities of sweet and starchy foods than other metabolic types. But you, too, will be burdened with weight gain and food cravings—and more serious problems down the road—if you consistently eat these foods to excess.

Frequently Asked Questions for *Mixed Types*

Should I mix foods from the protein and the carbo food groups at each meal or eat them separately?

On any given day, try to get a good balance between protein and Carbo Type foods and try not to emphasize one group over the other. It's not necessary at every meal to divide food equally between the two groups. Just make sure your overall food intake for the day is fairly equal. For example, if you make a salad, try to choose vegetables from both groups. Or, if you have, say, only two steamed vegetables with your lunch and they're both from the Protein Type list, be sure to emphasize Carbo Type vegetables for the evening meal. However, you may find it easiest to strike a balance at each meal rather than trying to keep track of your food balance over the course of a day.

Is it possible that I lean heavily toward either the Protein Type or the Carbo Type?

Yes, it's possible that a Mixed Type could have a strong tendency toward either a Protein Type pattern or a Carbo Type pattern. This situation illustrates the great value in learning how to fine-tune your diet and understand your body's way of communicating how it is doing. You should start your Mixed Type diet by eating a good balance of foods from the allowable foods lists for both groups. Next, follow the twelve steps to identify your personal fuel mix (still using a balanced mixture of foods from both groups). If this doesn't seem to work for you, stick to the same basic macronutrient ratio (appropriate for Mixed Types), but try experimenting with either more Protein Type foods or more Carbo Type foods. Use the Fine-Tuning Mini-Quiz in Chapter 9 to clarify what's right for you.

If I am a Mixed Type, does that mean I am healthier than the other two types because I am more balanced, meaning more in the middle? Am I more likely to stay a Mixed Type because I am more balanced?

All three types have the potential to be either healthy or unhealthy. An Eskimo (Protein Type) is not necessarily more or less healthy than a vegetarian East Indian (Carbo Type). Nor is a Mixed Type necessarily any better off than the others. The only real question is whether an individual (of any type) is acquiring all the nutrients for which he or she has a genetically based need. The question of whether you're likely to stay a Mixed Type is more an issue of whether your functional type (FT, the type you are now) is the same as your genetic type (GT, the type you were born to be). This applies to all three types. If your FT is the same as your GT, there is little likelihood you will change types unless you begin to eat improperly for an extended period. However, if your FT is different from your GT, there's a good chance you will change types at some point. Whether or not you change types isn't all that important. What is important is that you eat properly now to balance your body chemistry, improve your metabolic efficiency, and build your health.

Chapter

FINE-TUNING YOUR DIET

A Broad Spectrum of Dietary Needs

Here's a simple way to understand your unique dietary needs in relation to those of other people: Imagine the AM band on a radio. As you may know, the AM dial on a radio runs from 525 to 1625 MHz.

Imagine dividing your radio dial into three equal parts—each part corresponding to one of the three metabolic type categories.

For example, let's say that the Protein Type category runs from 525 to 892 on the dial, the Mixed Type from 893 to 1258, and the Carbo Type from 1259 to 1625.

Each individual point along the radio dial can be thought of as a distinct metabolic type, even though there are only three main metabolic categories. This will give you an idea of just how much physiological

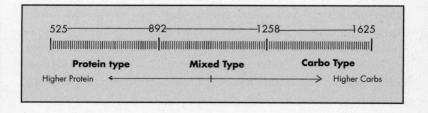

diversity actually exists among people, and, in turn, the broad spectrum of human dietary needs.

In this analogy, the farther you are on the left of the "radio dial," the greater your need for protein and fat, and the lower your need for carbohydrate. Protein types need the highest ratio of protein and fat to carbohydrates, while Carbo Types need just the reverse—the highest ratio of carbohydrates to protein and fat.

Note the variation that exists within each category on the radio dial. This shows how highly individualized your nutrient requirements really are. For example, even though you share the same allowable foods list as other people of the same metabolic type, your need for specific *combinations* of foods (your personal fuel mix, or macronutrient ratio) is likely to be *very different* from others in your metabolic category.

So in order to feel well, achieve your ideal weight, and enjoy robust health and fitness, you'll want to refine, or "fine-tune," your diet as much as possible—after you've identified your basic metabolic type.

Almost like "tuning in" to a radio station, you'll need to "listen" to your body, and use the information you receive to "pinpoint" a diet that's customized to your unique biochemical makeup.

Listening to Your Body

Make no mistake, your body knows what it needs. It will let you know at every turn whether or not you're eating the right foods, and in the right proportions.

The answers you seek are all within you. There's no diet/nutrition expert, health professional, or medical authority who can compete with your body's own built-in intelligence.

In this chapter are more techniques for tapping into this remarkable intelligence and understanding your own unique nutritional needs with unprecedented levels of precision and specificity.

The tools provided in this chapter can be thought of as "extensions" or "add-ons" to the twelve steps in Chapter 7—where you learned to identify your personal fuel mix, i.e., to tailor your macronutrient ratio to your own particular needs.

So, before you use any of the additional tools provided here, it's very important that you spend adequate time identifying the macronutrient ratio that works best for you. It's an essential technique that you need to learn before you move on to use the dietary customization tools that follow.

For some people, the twelve steps are easy to master, and they can rapidly and easily identify their ideal personal fuel mix. For other people, it takes considerable time and experimentation. Everyone's experience is different.

If you have any difficulty with the twelve steps, don't feel the need to rush through it. Just take your time, go at your own pace, and don't get discouraged. Use a notebook to record any incremental adjustments you make in the way you combine proteins, carbohydrates, and fats—until you hit upon a combination that consistently produces a distinct improvement in the way you feel after meals and snacks.

Remember that your allowable foods list and the twelve steps are the foundation of the process of customizing your diet. These two interrelated tools provide you with the core of what you need to know—they tell you what specific foods to eat and in what proportions.

In fact some people do so well just by sticking to their allowable foods list and mastering the twelve steps that they don't necessarily feel compelled to charge ahead right away and make use of the additional customization tools provided in this chapter.

Other people continue to experience problems such as fatigue, food cravings, and irritability even after they've spent a fair amount of time adhering closely to their allowable foods and following the twelve steps.

So, if you've already done a good job of implementing the techniques you learned in Chapter 7, but are still having problems—either negative reactions after eating or just in general failing to experience a distinct improvement in the way you feel—one or more of the fine-tuning techniques in this chapter are likely to offer an effective solution.

All the following tools, or self-tests, are simple to apply and can be used either separately or in combination. As you will see, each has a distinct purpose, yet all are designed to expand your awareness of what your body needs to function at peak efficiency and refine your ability to tailor a diet to your own unique body chemistry.

Easy-to-Use Interactive Tools for Added Dietary Precision

In our modern era, the concept of "interactivity" has become synonymous with "customization." For instance, we once had to make do with mass-distributed, "one-size-fits-all" news and entertainment options, but interactive media such as Web sites and CD-ROMs and pay-per-view TV now allow us to obtain products and services that are tailored to our own special tastes and interests.

The term "interactive" is typically associated with electronic media, though it actually applies to any process that involves dynamic, two-way communication or "interaction."

The science of metabolic typing is now widely accessible through revolutionary new interactive tools that allow each individual health consumer to become the central participant in a dynamic two-way process of self-discovery.

These advanced but easy-to-use tools take the form of questionnaires, evaluations, and simple experimental procedures that enable anyone to utilize and interpret the wealth of available data each of us has on our own unique physiological status.

The feedback you obtain from these simple but powerful tests will forever change your perspective of the science of nutrition. You'll move rapidly to a whole new level of self-awareness, and you'll be amazed at the profound limitations of the generic, prescribed dietary solutions we've all been forced to utilize for so long.

Once you use the self-tests in Chapters 6 and 7, and the follow-up tests on the pages ahead, you'll begin to understand the extent of your own metabolic individuality and you'll never go back to old ways of thinking about nutrition. You'll certainly never again be stuck in a never-ending search for answers. What you've needed all along are techniques, like these, that are both practical and scientific—methods that provide a testable, repeatable, verifiable means of identifying your individualized dietary needs.

Here's a brief summary of the self-tests you'll find in this chapter:

The Fine-Tuning Mini-Quiz,
page 263

This is an essential tool that is especially useful when used in conjunction with the twelve steps in Chapter 7. It will help you become very skilled at reading your own "body language" and identifying your ideal macronutrient ratio.

The Circadian Rhythm Indicator,
page 266

This is a simple test that can be used in conjunction with *both* the twelve steps and the Fine-Tuning Mini-Quiz. Many people's metabolisms shift throughout the course of the day, because of their own unique "biological clock." If these fluctuations affect you, this test will identify any resulting variations in your dietary requirements.

The Glycemic Index Evaluation,
page 270

This is an indispensable tool that will give you a very clear understanding of what kinds of carbohydrates you can tolerate. You'll learn how to avoid the onset of negative reactions to meals—including food cravings, fatigue, irritability, and emotional imbalance. It's an important tool for every metabolic type, but it's especially useful for Protein Types or anyone interested in weight loss.

Your Blood Type/Foods-to-Avoid Test, page 277

This test enables you to identify and avoid specific foods that may trigger negative immune responses in someone with your particular blood type. Certain foods contain lectins, substances that can cause digestive disorders, headaches, food allergies, and a host of other problems. Since various lectins react only with certain kinds of blood type cells (A, B, O, or AB), you can easily determine which foods may cause problems for you.

The Food Combining Assessment, page 280

This test enables people to determine if they should pursue some of the classic rules of "food combining." These rules are an extension of the food-combining approach already built into the twelve steps in Chapter 7. This approach is especially useful for people with certain kinds of persistent digestive disorders and weight loss issues.

THE FINE-TUNING MINI-QUIZ

When to Use It

The Fine-Tuning Mini-Quiz can be used any time you need to clarify or clearly define your reactions to a given meal. It's a very simple self-test that takes just minutes to complete. Once you've used it a number of times, you'll begin to develop a finely tuned awareness of exactly how you are affected, both physically and mentally, by specific foods and food combinations. It will enable you to identify your ideal macronutrient ratio with maximum speed, accuracy, and efficiency. The quiz can also be used intermittently to detect any changes in your metabolism and dietary needs resulting from stress, illness, hormonal changes, sports activities, exercise routines, environmental changes, and even seasonal changes.

Instructions

1. Make twenty or thirty photocopies of the Fine-Tuning Mini-Quiz and always keep a copy available at mealtime when you're trying to identify your ideal macronutrient ratio, or adjust it because of shifts in your metabolism.

2. Within one to three hours after a meal, take a few moments to fill out the quiz.

3. Add up the number of check marks in each column and fill in the totals as indicated.

4. If you have more "wrong" answers than "right" answers, your body is telling you that you didn't get the right protein-to-carbohydrate ratio at that meal.

5. Keep adjusting your protein-to-carbohydrate ratio until you get more "right" answers than "wrong" answers.

6. Use the twelve-steps in Chapter 7 as a guideline for adjusting your protein-to-carbohydrate ratio.

7. As you do the twelve steps, use a three-ring binder as a food diary and jot down what you have for breakfast, lunch, and dinner each day. Then put each completed Fine-Tuning Mini-Quiz in the three-ring binder as well, and mark down the specific time and date of the corresponding meal on each quiz form. This is a simple means of tracking what you've been eating and any improvements in the way you feel.

Hints

- Achieving your ideal fuel mix each time you eat will maximize your performance physically, mentally, and emotionally.

- More often than not, illness and increased stress of any kind will increase your need for protein.

- If you have a meal but don't feel a distinct and sustained energy boost, an improved sense of well-being and emotional stability, a sense of fullness and an end to food cravings (especially for sweets), the most likely explanation is that you're combining proteins and carbohydrates incorrectly. But if you've tried hard to fine-tune your macronutrient ratio, yet no combination seems to work and you still don't feel well after eating, here's what to do:

  - Review your allowable foods list and make sure you're sticking to it.
  - Make sure you're avoiding any foods to which you might be allergic.
  - Try the other tests in this chapter.

DIETARY FINE-TUNING MINI-QUIZ

Within one to three hours after a meal, place a check in the box next to any selection that applies to you. Tally your answers at the bottom of each column.

CATEGORY	RIGHT PROTEIN/CARB RATIO	WRONG PROTEIN/CARB RATIO
Appetite Fullness/ Satisfaction Sweet Cravings	❑ Feel full, satisfied ❑ Do not have sweet cravings ❑ Do not desire more food ❑ Do not get hungry soon after eating ❑ Do not need to snack before next meal	❑ Feel physically full, but still hungry ❑ Don't feel satisfied; feel like something was missing from meal ❑ Have desire for sweets ❑ Feel hungry again soon after meal ❑ Need to snack between meals
Energy Levels	❑ Energy is restored after eating ❑ Have good, lasting, "normal" sense of energy and well-being	❑ Too much or too little energy ❑ Became hyper, jittery, shaky, nervous, or speedy ❑ Feel hyper, but exhausted "underneath" ❑ Energy drop, fatigue, exhaustion, sleepiness, drowsiness, lethargy, or listlessness
Mental/ Emotional Well-being	❑ Improved well-being ❑ Sense of feeling refueled and restored ❑ Uplift in emotions ❑ Improved clarity and acuity of mind ❑ Normalization of thought processes	❑ Mentally slow, sluggish, spacey ❑ Inability to think quickly or clearly ❑ Hyper, overly rapid thoughts ❑ Inability to focus or hold attention ❑ Hypo traits: apathy, depression, or sadness ❑ Hyper traits: anxiety, obsessiveness, fearfulness, anger, short temper, or irritability, etc.
Score		

What It's All About

Life as we know it is largely dependent upon cycles and biological rhythms. The ocean tides are an example of cycles, as are the seasons and the endless shifts of day into night and night into day. Our planet has its own yearly cycle during which it makes a complete revolution around the sun. Events that take place repeatedly over a twenty-four-hour period are called circadian cycles, and the ebb and flow of our own internal body chemistry is known as our circadian rhythm.

In the same way your genetic makeup has influenced your unique dietary requirements, hereditary factors have created a kind of biological rhythm that is unique just to you. This is yet another facet of your metabolic individuality. In essence, your cells are programmed to function according to your own internal "body clock."

Have you ever noticed that some people are naturally able to function well at night (the proverbial "night owls") but can't function well in the morning? While other people ("morning people") are sharp, alert, and energetic at the crack of dawn, yet are unable to stay awake very far into the evening? These behavioral patterns are more than just arbitrary habits. And this is just one example of how all your physical and mental patterns and capabilities—your moods, the ability to think or learn or engage in athletic events or digest food—are heavily controlled by your biochemistry.

This means that your dietary needs are not only different from everybody else's, but your own needs may also vary according to the time of day.

For years, "one-size-fits-all" diet books have offered up confusing, contradictory advice on what to eat at specific times of the day. As an example, some experts say that "breakfast is the most important meal" and advocate heavy, protein-rich meals in the morning. Others recommend eating nothing but fruit until noon. But the truth is, you can't possibly adhere to these kinds of generic guidelines and expect to get the results you're after, except by chance. What it is that you need at any given time of day is a question only your body can answer.

When to Use This Self-Test

If you've identified your ideal macronutrient ratio and it works well for you some of the time but at other times you feel fatigued, lethargic, or irritable, it could be due to a variability in your fuel mix requirement over the course of a day. Some people do very well by adhering to the very same protein/carbohydrate balance at breakfast, lunch, and dinner, while others need one macronutrient balance in the morning, another at midday, and still another in the evening.

This simple test will indicate if your needs are consistent throughout the day or if they vary. If they do vary, all you need to do is use the twelve steps and the Fine-Tuning Mini-Quiz to identify what specific macronutrient ratios you need at different times of the day. Maybe you have a very high need for protein at breakfast and dinner but not at lunch. Or perhaps you do best on a higher amount of carbohydrates in the morning. Anything is possible and everyone is different.

Instructions

1. Make three or four photocopies of the Circadian Rhythm Indicator form.
2. Fill in one of these forms over the course of a day.
3. Before each meal, circle the number (one through five) on the rating scale that most accurately reflects your appetite, energy level, and food preference for that time of day.
4. Then add the three numbers you circled in column B and write the totals in column C. For example, if you circle 4 on the Appetite Scale, 2 on the Energy Scale, and 5 on the Food Preference Scale, write 11 in the appropriate slot in column C.
5. At the end of the day, compare your three circadian scores in column

C. If the numbers are very close, you likely have a consistent macronutrient ratio, but if the numbers are quite different, you may have a variable macronutrient ratio. If that's the case, use the twelve steps and the Fine-Tuning Mini-Quiz to identify the specific food combinations that will optimize your performance throughout the day.

Hints

• Try repeating the test a few times over the course of a few days, in case your appetite or energy pattern is different from usual on any given day.

• Be sure to fill in your responses three times each day, just *before* each meal—not after.

CIRCADIAN RHYTHM INDICATOR

A	B	C
TIME OF DAY	**TESTS**	**SCORES**
Breakfast	**Appetite Scale** — Weaker ← 1 2 3 4 5 → Stronger **Energy Scale** — Lower ← 1 2 3 4 5 → Higher **Food Preference Scale** — High Carbs ← 1 2 3 4 5 → High Protein/Fat	Breakfast Total
Lunch	**Appetite Scale** — Weaker ← 1 2 3 4 5 → Stronger **Energy Scale** — Lower ← 1 2 3 4 5 → Higher **Food Preference Scale** — High Carbs ← 1 2 3 4 5 → High Protein/Fat	Lunch Total
Dinner	**Appetite Scale** — Weaker ← 1 2 3 4 5 → Stronger **Energy Scale** — Lower ← 1 2 3 4 5 → Higher **Food Preference Scale** — High Carbs ← 1 2 3 4 5 → High Protein/Fat	Dinner Total

Before each meal, circle the number on each scale that best applies to you. For example, on the Appetite Scale, select 1 if you have little or no appetite and 5 if you are ravenous. For the Energy Scale, choose 1 if you have very little energy and 5 if you feel vigorous. On the Food Preference Scale, select 1 or 2 if you prefer fruits, vegetables, or grains, and 4 or 5 if you would like protein or fatty foods.

THE GLYCEMIC INDEX EVALUATION

What It's All About

The glycemic index ranks foods in terms of their ability to raise your blood sugar within two to three hours after eating. It was developed by food scientists in the early 1980s, and has become an invaluable reference for nutritionists. The index pertains mainly to carbohydrates such as vegetables, grains, and fruits, since proteins and fats do not raise the blood sugar significantly. It ranks foods on a numerical scale, comparing their glycemic value to that of sugar, which has a value of 100.

Prior to the development of the index, scientists assumed that simple sugars (such as table sugar, corn syrup, and fructose) hit the bloodstream much faster than complex carbohydrates such as whole grains. Surprisingly, however, we now know that this is not always the case, and that complex carbohydrates are all very different in terms of how quickly they break down during digestion.

For example, some foods like barley break down very slowly and therefore release glucose in a very gradual manner into the bloodstream. Other complex carbohydrates like potatoes, dates, and pineapple break down even faster than table sugar and thereby often cause problems by inducing rapid surges in blood sugar levels.

When to Use This Self-Test

This is a very simple test designed to show you how foods with varying glycemic index ratings impact the way you feel and your ability to function. It will also familiarize you with the index—a great reference device to assist you in preparing healthful meals and keeping your blood sugar on an even keel. You should use this test if you find that you don't feel well within two hours after meals, even though you're adhering to your allowable foods and your correct macronutrient ratio. It's possible that you're inadvertently consuming too many foods with high glycemic values. If you happen to be a Protein Type or even a Mixed Type, you're likely to be especially sensitive to foods with high GI values and prone to negative symptoms related to blood sugar disruptions.

This test is also an important tool for anyone trying to lose weight, since foods high on the glycemic index provoke rapid insulin secretions, which encourages fat storage and interferes with the conversion of fat into energy.

Hints

- If you're a Protein Type, you should eat sufficient protein and fat at the same time that you eat foods with high glycemic values. This will slow down the rate of glucose elevation in your blood.
- If you're a Carbo Type, you should eat a sufficient amount of your allowable (light) proteins at the same time—especially if you have blood sugar problems.
- If you're a Mixed Type, you'll want to eat whatever variety of protein and fat is best suited for you at the same time you eat any foods high on the GI.

GLYCEMIC INDEX CHART

	INDEX	SUGAR	DAIRY	FRUIT	GRAIN	VEGETABLES
	100 +	110 maltose 110 beer 110 alcohol		103 dates		101 parsnip
High-Glycemic-Index Foods	90–100	100 glucose 95 glucose drinks 95 sport drinks			91 instant rice 90 puffed rice	
	80–90	83 jelly beans			89 Rice Chex 88 white rice 85 pretzels 82 Rice Krispies 80 cornflakes 80 rice cakes	88 potato, baked 86 potato, instant mashed
(rapid insulin inducers)	70–80	73 Life Savers 70 jams		75 watermelon	75 wheat cereals 75 graham crackers 74 Cheerios 72 bagel 72 whole-wheat bread 72 white bread 72 saltine crackers 71 millet 70 pancakes, waffles	78 french fries 78 pumpkin 77 corn chips 75 rutabaga

GLYCEMIC INDEX CHART

	INDEX	SUGAR	DAIRY	FRUIT	GRAIN	VEGETABLES
Medium-Glycemic Index Foods (moderate insulin inducers)	60–70	68 soft drinks 65 corn syrup 65 sucrose (table sugar) 61 honey	61 ice cream	68 cantaloupe 67 pineapple 66 raisins 62 bananas 60 apricots	65 Rye-Krisp 67 shredded wheat 67 grape nuts 67 couscous 66 brown rice 66 Cream of Wheat 67 brown rice pasta 66 muesli	68 cornmeal 66 potato, mashed 66 beets
	50–60	51 chocolate	52 ice cream, low-fat	55 mango 52 kiwi	59 sweet corn 59 pastry 53 oatmeal 51 buckwheat 51 All-Bran 65 rye bread	59 corn 58 popcorn 56 sweet potato 53 yam 51 carrots 51 green peas 51 potato chips

GLYCEMIC INDEX CHART

Low-Glycemic-Index Foods (slow insulin inducers)

INDEX	SUGAR	DAIRY	FRUIT	GRAIN	VEGETABLES
40–49	43 lactose 41 Snickers bar		46 orange juice 45 grapes 41 apple juice 40 oranges	49 oatmeal 49 wheat bran 47 bulgur 46 whole-wheat pasta 46 sponge cake 43 white spaghetti 42 whole-wheat spaghetti 65 rye bread 40 spaghetti	48 dried peas 42 pinto beans 40 baked beans (canned)
30–40		36 flavored yogurt 27 milk, whole 32 milk, low-fat 30 butter	38 apples 36 pears 32 strawberries 30 bananas, unripe	34 rye	38 tomato soup 38 navy beans 36 chick peas 36 lima beans 33 blackeyed peas 32 split peas 30 black beans
<30	20 fructose		29 peaches 26 grapefruit 25 plums 23 cherries	22 barley 19 rice bran	29 kidney beans 29 lentils 23 dried peas 15 soy beans 14 green vegetables 13 peanuts

GLYCEMIC INDEX EVALUATION

- Select your test lunches as per your metabolic type.
- Eat as much as you want to eat.
- Eat a low-glycemic lunch the first day.
- Eat a high-glycemic lunch the second day.
- Check or record any adverse symptoms noted within three hours after eating each lunch.
- Compare the results of the two test diets in terms of your performance.

GLYCEMIC INDEX EVALUATION

	PROTEIN TYPE TEST LUNCHES		MIXED TYPE TEST LUNCHES		CARBO TYPE TEST LUNCHES	
	Low Glycemic	*High Glycemic*	*Low Glycemic*	*High Glycemic*	*Low Glycemic*	*High Glycemic*
	Steak, asparagus, cauliflower, celery small amount barley	Steak, steamed carrots and peas, winter squash, white rice, dessert	Roast beef, green salad, steamed cabbage, broccoli, barley	Roast beef, steamed rutabaga and potatoes, rice cakes, dessert	Chicken breast, steamed zucchini, broccoli, green salad, barley	Chicken breast, baked potato, steamed parsnips, white rice, dessert
	☐ energy drop ☐ negative emotions ☐ sweet craving ☐ thirst ☐ hunger ☐ sleepiness ☐ poor concentration ☐ irritability	☐ energy drop ☐ negative emotions ☐ sweet craving ☐ thirst ☐ hunger ☐ sleepiness ☐ poor concentration ☐ irritability	☐ energy drop ☐ negative emotions ☐ sweet craving ☐ thirst ☐ hunger ☐ sleepiness ☐ poor concentration ☐ irritability	☐ energy drop ☐ negative emotions ☐ sweet craving ☐ thirst ☐ hunger ☐ sleepiness ☐ poor concentration ☐ irritability	☐ energy drop ☐ negative emotions ☐ sweet craving ☐ thirst ☐ hunger ☐ sleepiness ☐ poor concentration ☐ irritability	☐ energy drop ☐ negative emotions ☐ sweet craving ☐ thirst ☐ hunger ☐ sleepiness ☐ poor concentration ☐ irritability
	Add your own symptoms ☐ ☐ ☐ ☐	*Add your own symptoms* ☐ ☐ ☐ ☐	*Add your own symptoms* ☐ ☐ ☐ ☐	*Add your own symptoms* ☐ ☐ ☐ ☐	*Add your own symptoms* ☐ ☐ ☐ ☐	*Add your own symptoms* ☐ ☐ ☐ ☐

What It's All About

In our experience, compared to the primary regulatory influence of the fundamental homeostatic controls, the influence of blood type on dietary requirements is a secondary factor. However, it does have a role to play and can make a significant difference in some people.

But your blood type actually has far more to do with what foods you should avoid than what foods you should eat. This is due to the presence of dietary lectins—protein substances that are found in small quantities in about thirty percent of our foods. Although cooking and digestion inhibit the activity of lectins to some extent, many find their way into the bloodstream where they act as antigens, or foreign invaders. Like little strips of Velcro, certain lectins bind to the surfaces of certain kinds of blood cells (A, B, O, or AB).

Lectins frequently cause agglutination (clumping) and subsequent lysing (destruction) of blood cells. They can also interfere with digestion and absorption and cause a host of additional problems, including: nutrient deficiencies, food allergies, inflammatory bowel disease, diabetes mellitus, rheumatoid arthritis, psoriasis, infertility, intestinal gas, immune deficiencies, fatigue, headache, achiness, diarrhea, irritability, and anemia.

The good news is that many lectins are blood-type specific, which means that they can cause negative effects only in people with specific blood types. You can avoid the harmful effects of lectins by limiting your consumption of foods known to contain the kinds that react with your specific blood type.

When to Use This Self-Test

If you've been following all the dietary instructions in Chapter 7 for a considerable time, and have implemented the Fine-Tuning Mini-Quiz, Circadian Rhythm Indicator, and Glycemix Index Evaluation but still don't feel well, try this simple test. Dietary lectins may be contributing to your poor health, especially if you're suffering with any of the problems or symptoms listed in the section above.

Instructions

1. Obtain a home blood typing kit. They're inexpensive (generally cost around $12) and extremely easy to use. One source is Ultra-Life, (800) 323-3842.
2. Once you've identified your blood type, simply check the chart on the following page to avoid the foods that contain lectins known to react with your specific blood type.

FOODS TO AVOID
ACCORDING TO YOUR BLOOD TYPE

BLOOD TYPE A	BLOOD TYPE B	BLOOD TYPE AB	BLOOD TYPE O
blackberries	bitter pear melons	blackberries	blackberries
brown trout	blackeyed peas	blackeyed peas	chocolate
clams	castor beans	brown trout	cocoa
cornflakes	chicken	clams	French mushrooms
French mushrooms	chocolate	cocoa	(amanita muscaria)
(hygrophorus hypothejus)	cocoa	cornflakes	halibut
halibut	French mushrooms	French mushrooms	flounder
flounder	(hygrophorus hypothejus,	(hygrophorus hypothejus)	sole
lima beans	marasmius orcades)	halibut	sunflower seeds
Product 19	pomegranates	flounder	
snow white mushrooms	salmon	lima beans	
sole	sesame	pomegranates	
soybeans	sunflower seeds	Product 19	
soybean sprouts	soybeans	salmon	
string beans	tuna	sesame	
tora beans		snow white mushrooms	
Total		sole	
		soybeans	
		soybean sprouts	
		string beans	
		sunflower seeds	
		Total	
		tuna	

What It's All About

Food combining is a dietary approach that seeks to enhance digestion and assimilation by limiting each meal or snack to foods that are known to be compatible in the digestive tract. Many of the rules are just common sense.

For example, it's not a good idea to eat a piece of fruit and a piece of meat at the same time because they pass through the digestive tract at different rates and require different kinds of enzymatic secretions from the stomach and other digestive organs. It's also generally not a good idea to overwhelm the digestive tract by combining meat and dairy at the same meal—for example, by having a glass of milk or a big helping of cottage cheese with a roast beef dinner.

You can benefit greatly by having a familiarity with these and other rules of food combining, though you certainly don't have to take them to an extreme. For instance, the ideal way for your system to digest and assimilate food would be to eat just one food per meal—but that's obviously not practical! Nonetheless, if you have a general awareness of how to avoid eating highly incompatible foods at the same time, you can certainly minimize any undue stress on your digestive tract.

When to Use This Self-Test

If you have persistent digestive disturbances that are not alleviated by eating according to your metabolic type and implementing the other tests in this chapter, it's possible that your problems are related to poor food combining.

For example, if you have chronic abdominal pain or discomfort after eating, intestinal gas, bloating, constipation, belching, a coated tongue, bad breath, a loss of appetite, undigested food passing through your system, colitis, or even insomnia, the following self-test might help your body deal with these problems.

Weak digestion is one of the most common problems in modern industrialized societies. And people of all metabolic types can and do suffer with weak digestion. Of course, everyone is different. There are people with very strong digestion who can eat very poor food combinations all the time and still do fine. Then there are others who have such weak digestion that they require digestive aids even on those occasions when they might be eating just one easy-to-digest food item—like yogurt, for example.

Regardless of the strength of your digestion, you might want to familiarize yourself with the following list of simple rules for food combining, and try to adhere to them when you can. Many are very easy to apply. If you have strong digestion, these tips can help prevent the onset of any digestive problems in the future.

If you have weak digestion, you'll want to pay stricter attention to the following rules and then move on to the simple self-test that follows.

Note that food combining can also be a useful tool if you are seeking to lose weight. This is due to the fact that poor digestion leads to a form of cellular "starvation," which in turn lowers your metabolic rate and increases fat storage.

SIMPLE RULES OF FOOD COMBINING

Remember that not everyone needs to be equally concerned with all the rules of food combining! They're primarily for people with severe or persistent digestive problems who have not found relief through other dietary approaches.

1. Try to Eat Protein with Nonstarchy Vegetables.

Meat dishes are particularly compatible with nonstarchy vegetables of all kinds, whereas grains and beans and starchy vegetables are most easily digested when they're eaten without meat or dairy products. Of course, this isn't always feasible, especially if you're a Protein Type, and you really need protein along with carbohydrates. So, here's a trick: Try eating any grains or starchy vegetables at the *start* of a meal. Then, thirty minutes later, eat your meat along with any nonstarchy vegetables.

2. Eat Fruits Between Meals.

Fruits don't go well with flesh foods or heavy meals of any kind. They're best combined with dairy products or nuts. Or, if you're a Carbo Type, you can probably eat fruit all by itself between meals with no adverse effects.

3. Avoid Milk and Meat at the Same Meal.

If you must eat a fast-food burger, definitely hold the milk shake! And don't have a slab of cheesecake if you're having a T-bone steak. This combination is too taxing for most people's digestive tracts and tends to cause a severe slowdown in normal intestinal activity and a toxic buildup in the colon.

4. Eat One Protein Per Meal.

If you have chronic indigestion, you can ease up on your digestive tract by eating only one protein per meal. For example, don't eat steak and seafood at the same time. If you're a Protein Type, you may do well with combinations like eggs and sausage at breakfast, unless your digestion is very weak, in which case you should eat these foods separately.

5. Eat Melons Alone.

If your metabolic type can handle melons, it's best to eat them between meals or at the start of a meal, since they digest very quickly. Don't eat them as dessert, especially at the end of a heavy meal, and never eat them with meat or raw vegetables.

6. Don't Combine Fruits and Vegetables.

This applies to all fruits and vegetables for the most part, but particularly raw fruits and vegetables. However, some experts believe it's okay to combine acid fruits with nonstarchy vegetables. Experience is your best gauge in cases like this.

7. Avoid Mixing Starches and Citrus Fruits.

Grapefruit and cereal for breakfast, although typical, is not a good combination for people with digestive problems.

FOOD COMBINING ASSESSMENT

This test is very simple. Just eat as you normally do for four days and record your symptoms in this log. Then use the rules of food combining for ten days and see if your symptoms improve. See the sample menus on the following page for tips on meals. Each day, use the rating scale below to record the severity of your symptoms. Then compare your results and look for improvement in your digestive problems.

Rating Scale: 1 = Very poor, much worse. 2 = Poor, worse.
3 = Average, no change. 4 = Good, better. 5 = Very good, much better.

Symptoms	Regular Diet							Food Combining Diet						
	1	2	3	4	5	6	7	8	9	10	11	12	13	14
Intestinal gas														
Burping														
Heartburn														
Undigested food														
Constipation														
Diarrhea														
Abdominal bloating														
Coated tongue														
Bad breath														
Colitis														
Insomnia														
Energy														

SAMPLE FOOD COMBINING MEAL SUGGESTIONS

MEAL	PROTEIN TYPE	MIXED TYPE	CARBO TYPE
BREAKFAST	old-fashioned oatmeal, *30 minutes later* steak, asparagus	whole wheat toast with butter, apple, *30 minutes later* egg(s)	fruit, whole-grain toast with teaspoon butter, *30 minutes later* low-fat cottage cheese or plain, low-fat yogurt
LUNCH	pea and mushroom sauté, slice of toasted 100% rye, sprouted bread with butter, *30 minutes later* broiled salmon	steamed green beans, wild rice and butter, romaine lettuce, chopped cucumber, green pepper, olives, tomato, with fresh lemon juice and olive oil, *30 minutes later* broiled trout	steamed beets and beet greens, sliced tomato, and cucumber spelt toast with garlic butter *30 minutes later* chicken breast
DINNER	wild rice with butter, steamed spinach, *30 minutes later* broiled lamb chops	steamed zucchini, sweet potato and butter, *30 minutes later* broiled pork chops	yam, coleslaw with chopped scallion and green pepper with vinaigrette dressing *30 minutes later* baked Cornish game hen

10

Chapter

CUSTOMIZED
WEIGHT LOSS

The Boomerang Effect

I remember, as a ten-year-old child, being thoroughly fascinated when an uncle gave me a simple but endlessly entertaining birthday gift—a boomerang. The odd-looking angular toy quickly became one of my most prized possessions. My friends and I spent countless hours marveling at the way it would soar in flight when we tossed it into the air, then slowly turn and make its way back to us. What was baffling about it was that no matter how hard or how far we managed to throw the boomerang, it always came right back to the place from which it had taken off. We were too young at the time to understand that natural law, not magic, was responsible for the "boomerang effect."

Does this phenomenon sound familiar? If you're one of the many millions of overweight Americans, perhaps you have some experience with a similar kind of boomerang effect. As you know, the only thing more difficult than losing weight is keeping it off. Many of us invest extraordinary amounts of time, energy, and money in an effort to shed excess pounds. But no matter how hard we try or how much initial success we might achieve, more than ninety percent of the time, all the weight comes right back again. It's a very frustrating experience and a very puzzling phenomenon. Or . . . is it?

Actually, the laws of physics and the principles of aerodynamics can easily explain what otherwise might be viewed as the mysterious phenomenon of a boomerang in flight. Similarly, there are fundamental laws of physiology and biochemistry that explain why so few people who fight the battle of the bulge manage to maintain their ideal weight on a permanent basis.

For people who are serious about losing weight, it's generally not too difficult to find a way to drop a significant number of pounds. They may have to experiment with lots of different approaches, but if people persevere long enough, they usually stumble across something that seems to work. This is because there are plenty of crash dietary techniques one can use to effectively trick the body into an artificial weight loss mode.

The only problem is—it's not easy to fool the body for very long. In an overwhelming majority of cases, not only do people gain back all the weight they managed to lose, they also add even more pounds than they carried in the first place.

If you're lucky enough to be thin and are not personally familiar with this phenomenon, perhaps you've noticed it among friends and acquaintances. A variation on the boomerang effect is the yo-yo effect—when weight goes up and down, up and down, over and over again.

The reason people can't keep weight off is this: They assume it's somehow possible to force weight off the body in an arbitrary, unnatural manner, using one-dimensional approaches such as liquid diet drinks, diuretics, appetite suppressants, diet pills to speed up their metabolism, low-calorie and other restriction diets, or extreme exercise regimes.

People mistakenly view obesity as a problem unto itself rather than seeing it for what it really is—a symptom of poor health, and underlying disturbances with the metabolism of protein, fat, and carbohydrate.

If you view obesity as an isolated problem rather than an outward manifestation of deeper and more complex imbalances, it's natural to assume that a "quick and dirty" diet of some kind may actually succeed over the long haul.

But forced weight loss is no more a solution to chronic obesity than antihistamines are a solution for chronic allergies. Crash dieting, and the accompanying rapid weight loss, is the equivalent of any other medicinal quick fix—a temporary measure that merely sweeps symptoms under the rug while missing the real problem entirely.

The truth is, there's only one way to achieve lasting weight loss, and that is within the context of building health.

If you're overweight, you're bound to have other physiological problems and nagging ailments of one kind or another. They may not be as noticeable or as bothersome as your weight, but they're every bit as significant. That's why you need to address all your health problems at a foundational level, and in a comprehensive way.

By treating your weight as an issue that's separate from your health, you'll never be able to achieve or maintain your ideal weight. But if you focus on balancing your body chemistry with a diet that supports your metabolic individuality, you can solve multiple health problems all at once, including excess weight and obesity.

The good news is that weight loss is not an endless, futile struggle when it's approached logically, within the larger context of the pursuit of health. What happens then is that the weight drops off naturally and effortlessly, and it stays off, simply as a side effect of building health from the ground up.

Fat Burning vs. Weight Loss

As you know, the primary function of food is to supply you with enough energy to support the many functions of your body at work or at play. All the macronutrients can supply energy, but of the three, fat is the most concentrated source; it furnishes more than twice as much energy as comparable amounts of either carbohydrate or protein.

The unit that's used to measure the amount of energy contained in food is the calorie. When you eat foods that contain more energy or calories than you need, the excess energy gets stored in the body, primarily as fat. Later, when you need more energy for any reason, your body taps into its most plentiful and efficient energy resource—fat stored in fat cells and adipose tissue—and mobilizes it to where it's needed.

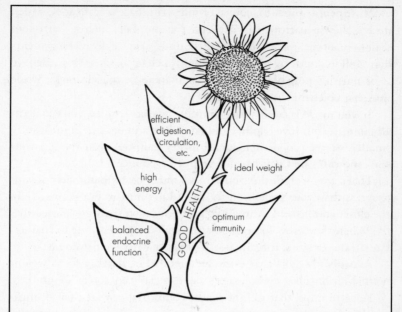

Weight normalization is simply a component or a side effect of a much broader picture, involving balanced and efficient metabolism at every level within the body. That is why the secret of achieving permanent weight loss is to address it within the context of a program designed, first and foremost, to build health.

Even though all the cells and tissues in your body use fat for energy, your muscles, which are always contracting and moving, require significantly greater amounts of energy than other tissues. They're "energy hogs" due to the active and strenuous nature of the work they perform.

Your muscle cells can also be thought of as miniature fat furnaces. They're unsurpassed in the way they burn calories—at least eighteen times faster than fat cells, for example. That's why it's important to exercise and have well-developed muscle tone. When you build lean body mass (muscle tissue), it becomes a fat-burning powerhouse, thus allowing you to eat more without growing fat.

With this in mind, here's something else that's very important for you to understand: the distinction between fat loss and weight loss.

Most people pursue a course of indiscriminate weight loss, which means they're narrowly focused on the numbers on the bathroom scale—in other words, dropping pounds. Yet scale measurements don't tell us anything at all about how much fat has been lost. Believe it or not, it's possible to burn fat and increase muscle mass, while showing no change in scale weight.

Since muscle is twenty-two percent heavier than fat, you can actually lose all your love handles and fat bulges and become significantly smaller, better proportioned, and nicely sculpted even though your scale indicates that you haven't dropped a pound!

That's why weight distribution is a much better barometer of your progress than your scale. In fact, it wouldn't hurt to put your scale in the closet and instead focus all your attention on the way your clothes fit. When they grow loose and baggy and you get to shift to smaller-size dresses or suits, it really doesn't matter what your scale says.

Actually, the goal that everyone ought to be striving for is weight normalization, not weight loss per se—especially not forced weight loss.

Keep in mind that weight can be comprised of water, fat, or muscle. For example, if you have excess water weight, you could take a diuretic and look significantly thinner for a while, but the metabolic imbalances that are causing the fluid buildup in your body tissues would remain unchanged. Your excess body fat would also remain untouched.

Or if you were to pursue some type of restriction diet and didn't get adequate macronutrients—especially proteins and fats, for example—you might lose weight initially, but you'd also tear down muscle mass and would lack the raw materials necessary to rebuild it. This would leave you without the very tissue that's most essential for burning fat.

As you can see, these sorts of narrowly focused weight loss strategies work only to ensure that you remain stuck in a yo-yo diet mode. They can't help you keep weight off for any length of time, and they do nothing whatsoever to enhance your health.

On the other hand, the right kind of nutritional regime—one that has the restoration of your biochemical balance and your overall health as its primary goal—can solve both your health problems and your weight problem simultaneously.

If you're carrying excess water weight, for example, you can't just pop a pill and expect the condition to be permanently solved. The only logical way to remedy the situation is to identify your genetically based dietary needs and then eat accordingly. You won't get the same instantaneous result you'd get from a diuretic, but a sound nutritional approach can solve your problem in a healthful, long-lasting way.

Ultimately we all need to realize that there are no diet plans or packaged meals or pills or drinks or gimmicks that can ever begin to compete with our bodies' own built-in intelligence. That's why you don't see weight loss industries in cultures where people enjoy the highest levels of health and fitness.

So the best possible weight loss strategy is to stop investing your time, attention, and resources in modern fad diets or superficial stop-gap measures, and to start thinking in much simpler and more basic (yet bigger picture) terms about your body's fundamental nutritional requirements.

Remember—the real secret to staying thin is no different from the secret to staying healthy. What you need to do first is to identify the specific raw materials that will support your body's unique biochemical requirements, and then supply them in the right combinations. Then simply step aside and let your body repair, rebuild, and regulate itself.

Add a little bit of easy, enjoyable exercise and—*voilà*—you'll have the lean, svelte appearance you've always wanted, as just one among the many benefits of robust good health. If you make a decision to become healthy, weight loss just naturally follows.

Building and Stoking Your Fat Furnaces

Your metabolic rate is one of several important factors that determine your weight. It refers to the rate at which your body burns calories or utilizes energy.

Technically speaking, your basal metabolic rate is defined as the amount of oxygen your body uses when your system is totally at rest—twelve hours after eating, in a comfortable temperature, and not engaged in exercise, physical activity, or emotional excitement of any kind.

If you have a fast metabolic rate, you'll tend to be thin because you'll need to take in lots of calories just to keep up with the rate at which your body churns out energy.

If you have a slow metabolic rate, your caloric demand for energy is not very high, so it will be very easy to eat more calories than your body needs to maintain itself, and any excess calories will be stored as fat. What's worse is that the existing calories you already have stored away as fat will rarely need to be mobilized and converted to energy.

So, if you're overweight, it's essential for you to speed up your metabolic rate. How do you do that? It's simple, really. All you need to do is to build up your lean body mass (your muscle tissue, or "fat furnaces"). There are two ways to do this: 1) by eating a metabolically appropriate diet, and 2) by doing some exercise.

Your basal metabolic rate is directly proportional to your lean body mass. In other words, the more muscles you have, the higher your metabolic rate, and the greater your body's need for energy.

Increasing your metabolic rate will give you the freedom to eat more than you do now—while at the same time staying thin and avoiding the boomerang effect. You'll be surprised how much more food you can eat once you build up your muscle tissue.

As we grow older, it's particularly important to maintain lean muscle mass. After age forty, muscles tend to diminish at the rate of one third of a pound a year. Generally speaking, men naturally maintain more muscle than women, although it's important for everyone to make an active effort to develop muscle tissue.

Here's a simple analogy that may be helpful: To get fit and trim, and to stay that way, what you need to do is build and stoke your fat furnaces.

You build fat furnaces throughout your body by building and maintaining muscle tissue. And you stoke your fat furnaces by consuming the right kind of body fuel.

The combination of a metabolically appropriate diet and a little of the right kind of exercise will effectively build your lean body mass and automatically raise your metabolic rate, with the inevitable result being a slender new you.

Sometimes women get concerned when they hear all this talk

about muscle mass. They're eager to drop fat, and they understand the critical importance of exercise and lean body mass, but they certainly don't want to wind up looking like Arnold Schwarzenegger.

But there's no need to worry, because Arnold has something women don't: male hormones. For hormonal reasons, women simply don't get bulging, rippled muscles no matter how hard they work out. The women we see in body-building magazines don't get that way without the use of extreme measures, even the use of steroids in some cases.

So if you're a woman who's considering a course of exercise to build up those fat furnaces, rest assured that you won't look remotely like a female body builder even if you exercise extensively. Your muscles will simply become denser, not larger. Any flabby, atrophied muscle tissue will be replaced by smooth, taut, younger-looking body tissue on your arms and legs and torso. Your body will become smaller and firmer and nicely sculpted, but in a feminine way.

Maintaining Lean Body Mass

Now the inevitable question arises: How exactly does one go about building these fat furnaces, this muscle tissue? Well, with exercise, of course—though not just any exercise. As you know, there are two basic kinds of exercise: aerobic and anaerobic.

Aerobic exercises such as running, swimming, bicycling, or playing tennis use up lots of oxygen and burn up lots of calories and fat. Whereas anaerobic exercises like weight lifting and various forms of resistance training use relatively little oxygen and do not immediately burn off a lot of calories and fat.

However, anaerobic exercises such as weight lifting are by far the best way to build strength and muscles, which means they provide long-term fat-burning benefits. That's why it's best for you to incorporate both aerobic and anaerobic exercises into your day-to-day activities.

The good news is you don't necessarily have to join a gym, hire a personal trainer, or be the slightest bit athletically inclined to reap enormous rewards from exercise. In the aerobic category, for example, lots of health experts worldwide believe that a low-intensity pastime like walking is one of the very best exercise options for people of any age.

Believe it or not, when you engage in high-intensity aerobic routines, you often use up less stored fat than you would with a low-intensity exercise like walking. Because when you begin exercising too hard, your muscles frequently can't efficiently acquire enough stored fat from your adipose (fat) tissue, so they switch to the alternative energy source: the carbohydrate that's stored right within the muscle tissue. That's why many people find it more beneficial to exercise less intensively for longer periods of time.

It's best to do at least thirty minutes of brisk, uninterrupted walking each day. If you live in an urban area, head for a park where you can walk continuously without having to stop and wait for traffic each time you cross the street. Hiking is another good option.

If possible, take an hour-long walk or supplement your thirty-minute walk with an extra twenty to thirty minutes of some other form of aerobic exercise, such as walking briskly on a treadmill, running in place on a rebounder (miniature trampoline), or working out on a stationary bike or rowing machine. Rebounders are fun to use and ideal for people who like to jog but want to avoid knee damage or any harsh, jarring impact on the joints or internal organs.

Just pick something you find easy and enjoyable, and something that fits easily into your lifestyle, that you know you can stick to. Remember that exercise doesn't have to be boring. In fact, for many people, it's a wonderful break they eagerly look forward to each day. You can walk the dog or listen to music or watch TV or listen to interesting tapes while you build up your cardiovascular strength and burn off calories and fat.

You'll get plenty of other "sweat benefits" from aerobic exercise as well. It's a vitally important way to continuously eliminate toxins from your body (the result of normal metabolic processes as well as environmental pollutants), and to help maintain circulation within your lymphatic system.

Here's another reason aerobic exercise is essential: It effectively neutralizes the negative effects of stress hormones.

In primitive times, if someone encountered a bear or a tiger, his body would start producing anabolic (stress) hormones so he'd be physically prepared to engage in "fight or flight." For modern man, the very same mechanism is at work as a response to the subtler but more consistent stresses each of us encounters on a daily basis.

Stress hormones need to be kept in check because they encourage anabolic processes like fat storage. They also play a role in the development of degenerative diseases, including cancer and heart disease. So the neutralization of stress hormones is yet another way in which aerobic exercise can keep you healthy and fit.

Aerobic exercise is also essential if you expect to feel well! No matter how carefully you manage your diet, you'll feel a whole lot better both mentally and physically if you devote a little time each week to some simple aerobic activities.

But don't forget to include anaerobic exercise in your weekly regimen. Lifting weights for even five to ten minutes each day is a great way to build strength and muscle mass, strengthen the joints, build bone density, and prevent osteoporosis.

Weight training also helps reduce fat storage by reducing elevated insulin levels and promoting the release of growth hormone, a substance that produces multiple health and fitness benefits. Growth hormone stimulates the development of lean body mass and the growth and repair of body tissues, encourages the use of fat as a fuel source, and mobilizes fat stores.

Growth hormone is what keeps children and teenagers thin and gives them an abundant supply of energy. It's stored in the brain and is readily released into the systems of children. Adults have adequate supplies of growth hormone, but it's not as readily accessible. Besides exercise, there are a number of factors that encourage the release of growth hormone, including stable blood sugar and adequate sleep.

Some researchers believe that the release of growth hormone is enhanced by exercising on an empty stomach, and in particular avoiding the consumption of high-carbohydrate foods or beverages (such as sports drinks or nutrition bars) before or after exercising.

However, other researchers believe that exercising on a completely empty stomach lowers the metabolic rate and keeps it low throughout the rest of the day (thereby compromising the fat-burning value of the exercise). So you may find that a snack of some kind thirty minutes before you exercise enhances your performance.

Ultimately your body will let you know what you need. If you don't eat anything and you feel very weak and lacking in stamina while exercising, it's a sign that your metabolism has slowed and you needed some food before getting started. So what you can do is experiment with various kinds of snacks appropriate to your metabolic type. Listen to your body and you'll inevitably find what works best.

Here are some easy-to-follow but effective how-to materials:

Books on Weight Training

Dr. Bob Arnot's Guide to Turning Back the Clock, by Bob Arnot, M.D., Little, Brown, 1996.

Weight Training for Dummies, by Liz Neporent and Suzanne Schlosberg, IDG Books, 1997.

Strong Women Stay Young, by Miriam Nelson, Bantam, 1997.

Video and Audio Tapes on Aerobic Exercise

Jane Fonda's Low-Impact Aerobic Workout (video)

Kathy Smith's WALKFIT Plus Lean Walk System (audio)

Reset Your Fat Thermostat

Here's a very typical diet scenario: You decide you need to lose 10 or 15 pounds in a hurry, maybe for a class reunion or a wedding or some other social event. Or simply because you're tired of trying to squeeze into all your clothes. To take off the weight quickly, you decide to go on a very low calorie diet for a few weeks. You cut your food intake way down for a month or so by skipping meals frequently and eating very sparingly the rest of the time. The plan works and the weight peels off.

But before long, all the fat you lost stealthily creeps back. Although you tried your best to maintain your new leaner figure, it proved to be impossible. You're not sure why, though, since you never indulged in bingeing. In fact, you were very careful about what you ate and seemed to be doing a good job of staying in a maintenance mode.

Oddly, your weight boomeranged back to the exact same level it was before you went on the crash diet. Though you managed to drop 15 pounds in a hurry, 15 pounds is precisely what you put back on again. Now your weight just seems to be hovering steadily at that level. It almost seems as though your body is programmed to hang on to that 15 pounds, to stay at a specific weight regardless of what you do.

Believe it or not, your body *is* programmed to stay at a specific weight. This phenomenon has a name—it's called your setpoint. It's actually a survival mechanism, a biological holdover from primitive times. People in hunter/gatherer societies needed a way to conserve body fat during periods when food was scarce, and this mechanism worked very well. It's still very functional in modern man.

The only trouble is, if you suddenly decide to cut your food intake way down, your body doesn't know the difference between dieting and starving. Your body can very easily interpret your greatly reduced food intake as a sign that you are in a starvation mode. So your setpoint mechanism will kick in, in order to protect you.

The brain sends a message instructing your metabolism to slow down and your appetite to pick up. If you truly are in a starvation mode, you'll need to have a decent appetite so you'll be motivated to eat and revive yourself whenever food does become available. If you're just dieting, however, the increased appetite will just make it more difficult.

Your setpoint mechanism works in the other direction as well. If you suddenly add weight, your metabolism speeds up and your appetite decreases. That's why some experts think of the setpoint as a kind of fat thermostat. In the same way a regular thermostat automatically regulates the temperature in a room, your setpoint automatically regulates your body fat.

In a 1995 study at Rockefeller University, researchers found that the metabolic rates of adults who had lost 10 percent of their body weight on an 800-calorie-a-day diet plan (a very low calorie diet) also decreased their metabolic rate by at least 10 percent. Conversely, those who gained 10 percent of their body weight had a metabolic increase of 10 percent.

Of course, your metabolic rate and appetite control centers are governed by a range of factors, including genes and hormones, not just the setpoint. And the setpoint is also influenced by genetics; it's not simply a matter of eating behavior. For hereditary reasons, each of us tends to gravitate toward a particular weight level.

Nonetheless, none of us is a slave to a fixed setpoint. We can all raise or lower our setpoint to some extent, within certain genetically determined boundaries. If you're overweight and you want to lower your setpoint, here are two things you need to remember:

1. To prevent your metabolic rate from slowing down too much, avoid low-calorie diets. And remember that when you use a metabolic typing approach to weight loss, you really don't need to be concerned about counting calories at all. But if you're a very calorie-conscious person and you really want to reduce your caloric intake, be sure to do it gradually and only moderately. Bear in mind that if you cut your food intake too much, the pounds you shed will be composed not only of fat, but of lean muscle as well. And of course lean muscle is what you need to burn fat. It's hard to say exactly how many calories one should cut to avoid a severe metabolic slowdown, since everyone is different. Some experts recommend that you figure out how many calories you're eating now, and reduce that number by no more than 500 calories per day. But never go below 1,200 calories per day.

2. Increase your metabolic rate with aerobic exercise and supplement this with a little weight training (anaerobic exercise).

Managing Your Insulin/Glucagon Balance

As you know, hormones regulate virtually every activity that takes place in the body. Two hormones in particular—insulin and glucagon—play central roles in determining your weight. They function as complementary opposites with respect to fat. Glucagon is known as the fat-burning hormone and insulin is known as the fat-storage hormone.

Each of these hormones is activated by shifts in blood sugar levels. Insulin's primary task is to keep the blood sugar from rising too high, while glucagon's chief task is to keep the blood sugar from dropping too low. Whenever your blood sugar goes up, your insulin level goes up as well. Conversely, when your blood sugar falls, your insulin drops and glucagon rises.

In order to keep the fat away, what we need to do is eat in a manner that stimulates the fat-burning hormone and limits the activity of the fat-storage hormone.

Although you can't influence the secretion of these hormones in a *direct* way, you can certainly manage them in an *indirect* way—by controlling the blood sugar. The goal, of course, is to eat the kinds of foods and the combinations of foods that will keep blood sugar on an even keel and thereby limit the secretion of insulin.

Excess insulin is secreted by the pancreas (the beta cells of the islets of Langerhans) whenever your blood sugar rises too high or too quickly—as a result of eating too many carbohydrates or high-glycemic carbohydrates or too many carbohydrates in proportion to protein and fat.

It's important to avoid elevated levels of insulin, because when this happens, the body is forced to burn carbohydrates as a fuel source and prevented from using stored fat as a source of energy. Insulin also converts and stores any excess glucose as body fat, and in general shifts the whole body into a fat-storage mode.

The fat-storage processes set in motion by insulin are brought to a halt by glucagon, which is secreted by the alpha cells of the pancreas, primarily as a response to an adequate intake of protein. Glucagon reverses the effects of insulin and shifts the metabolism into a fat-burning mode. It mobilizes the release of fat directly into the bloodstream. From there the fat is made available to the muscle cells, which use it as their preferred source of energy.

Both insulin and glucagon are present in the blood all the time. The trick is to keep them in balance and prevent one from assuming dominance over the other. The way to do this is by eating meals and snacks composed of the right proportions of proteins, carbohydrates, and fats. When you get your macronutrient ratio right, your blood sugar will remain at a stable level, and insulin and glucagon will maintain a harmonious balance.

So the obvious question for overweight individuals is: What's the right combination of macronutrients that will keep my insulin/glucagon levels in balance?

Different nutrition experts have different responses to this question. For instance, one very popular school of thought is based on the idea that a "40-30-30" diet (i.e., meals composed of 40 percent carbohydrate, 30 percent protein, and 30 percent fat) is the ideal way to produce the desired hormonal balance. And there's no question that this approach works very well for some people.

Other experts advocate different macronutrient combinations, involving varying percentages of protein and carbohydrates. These approaches also work well for some people.

But contrary to what the nutrition experts claim, there is no single macronutrient ratio that will effectively balance everyone's insulin/glucagon levels. Proof of this lies in the fact that some people lose weight on 40-30-30 diets, others lose weight on high-carbohydrate diets, still others lose weight on high-protein diets, and so on. And with each of these approaches, some people actually gain weight as well.

For genetic reasons, different people have different insulin responses than others. As an example, let's say you and a friend go on a two-week cruise and you each order the same dinner every night. Perhaps your meals include rolls, starchy vegetables, and desserts. Let's say that you pack on the pounds this way, while your friend barely gains an ounce.

What this means is that your friend has a higher insulin-triggering threshold than you do. Thus she has a natural hereditary ability to tolerate larger amounts of glucose in her blood before her body senses that there's too much and alerts her pancreas to start pumping insulin to keep it in check.

But there's more to it than that. For instance, in this example, you're likely to be a Protein Type, while your friend is probably a Carbo Type. This means not only that she can get away with a higher carbohydrate-to-protein ratio, but her metabolism actually *requires it* in order to be balanced and healthy, and to enable her to stay lean.

Ultimately there is no set formula for balancing your insulin/glucagon levels any more than there is a standard macronutrient ratio for balancing your autonomic, endocrine, or oxidative systems. The only way you can be sure to keep your insulin levels in check is to eat according to your metabolic type—which involves identifying a macronutrient ratio that is customized to your unique body chemistry.

Real-World Success Stories

Over the years, my consultations with athletes have revealed a great deal about what works and what doesn't work in the area of weight management. Since athletes are so well conditioned and so carefully attuned to their own bodies and performance capabilities, it's always glaringly apparent when they're eating in a way that undermines their health and fitness.

When athletes get fat, you know it's not due to a sedentary lifestyle or their failure to engage in adequate exercise. Similarly, it's never an isolated problem. There are always other, readily observable symptoms—such as a loss of strength and endurance, and an inability to build and sustain lean body mass.

By observing the lifestyles, diets, and physical capabilities of athletes, one gets a very clear and immediate sense of the importance of eating according to one's metabolic type and the disastrous effects of "one-size-fits-all" diets.

Football player Carl Zander is an interesting case in point. I first had the pleasure of meeting Carl in July 1990. He phoned me from a training camp, where he was preparing for the upcoming pro football season.

For years prior to the summer of 1990, Carl had been in peak condition and was enjoying exceptional career success. In the previous season, 1989, he played in the Super Bowl as starting middle linebacker for the Cincinnati Bengals.

But now, for some mysterious reason, he was experiencing dramatic physical deterioration. Carl was rapidly losing muscle mass all over his body, and, with it, the ability to burn fat. He was struggling with other serious problems as well: a loss of strength, endurance, speed, reaction time, and agility. His recovery time from bruises and contusions had also become much slower than normal. Needless to say, all these problems were having a very adverse impact on his athletic performance.

Carl also suffered with extreme fatigue both during and following practice sessions. Since he felt so exhausted by the time he went home each day, he had no time for family or friends. All he could do was eat and go to bed early, only to awaken the next day feeling almost as tired as when he went to bed the night before. He was doing the best he could to hide his real condition from his coaches and teammates, but he knew it was just a matter of time before he would lose his starting position with the team.

He asked if I could help him, and I said there was a good chance that I could, but that we would first need to determine his metabolic type. I explained that the goal would be to identify specific imbalances in his fundamental homeostatic control mechanisms. From there I'd be able to recommend a nutritional protocol to help restore balance and efficiency to his metabolism. But Carl said he couldn't last the two weeks it would take to complete the metabolic evaluation process. His health was unraveling much too quickly, and he needed help right away.

I was very reluctant to give him any immediate dietary recommendations, since I knew almost nothing about him. But we talked further and he revealed an interesting clue: He reported that the camp coaches were big advocates of carbohydrate loading. Before practices each day, players were strongly encouraged to load up on carbohydrates to sustain their energy through the grueling training sessions.

This was particularly interesting in light of other things Carl began to tell me about himself and his dietary history. It sounded as though he might be a parasympathetic dominant—in other words, a Protein Type. If this was the case, he could never hope to function well without significant quantities of heavy proteins and fat, and relatively small amounts of carbohydrates.

So I suggested he forget about carbo loading and, while his teammates were wolfing down pasta and bagels, he should eat all the red meat and butter his appetite could handle. Carl was skeptical about this approach, since all the "experts" around him were firm believers in the dangers of red meat and saturated fats. Nonetheless, he'd run out of options and had little choice but to implement my suggestions immediately.

I pointed out to Carl that if he were a Protein Type, all the high-carbohydrate meals he was eating would wreak havoc on his blood sugar balance and cellular oxidation. This would explain why his body was storing fat and unable to burn it. A lack of adequate protein was also likely to be causing the breakdown in his muscle tissue, along with disturbances in his adrenal and thyroid function and a lowered metabolic rate. Seen in this light, all his symptoms, including his profound fatigue, made perfect sense.

A few weeks later, Carl called to report that all his physical problems were rapidly reversing. To his surprise, his fatigue disappeared almost immediately on a high-protein, high-fat diet. Shortly thereafter, his muscle tissue began to restore itself, his metabolic rate picked up, and he was clearly on the way to becoming lean and fit once again. His ability to recover rapidly from bruises, muscle strains, and other injuries was also returning.

He wasn't cut from the team and didn't lose his starting position. Best of all, he was able to enjoy his family and friends and personal life once again. Carl has since retired from pro football but remains committed to optimizing his health and maintaining his weight by eating according to his metabolic type.

Note that many of Carl's teammates were able to stay fit and trim and enjoy peak physical performance on the *very same diet* that caused Carl to gain weight and brought him to the brink of a complete physical collapse.

I see this metabolic diversity among athletes all the time. They have highly individualized needs, yet for many years they've all been pushed toward a narrowly conceived, "one-size-fits-all" dietary strategy of one sort or another.

As an example, a few years before meeting Carl, I was approached by an all-star, record-setting quarterback from another NFL team.

This individual (I'll call him Sam, though that's not his real name) had symptoms virtually identical to Carl's, including debilitating fatigue. But unlike Carl, Sam had been in retirement from pro football for a number of years. He was no longer doing rigorous physical training and exercise, and his weight had ballooned up to 60 or 70 pounds above what it should have been.

Tests revealed that Sam was a sympathetic dominant, or a Carbo Type. What he needed was a diet low in protein and fat and higher in carbohydrates. At the time, he was living on a high-protein diet. Thus he had the same problems Carl had—but in reverse.

Because he wasn't getting adequate glucose, Sam's body was tearing down (catabolizing) his muscle tissue for desperately needed fuel. He also had disturbed adrenal and thyroid function, which was contributing to his fatigue and sluggishness. All these factors helped slow his metabolic rate way down, and disruptions in his cellular oxidation were causing him to store rather than burn fat.

Much to my surprise, Sam told me something that he said no one really knew about his playing days. During his era, high protein was the rule at football training tables—just the opposite of the carbohydrate loading that was in vogue when Carl played. So Sam ate the high-protein fare before each game, just like all his teammates.

Sam confessed that he always felt terrible for the first half of the game, and it wasn't until the third quarter that he began to feel somewhat normal and energetic. It's amazing that he set as many records as he did. He remarked to me that he wonders what he could have done had he not been so wiped out during the first half of every game.

Once we got him on the right diet, Sam regained his energy and muscle strength. Over a period of about eight months he also dropped close to 50 pounds. Needless to say, he looked and felt great, and he stayed that way. The weight never came boomeranging back.

Here's a very important point: Sam didn't come to me with weight loss as his number one priority. He was primarily interested in feeling better and doing whatever he could to optimize his health and his ability to enjoy life. The weight came off as a natural by-product of Sam's broader agenda and health-building protocol. And he never deprived himself of the foods he enjoyed. He could eat until he was full and never had to endure food cravings or continuous hunger.

Recently, I consulted with a young woman athlete who had problems very similar to Carl's and Sam's. When she contacted me in 1998, Rebecca was a freshman who'd been awarded a volleyball scholarship to a major university on the East Coast. Prior to coming to the university, Rebecca was happy, excited, and brimming with confidence, because she'd gotten herself into the best shape of her life—with low body fat, high lean body mass, and excellent strength, speed, and agility.

Although she was in great condition when she first arrived at school, within just a few months Rebecca underwent a dramatic physical breakdown. She packed on a lot of fat and lost a great deal of muscle and strength. She no longer had the requisite energy or stamina to keep up with her teammates or last through the games, much less perform well.

Rebecca was on the verge of not only losing her starting position on the team, but of being dropped from the team entirely. Even worse, her self-confidence had been shattered and she'd developed severe depression. When we first spoke, she was weak and lethargic and was having a lot of trouble staying focused and motivated enough to try to resolve her serious dilemma. She was also frightened and confused and didn't understand what had happened to her or what to do about it.

After we talked for a while, I discovered that Rebecca's athletic department had taken a keen interest in nutrition. With the intention of assisting and enhancing the performance of the athletes, the coaches and team managers had adopted a strict training table based on a 40-30-30 dietary approach (40 percent carbohydrate, 30 percent protein, 30 percent fat). While many of her teammates did extremely well with this formula, it was obviously having a devastating impact on Rebecca.

Sure enough, tests revealed that the 40-30-30 mix was very wrong for Rebecca's metabolism. She turned out to be a slow oxidizer, or a Carbo Type. This meant that the 40-30-30 diet was overfeeding her protein and fat and failing to provide her with enough carbohydrate. As a result, she couldn't efficiently convert her food to energy.

This produced a cascade, or chain reaction, of negative biochemical events. Because she was eating too few carbohydrates, her body was starved for glucose. To get more, and to fulfill the especially urgent priority of making glucose available to her brain cells, Rebecca's body was actually cannibalizing itself (i.e., breaking down muscle tissue).

Rebecca's inability to get the right macronutrients—in the right proportions—prevented her from effectively metabolizing proteins, carbohydrates, or fats. This slowed down her metabolic rate, caused her to store fat rather than burn it, and severely undermined her body's ability to build muscle tissue. It also created an alkaline shift in her body and suppressed her adrenal and thyroid function. These and other factors contributed to her depression, lowered energy, lack of motivation, and lowered metabolic rate.

As you can see, there is no specific dietary formula for staying thin and fit. Some of the dietary approaches now on the market work well for some people. For others, they are ineffective at best, and, at worst, disastrous. The following chart provides a brief summary of some of the key benefits and limitations of the most popular current dietary systems.

COMPARATIVE BENEFITS AND LIMITATIONS OF "WEIGHT LOSS" DIETS

DIET	BENEFITS	LIMITATIONS
High-Carb/ Low-Fat Diets	*facilitate weight control, but only for certain metabolic types:* • sympathetic dominants • slow oxidizers ("carbo types")	*in protein types and mixed types:* • increase fat storage by: ✔ increasing insulin levels ✔ disturbing cellular oxidation • lower metabolic rate by: ✔ breaking down muscle tissue due to insufficient protein ✔ accelerating parasympathetic output ✔ disturbing adrenal and thyroid function
High-Protein/ High-Fat Diets	*facilitate weight control, but only for certain metabolic types:* • parasympathetic dominants • fast oxidizers ("protein types")	*in carbo types and mixed types:* • increase fat storage by: ✔ disturbing cellular oxidation • lower metabolic rate by: ✔ creating a shortage of glucose, causing the body to catabolize (tear down) its own muscle tissue for desperately needed fuel ✔ disturbing adrenal and thyroid function, causing fatigue and impaired performance
40-30-30 Diets	*facilitate weight control, but only for certain metabolic types:* • balanced dominants • mixed oxidizers ("mixed types")	*in carbo types and protein types:* • increase fat storage by: ✔ disturbing cellular oxidation • lower metabolic rate by: ✔ creating a shortage of glucose in carbo types, causing the body to catabolize (tear down) its own muscle tissue for desperately needed fuel ✔ breaking down muscle tissue in protein types due to insufficient dietary protein
Metabolic Typing Diets	*facilitate weight control for all metabolic types*	*in all metabolic types:* • regulate blood sugar • minimize fat storage by balancing insulin/glucagon ratio • enhance lean body mass • increase metabolic rate • normalize weight

The following provides a quick reminder of things you can do to achieve and maintain your ideal weight. By following these simple guidelines, you will lose weight in an effortless, natural way, as a by-product of a broader health-building strategy. Making health your first priority is the only way to lose weight and keep it off *permanently*.

The most exciting aspect of this natural weight loss approach is that you never have to diet or deprive yourself in any way. Restriction diets that leave people feeling hungry and unsatisfied have proven not to work.

What does work is eating according to your genetically based nutritional requirements. When you eat the foods that effectively support your own unique engines of metabolism, weight normalization is the inevitable outcome. This means that if you are obese, you will lose weight, and if you're underweight, you will gain weight.

If you supplement a metabolically appropriate diet with other simple lifestyle changes such as a little low-intensity exercise, you won't have to struggle to achieve the results you desire. Remember that effective weight management is *not* about struggle or hard work. If you're struggling and not enjoying yourself, you're definitely doing something wrong!

First Things First

- *Eat the Right Foods for Your Metabolic Type*
Don't forget that the most fundamental priority in your effort to lose weight is to eat the foods that are right for your metabolic type. In this way you will balance your body chemistry, increase your metabolic efficiency, normalize your fundamental homeostatic controls—and in turn increase both your metabolic rate and your lean body mass.

- *Balance Your Macronutrient Ratio*

Eating the right foods for your type isn't enough. You must also identify what specific combination of foods (that is, the proportion of protein to carbohydrate to fat) is right for you. In this way you will balance your insulin/glucagon ratio, burn calories for energy instead of storing them as fat, and build lean muscle mass.

Don't Undereat

- *Forget About Skipping Meals*

When you skip meals, the risks are great and the rewards are nonexistent. It may seem like a good way to shed some fat, but just the opposite is true. In reality, skipping meals only pushes you further along on the road to obesity! All you do is disrupt your blood sugar, slow down your metabolic rate, and set yourself up for binges and sweet cravings.

- *Never Cut Your Caloric Intake Too Much*

Excessive caloric reduction is a big mistake. Your body will think you're starving and your metabolism will slow down. Next your body will start to break down muscle tissue for fuel, thereby destroying your fat furnaces and innate ability to burn fat. The lack of calories will also raise your setpoint, i.e., your body will be programmed to gravitate toward a higher weight.

Eat to Lose

- *Don't Go More Than Four Hours Without Eating*

It's a scientific fact: Eating raises your metabolic rate. Calorie reduction or starving yourself *lowers* your metabolic rate. Develop the habit of eating regularly and within three to four hours of your last meal.

- *Keep Your Blood Sugar Stable*

Low blood sugar creates an alarm reaction and throws your body into a compensation mode. This leads to exhaustion of the glands that ordinarily maintain your metabolic rate at a high level. It also elevates your insulin and throws your body into a fat-storage mode. To stabilize your blood sugar, eat at regular intervals and use the fine-tuning checklist in Chapter 9 to make sure you're eating the right proportion of protein to carbohydrate to fat.

- *Eat Before You're Hungry*
This is a secret known to many thin people! If you wait until you're hungry, especially if you get *really* hungry, chances are excellent that you'll overeat unnecessarily. So eat at regular times each day. Try eating smaller amounts of food but more often throughout the day.

Get Adequate Protein

- *Have Some Protein at Every Meal or Snack*
Protein stimulates glucagon, which mobilizes fat from storage and converts it to energy. What could be better? When you eat carbohydrate alone, without protein, you stimulate insulin and fat storage instead. So eat protein each time you eat. Also, try eating the protein portion of your meal or snack first. This will help control the amount you eat.

- *Build Lean Body Mass*
The more muscle you have, the faster your metabolic rate can be. The higher your metabolic rate, the greater your need for calories. Build muscle, burn fat. It's that simple. Without adequate protein intake, not only will you not build muscle, but your body will also tear down your existing muscle tissue to fulfill its need for protein.

- *Stimulate Your Sympathetic System*
Protein stimulates the sympathetic branch of your autonomic nervous system. Your sympathetic system is responsible for increasing your metabolic rate. Insufficient protein intake causes parasympathetic dominance "by default," which naturally slows the metabolic rate.

Listen to Your Body

- *Tune In to Feelings of Hunger and Fullness*

Your body knows what amount of food is right for you at any given time and always lets you know. You'll know you've had enough when your hunger feels completely satisfied, but in a comfortable way. This is very different from feeling physically "stuffed." Start to pay close attention to the difference between these two states.

- *Stop When You've Had Enough*

Note that your hunger always feels satisfied long before you get that stuffed feeling. But if you rush through meals, you can easily miss the point at which your hunger is sated and just keep eating unnecessarily. So just slow down and always eat very leisurely, at a snail's pace if you've got the time. That's what most thin people do. Besides, savoring each mouthful is a lot more enjoyable than gobbling your food. Try chewing each bite twenty to thirty times, or putting your fork down after each mouthful. Anything that slows you down will aid digestion and give your brain time to monitor your food intake and alert you to stop eating at the appropriate time.

- *Leave Food Behind*

Many of us are programmed to eat whatever food is around or whatever is put in front of us. Some people feels it's impolite (say, at a social gathering) or somehow ethically wrong (remember what your parents said about those starving children) to leave food on their plate. Wrong. Never eat anything just because it's in front of you or easily accessible or because you think it would be "wasteful" not to finish what's left on your plate. Always let your body call the shots about when to turn away from food.

Get the Facts About Fat

- *Remember, Fat Won't Make You Fat*

For years now, dietary fat has been blamed for the obesity epidemic, so people have been obsessed with avoiding it. Low-fat and no-fat food products and recipe books of every conceivable variety have taken over the shelves at supermarkets and bookstores. But guess what? Fat is definitely *not* the culprit we've all been programmed to think it is. Believe it or not, fat plays many vitally important roles in keeping you lean and fit, and most people don't get enough of the right kind of dietary fat.

• *Eat the Good, Restrict the Bad*

How much fat is good for you depends on your metabolic type and is covered in Chapter 7. Of course, there are good fats and bad fats, so regardless of your metabolic type, you need to stick to the good and avoid the bad. What you need to avoid are *trans fats*—processed fats found in hydrogenated oils and non-cold-pressed vegetable oils. Avoid these products, including those hidden in packaged foods. Never use margarine or butter substitutes. Instead, use butter or ghee (clarified butter), and cold-pressed olive oil or coconut oil for cooking.

• *Fat to the Rescue*

Without an adequate amount of dietary fat, your body can't manufacture hormones or carry on normal cellular oxidation and energy production. This slows the metabolism and interferes with the development of lean body mass. And unlike carbohydrates, fat doesn't trigger the insulin response. In fact, it actually helps slow down the conversion of carbohydrates into blood sugar. To stay lean and healthy, learn about the many benefits of fat.

• *Read All About It*

Check out *Fats That Heal, Fats That Kill: The Complete Guide to Fats, Oils, Cholesterol and Human Health,* by Udo Erasmus, Alive Books, 1999. Although the book does not include a discussion of fats in relation to metabolic typing, it's an invaluable resource that you don't want to be without.

Do a Little Exercise

• *Work Up a Sweat*

Each day, do at least thirty minutes of aerobic exercise to oxygenate your system and get your heart pumping and your circulation moving—and to raise your metabolic rate and burn calories and fat. Work up a sweat by walking, bicycling, playing tennis, swimming, or using a treadmill, rebounder, stationary bike, or other aerobic exercise equipment. You'll get thin, feel great, stay young, and ward off chronic illness. Check with your doctor before doing anything strenuous.

• *Lift Some Weight*

Don't forget to include a little bit of anaerobic exercise in your daily routine. Even a few minutes a day of lifting weights or a similar form of resistance training will give you the lean body mass (muscle) you need to raise your metabolic rate and burn fat on a continuous basis.

Be Focused and Realistic

• *Pace Yourself*

Don't expect to lose huge amounts of weight overnight. Have realistic expectations and reasonable goals. Remember that it's not biologically feasible to lose more than one to one and a half pounds of body fat per week.

• *Think Long-Term*

Strive for long-term metabolic shifts, not quick-hit, forced weight loss. After all, your body has its own health-building priorities; it knows far better than you do how to go about normalizing your weight, and on what schedule. Just eat for enhanced energy and a sense of well-being and to be free of hunger and cravings. Your body will take care of the rest.

- *Keep It Simple*

Don't count calories, don't weigh your food, and don't even be concerned with portions. Healthy thin people in native cultures throughout the world don't do this, and neither should you. Just focus on eating the foods that are right for your type and in the right proportions. Then you, too, will develop "native intelligence," i.e., you won't need higher math to figure out how much to eat, you'll just know.

General Dos & Don'ts

- *Cheat a Little*

As long as you're eating right 90 percent of the time, you can cheat a little with sweets, desserts, wine, or whatever it is that you love to eat.

- *Drink Lots of Water*

Be sure to drink plenty of water between meals. Any degree of dehydration adversely affects your metabolism and will interfere with your weight loss effort. Read about the importance of water in Chapter 11.

- *Don't Use Meal Replacements*

Protein shakes and nutrition bars are okay—but as snacks, not meal replacements. Look for products with quality ingredients. Protein powders made of whey protein are best. Select nutrition bars appropriate to your metabolic type, as they each contain different amounts of protein and carbohydrate.

- *Bypass Artificial Sweeteners and Diet Pills*

Never use drugs or herbal preparations designed to speed the metabolism, suppress the appetite, or block fat absorption. Also, avoid all artificial sweeteners such as those used in diet colas. Some of these chemicals are widely believed to cause brain damage and other serious health disorders. Use stevia instead, an all-natural herbal sweetener. See Chapter 12 for more information on stevia.

- *Consider Food Intolerances*

In some instances, hidden food sensitivities can interfere with weight loss. For example, food intolerances can sometimes disrupt blood sugar levels and the insulin/glucagon balance, and result in carbohydrate cravings. Food intolerances have also been found to create food addictions, possibly arising from a food allergy-induced seratonin deficit. This produces a need for greater and greater amounts of the sensitive foods. Edema, the accumulation of excess water weight, and autoimmune damage to the thyroid and other glands, have also been linked to food intolerances. Read *Your Hidden Food Allergies are Making You Fat*, by Roger D. Deutsch and Rudy Rivera, M.D., Prima Health, 1998. If you've been following a good diet/exercise regime but are not getting the results you seek, see Chapter 11 for information on the ALCAT food sensitivity test.

Chapter 11

KEY CONSIDERATIONS BEYOND DIET

The Riddle of Human Illness

What is it exactly that makes us ill? Since the dawn of civilization, people have been intensely preoccupied with the search for answers to the question of what makes us vulnerable to suffering and disease.

To our cave-dweller ancestors, sickness was a bewildering phenomenon and seemed to come and go entirely at random, purely at the whim of supernatural forces. Since people couldn't hope to understand the dark and mysterious nature of disease, the best they could do for thousands of years was to try to prevent it by appeasing the gods with rituals and sacrifices.

The ancient Egyptians believed that evil spirits were to blame, so sorcerers and exorcists were usually called upon to recite incantations over the bodies of the afflicted. Much later, in medieval Europe, very little had changed. Sickness was attributed to astrological and other cosmic influences, and medieval healers relied heavily upon amulets, charms, and magic spells.

As recently as the mid-1800s, people still had no realistic ideas about the origins of illness. In the Western world, a common assumption was that health disorders were caused by mysterious "vapors" drifting through the air. Religious fundamentalists were convinced that diseases were the result of God's wrath and angry judgment of the sinful.

Physicians in the nineteenth century had vague notions about "bad blood" being responsible, so they used "bleeding" (cutting patients' veins with lancets) and "purging" (administering toxic metals such as mercury to induce vomiting) in an effort to remove blood and other unspecified toxins from the body.

Microbe Hunting and Magic Bullets

A large portion of the riddle of human illness was solved once people learned about the remarkable unseen realm of the microbe. Bacteria, tiny one-celled organisms, were first discovered in the 1600s by Antony van Leeuwenhoek, a Dutch janitor who made a hobby of constructing microscopes in his spare time. Though scientists at the time took note when Leeuwenhoek found vast quantities of bacteria in human saliva and in rivers and lakes, no one suspected that these organisms might be a source of illness; rather, they were considered mere curiosities.

But nothing came of this discovery until the 1850s, when a French chemistry professor, Louis Pasteur, was hired by local wine makers to investigate why certain vats fermented and others did not. In the process, he discovered that yeast, a microbial type of fungus, was the organism responsible for producing alcohol. He also learned that certain kinds of bacteria could prevent fermentation and cause contaminated food to decompose. Shortly thereafter, Pasteur and other scientists throughout Europe began to see the connection between microbes and human disease.

Within a decade or two, other important discoveries helped launch the science of bacteriology. Robert Koch, a German physician, isolated the microbes associated with anthrax and tuberculosis and developed "Koch's Postulates," the classic scientific criteria used to identify infectious diseases.

Joseph Lister, a young British surgeon, showed that postsurgical infections could be dramatically reduced by the sterilization of instruments. Austrian obstetrician Ignasz Semmelweis demonstrated that the lives of childbearing women could be protected if attending physicians disinfected their hands. These and other developments bolstered the significance of Pasteur's work, and before long he rose to legendary status as the father of the new "germ theory" of medicine.

The germ theory has provided the conceptual foundation for modern Western medicine for almost 150 years. It's based on the idea that a given germ (i.e., a "single agent") causes the same disease in all patients under all conditions. In modern times, this basic concept has been expanded to accommodate noninfectious diseases as well. For example, many researchers now believe that diseases like cancer or Alzheimer's are caused by "single agents" in the form of viruses or malfunctioning genes.

In the latter half of the 1800s, the germ theory shed enormous light on the major health problems of the day: cholera, diphtheria, typhoid, and other infectious plagues that caused widespread terror, suffering, and premature death. Public health got a tremendous boost once people learned that sanitation could prevent the spread of disease through faulty sewage systems and polluted water supplies.

Pasteur and Koch and other early "microbe hunters" also set the stage for the growth and global expansion of the pharmaceutical industry. Because if a "single agent" like a microbe is responsible for a disease, then a drug designed to target and destroy the invading organism represents a sensible therapeutic approach.

The early microbe hunters facilitated the discoveries of people like Paul Ehrlich, a German researcher who dreamed of creating chemicals that would kill microbes or treat diseased organs in a highly specific way, while leaving other areas of the body untouched and free of harmful side effects. In 1910 Ehrlich coined the phrase "silver bullets" (also known as "magic bullets") to describe this vision of the future of drug design. His experiments in this direction, with chemicals designed to treat syphilis, earned him the enduring distinction of being known as the "father of modern pharmacology."

In many ways, the germ theory has yielded phenomenal medical triumphs. For instance, with the help of antibiotics and vaccines, infectious diseases have been largely eliminated in developed regions of the world. Today, all infectious diseases combined claim less than 1 percent of the lives of Europeans and Americans. On the other hand, vast numbers of scientists and physicians believe that the germ theory and the allopathic medical tradition it supports have profound limitations and may ultimately have created as many problems as they have solved.

As an example, in the 1993 book *Medicine at the Crossroads: The Crisis in Health Care*, medical historian Melvin Konner, M.D., Ph.D., points out, "The phrase 'magic bullet' is the way Ehrlich's concept has come down to us . . . but . . . there is not one yet, for syphilis or any other disease." Leading alternative medical expert and Harvard-trained physician Andrew Weil concurs, but offers sharper criticisms of a narrowly focused, drug-based health care system. In *Health & Healing,* he writes, "Here is the major practical failing of modern allopathic medicine: the kinds of drugs it favors and the ways it puts them into people are very dangerous."

The Never-Ending Germ vs. Host Debate

Today many critics contend that the enormous commercial value of the germ theory has enabled it to monopolize medical research for well over a century and effectively suppress other important medical philosophies and approaches.

For example, Pasteur's role as the chief proponent of the germ theory turned him into a household name and a major luminary in the realm of modern medical science. Medical history books are full of formulaic summaries of his work and unqualified praise for his achievements. What is heavily obscured, however, is the fact that some of Pasteur's contemporaries believed the germ theory was overly simplistic and failed to explain the multidimensional nature of disease.

Chief among Pasteur's critics was the physician Jacques Antoine Bechamp, who was one of France's most prominent and active researchers and biologists, with credentials and scholarly achievements that significantly overshadowed Pasteur's. In 1923 the British historian E. Douglas Hume chronicled the opposing medical perspectives of these two men, and their long and bitter professional feud, in the book *Bechamp and Pasteur: The Lost History of Biology* (Kessinger Press, 1997).

Bechamp disputed Pasteur's claim that microbes are the primary causes of disease. He believed that the overall condition of the body, or the "host," was the primary determinant of the course of illness, and that diseases were "multifactorial" in nature, i.e., attributable to a range of environmental or physiological variables unique to each individual. The ideological battle between the two men captured a great deal of public attention in their day. Yet Bechamp's ideas, unlike Pasteur's, did not lend themselves to large-scale industrial solutions, so ultimately Bechamp's identity and contributions fell into obscurity.

What's most significant is that Pasteur and Bechamp ignited the "germ vs. host" debate. More than any other single topic, this one has come to represent the ideological rift between alternative practitioners and proponents of modern Western medicine. Interestingly, this concept has also been the source of countless hostile and extremely divisive controversies within the medical/scientific establishment itself for well over a century.

The latest incarnation of the germ vs. host debate is the intensely rancorous scientific battle over the cause of AIDS (acquired immune deficiency syndrome). Although it has rarely been reported in the mainstream media, the debate has become a huge international tug-of-war involving hundreds of "dissident" scientists who dispute the commonly accepted belief that AIDS is caused by a single infectious agent known as HIV (human immunodeficiency virus).

The rebel scientists—including physicians, Nobel laureates, internationally renowned researchers, and tenured professors at leading universities—believe that AIDS is more likely a multifactorial syndrome caused by a variety of environmental influences such as toxic pharmaceuticals, recreational drugs, malnutrition, and a range of other factors known to suppress the human immune system.

They claim that the concept of HIV as the "lone virus" causative agent in AIDS is weak and simplistic, and leaves many critical scientific questions unanswered. Health officials worldwide dismiss these ideas as nonsensical, irresponsible—even dangerous. Yet the dissidents continue to insist, as they have for a decade, that HIV's role in

AIDS has far more to do with political and economic imperatives (e.g., the race for blockbuster antiviral drugs or vaccines) than it does with sound scientific reasoning.

One of the most controversial dissenters is Peter Duesberg, a professor of molecular biology at the University of California at Berkeley and an eminent virologist. For many years Duesberg was a highly respected, top-ranking researcher within the scientific establishment. His rigorous and prolific investigative efforts were widely admired worldwide, and generously funded on a routine basis by the National Institutes of Health.

In the mid-1980s, however, Duesberg took a very unusual step. He began to question the validity of the large and prestigious arena in which he himself had long been a superstar—virology-based cancer research. For fifteen years the United States government had spent vast sums of money on research programs based on the idea that some forms of cancer are caused by retroviruses, a special category of viruses not typically associated with human illness. By 1986 Duesberg believed that the long-term research efforts had run out of steam and had failed to establish any connection between viruses and cancer.

Then, in 1987, he published a paper in the journal *Cancer Research* that went even farther by challenging the notion that either cancer or AIDS is caused by a retrovirus. The paper raised scores of provocative questions related to both epidemics (e.g., if cancers are caused by viruses, why are they not contagious?). These issues posed a significant potential threat to the stability of the virology infrastructure, especially since they were raised by a scientist of Duesberg's stature. Not surprisingly, he soon became the ultimate scientific pariah— shunned by colleagues, stripped of all research money, banished from professional conferences, and cast out of the elite upper echelons of academic research.

Throughout the 1990s, large numbers of independent scientists and physicians joined in the HIV/AIDS debate. They formed an international coalition (www.virusmyth.com) to protest the direction of AIDS research, which they view as the most egregious current example of a bloated worldwide scientific establishment driven by commercial interests and ruthless politics, as opposed to public health concerns.

A Multicausal Perspective

For alternative medical practitioners, there are seldom any quick or easy answers to the question "what's causing me to be sick?" Disease is viewed as a complex phenomenon—the result of any number of influences unique to each individual's internal status and external environment. This "multicausal" perspective on the origins of illness was undoubtedly best articulated by Hans Seyle, M.D., who in the 1950s published the classic book *The Stress of Life* (McGraw-Hill, 1956, 1978).

Over the course of many years of meticulous research, Seyle developed a comprehensive model to explain disease processes in human beings. It's based on the concept of "stress and adaptation." Seyle believed that health is largely determined by how well a person can adapt to the cumulative effects of any and all the stresses he or she encounters—job-related stress, family pressures, negative emotions, toxic environmental exposures, dietary deficiencies—that is, a virtually unlimited range of influences.

Seyle showed that stress can trigger a three-stage adaptation syndrome. The first stage is the "alarm reaction." At this point the body mobilizes its defenses to battle a given "stressor" or combination of "stressors," and if the effort is strong enough, the body wins and the stress is resolved and biological equilibrium (homeostasis) is reestablished.

But if Stage 1 proves inadequate and the stress is *not* resolved, the body moves into the "stage of resistance." This is a kind of "standoff" phase in which neither the body nor the stress initially has the upper hand. If the body manages to seize the upper hand, there is a return to Stage 1, in which the body has a strong ability to neutralize the stress.

However, if the body *cannot* resolve its problems in Stage 2, and the stress becomes chronic, the body's defenses eventually wear down, and the system moves into Stage 3, the "Stage of Exhaustion." This is the point at which chronic diseases can develop.

The science of metabolic typing incorporates the idea of "stress and adaptation." Like other holistic approaches, it too supports the notion that stress can come from any direction and impact the body in countless different ways. Similarly, it's a discipline that rejects the concept of "magic bullets" in favor of diet and lifestyle management.

What's unique about metabolic typing is that it expands upon the classic "stress and adaptation" concept by providing customized diet/lifestyle solutions that restore efficiency to the fundamental homeostatic controls, thereby optimizing a person's ability to neutralize stress and, in turn, avoid illness.

In the metabolic typing model, the fundamental homeostatic controls are the primary adaptive mechanisms. If they lose their efficiency or normal functional capacity, the body loses its ability to overcome stress, and a person then becomes vulnerable to either chronic or acute (i.e., infectious) health disorders. And if a homeostatic mechanism is unable to resolve stress, it can get "stuck" in a defensive response. The homeostatic response itself then becomes a problem because homeostasis is dependent upon these mechanisms remaining flexible, in turn allowing the body to shift into whatever mode it requires at any given time.

An unhealthy diet—especially a diet that's incorrect for your metabolic type—places enormous stress on your fundamental homeostatic controls, and is thus a primary cause of illness. But a poor diet is certainly not the only factor.

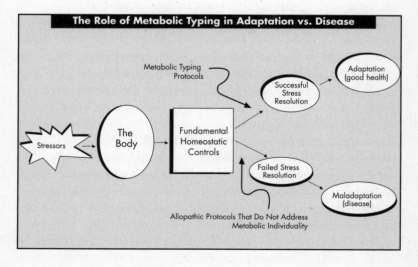

The Role of Metabolic Typing in Adaptation vs. Disease

There are many other forms of stress to which most of us are exposed on a routine basis. For the sake of ease and efficiency, I've organized these factors into four categories:

- psychological
- structural
- biochemical
- environmental

Illness can be caused by stressors from any one of these categories. Just as one example, allergies can be the result of a poor diet (biochemical stress) or a spinal misalignment (structural stress) or exposure to toxic chemicals (environmental stress) or emotional problems (psychological stress). Any of these factors can compromise your immunity.

Once a stress is encountered, your biochemistry will always be affected, regardless of the point of origin of the stress. That's why it's always important to make sure you eat a metabolically appropriate diet. However, in order to resolve the stress and any resulting health problems, the causal level must be addressed.

For instance, let's say you have a misaligned vertebrae that is causing irritation of your vagus nerve and overstimulation of your parasympathetic system. This is a structural stress that could easily produce hay fever, allergies, asthma, and all sorts of other health problems. Obviously you wouldn't be able to resolve these health issues just by eating the right diet. You would need to remove the cause of the problem by having a spinal adjustment.

Or let's say you're experiencing problems like chronic fatigue or headaches or depression as the result of a psychological stress such as a divorce from your spouse, or an environmental stress such as exposure to toxic chemicals at your job. Although diet could help alleviate your symptoms to some degree, you would not be able to fully resolve these problems just by optimizing your nutritional protocol. Instead you would want to take specific steps—like seeking counseling or getting a new job—to remove or neutralize these psychological or environmental causal factors.

The chart below provides a sampling of typical stressors that can either cause or contribute to the development of virtually any illness.

WHAT'S MAKING ME SICK?

CAUSAL FACTORS OF ILLNESS

Commonly Occurring Stressors

Psychological	Structural	Biochemical	Environmental
harmful beliefs, attitudes	cranial stress	wrong diet for metabolic type	mercury dental fillings
negative emotions	TMJ stress	sugar	other metal fillings
anger	spinal stress	alcohol	manufacturing pollution
fear	insufficient exercise	tobacco smoke	pesticides, herbicides
resentment	accident	preservatives	
worry	surgeries	synthetic foods	new building syndrome
traumatic events	falls	junk foods	allergens
marriage	blows to head	microwaved foods	work-related chemical exposure
divorce		tap water	
death of loved one		chemical food additives	paint fumes
death of pet		prescription drugs	lawn/garden chemicals
job stress or loss		caffeine	hair dyes
illness in family		hydrogenated fats/oils	chemical deodorant, perfume
financial loss		food allergies	dental root canals
relocating		menopause or andropause	
		fat restriction	electromagnetic pollution
		salt restriction	geopathic stress
		caloric restriction	parasitic infection
			lack of sunlight

Although diet provides an essential foundation for good health, it's not always the total solution. Many different types of stress also play a role in the development of illness. To optimize your health, follow a metabolically appropriate diet and minimize your exposure to the kinds of common stressors listed above.

If you've been following every aspect of your recommended nutritional protocol but have not yet achieved the results you desire, it may be time to investigate factors beyond diet. Or, if you're eating well and feeling great but want to ensure that you continue to maintain a high level of health, you'll definitely want to optimize other key aspects of your lifestyle as well.

The following pages contain many practical tips and essential information about how to avoid or minimize the risk of health problems due to structural, environmental, or psychological stress.

As you pursue these lifestyle considerations, however, please try to be consistent in maintaining the right kind of dietary regime, since it will optimize your body's ability to resolve structural, environmental, or psychological challenges. Conversely, a metabolically inappropriate diet can significantly worsen problems of nondietary origin.

Of course, if you have persistent health problems, it's advisable to check with your doctor. Needless to say, it's always a good idea to consult with physicians and other licensed health professionals who are very tuned in to the critical importance of diet and lifestyle considerations.

STRUCTURAL THERAPY

Staying Well with Chiropractic Care

The proper functioning of your nervous system is essential to the maintenance of good health. In turn, your nervous system is dependent upon a properly aligned spinal column and vertebrae. Here's a helpful analogy: If your body can be likened to a car, think of nutrition as the gasoline and your nervous system as the car's electrical system.

Your nervous system is the master regulator of your metabolism, but if the vertebrae in your spine are out of alignment, they can exert pressure on various nerves and inhibit their ability to function normally. And when the nerve flow to various internal organs is interrupted, all kinds of metabolic disturbances can develop. In this case, nutrition will be limited in what it can do for you, in the same way that gasoline would be of little help if your car's electrical system is malfunctioning.

Many things can cause misalignments in the spine (known as subluxations), including excess physical exertion, bad posture, poor muscle tone, genetic weaknesses, a sedentary lifestyle, nutritional deficiencies, or any kind of physical or emotional trauma. But a chiropractor can restore normal nerve function by adjusting the spinal joints to remove subluxations. When the vertebrae are properly aligned, the spine remains mobile, and electrical impulses from the brain can then travel freely to the internal organs and glands.

Because of its effectiveness in correcting back problems, traumatic injuries, head and neck stiffness and pain, and pains in the extremities—and its ability to resolve or improve many kinds of physiological problems—chiropractic is now the second-largest primary health care field in the world. Each year in the United States alone, many millions of people turn to chiropractors for a natural, drug-free treatment approach to curing common ailments. Since its emergence in the late nineteenth century, the chiropractic profession has gained broad acceptance, despite many years of controversy and political battles with the orthodox medical community.

There are many different types of chiropractic physicians, just as there are different kinds of specialists within medicine. Some chiropractors deal only with locating and correcting subluxations in the spine, while others adopt a more integrated approach by offering adjunctive techniques such as massage, diet and lifestyle counseling, heat therapy, electrical stimulation, and applied kinesiology.

Some chiropractors prefer to use "nonforce" techniques in which gentle pressure is applied to the spine, skull, and pelvis, and no "popping" sounds are heard when vertebral subluxations are corrected. Many also employ kinesiology as a diagnostic tool to detect weaknesses in internal organs and related spinal misalignments.

Various forms of massage, including deep tissue massage, are often a very important adjunct to spinal manipulation. When your muscles are functioning properly (i.e., free of tension and spasms and blockages), they help keep your spine in alignment. This is because your musculature is inextricably linked to your skeletal system. As a result, chiropractic adjustments tend to "hold" much longer when strained muscles are corrected through massage therapy.

There are many excellent chiropractors throughout the country. Often the best way to locate a good one is to ask knowledgeable friends or relatives whom they would recommend. For information on chiropractic, contact the American Chiropractic Association in Arlington, Virginia (703) 276-8800. For more information and resources on structural therapies, visit the Web site of Dr. June Wieder at: www.drwieder.com or call (877) 679-9978, ext. 158.

An Essential but Overlooked Factor: Cranial Balance

One of the most overlooked but vitally important systems in the body is the craniosacral system, which links the cranium (the bones of the skull) with the sacrum (the base of the spine). The system is comprised of the skull, vertebral column, brain, and spinal column, which all work together in a well-orchestrated, interdependent manner.

Few people realize that the cranial sacral system contracts and expands slightly, in a subtle rhythmic cycle, six to twelve times per minute. The twenty-two bones of the skull, which are held together by soft tissue sutures, are constantly being moved by the cranial rhythmic impulse, which in turn facilitates the constant flow of cerebrospinal fluid between the brain and the spinal cord.

The proper functioning or mobility of the bones in the skull is vitally important to the maintenance of good health. That's why some structural therapists specialize in cranial therapy, which involves gentle manipulations of the sutures of the skull bones to keep them flexible. If the cranial bones become stuck, jammed together, or "frozen in place," the entire spinal column, craniosacral system, and nervous system are negatively affected.

This can lead to any number of painful symptoms, metabolic disturbances, and chronic health disorders. Unfortunately, because of a generalized lack of public awareness and a shortage of skilled cranial therapists (also known as craniopaths or craniosacral therapists), health problems caused by cranial disturbances often go undiagnosed.

In modern society, cranial problems are extremely common. A primary reason for this is that malnutrition has been very prevalent now for several generations. As a result, many people have been born with defects in their skeletal system, especially underdeveloped facial and jawbones. This often creates very significant misalignments in the bite. And the bite, in turn, is what pushes the cranial bones into proper position. Without a properly balanced bite, the cranial bones are subject to distortion.

In isolated or primitive societies where nutrition is very adequate, people tend to be born with excellent, fully developed facial bones, jaw bones, and dental arches. This generally means that: 1.) their lower jaw "fits" properly into the upper part of their skull, and 2.) their teeth are well formed and properly aligned. As a result, people tend to have effectively balanced bites and well-functioning craniosacral systems.

However, poor bone structure is not the only factor that distorts the bite and interferes with cranial balance. Many kinds of dental procedures—such as tooth extractions and orthodontic procedures— also exert a powerful and immediate effect on cranial bones, often pushing them into a jammed or misaligned position. This is true even for people in modern society who happen to have good bone structure and balanced bites. Accidents or any form of head trauma can also push the cranial bones out of whack.

Fortunately, growing numbers of health professionals throughout the world today are becoming aware of the important interdependency between the bite and the cranial bones. This has created a very promising new clinical phenomenon in which dentists and chiropractors (those specializing in cranial therapy) are joining forces for the purpose of providing patients with integrated care.

The Vitally Important Cranial/Dental Link

Your lower jawbone is known as your mandible, and it is connected to, or swings into, the temporal bone in your head. That is why the joint that connects your jaw with your head is called the temporo-mandibular joint, and why imbalances in your bite are referred to as TMJ problems. Since TMJ is a very common problem, many dentists treat it with "splints" or "bite plates." These plastic retainer-like devices are usually worn at night and offer a temporary means of adjusting the bite in order to reduce head and neck pain and to prevent teeth grinding, typical TMJ symptoms. Dentists also routinely adjust the bite (dentists refer to the bite as "occlusion") by raising or lowering the height of the teeth in a permanent way.

Unfortunately, many dentists who treat TMJ or similar occlusion problems focus all their attention on only one aspect of the problem—the jaw. They're often unaware that an occlusion or bite problem is really a two-part problem: there is the jaw component and the cranial component. Many chiropractors address TMJ symptoms (i.e., head and neck pain) in a similarly one-dimensional way. They usually focus on vertebral adjustments or massage but don't get involved with the dental or cranial aspects of the problem. This leaves patients with relatively few places to turn for substantive solutions to dental/cranial problems and related metabolic disorders.

However, in some parts of the world—especially England and

Australia, and to a lesser degree in the United States—significant and growing numbers of dentists and chiropractors are collaborating with one another for the purpose of offering patients interdisciplinary solutions to the TMJ dilemma and related dental and structural problems. This dual approach is sometimes referred to as chirodontics. It's an exciting emerging field comprised of dental experts and structural therapists.

One of the world's leading experts in chirodontics is Dr. Robert Walker. He's based in Australia, although he regularly travels the globe to teach health professionals about the crucial synergy between dentistry and chiropractic and related disciplines. For more information on *chirodontics* and for referrals to American and European clinicians trained in this field, visit Dr. Walker's Web site at: www.chirodontics.com.

If you have TMJ problems, you may also want to investigate a company called Accu-Liner, at www.accu-liner.com. It manufactures a relatively simple diagnostic tool that is used to determine how people's bites need to be modified, from a cranial perspective as well as a jaw perspective. If your dentist is already using the Accu-Liner tool and/or works in tandem with a cranial therapist to address TMJ problems, it's likely that he/she is up to speed in the rapidly evolving area of chirodontics. The Accu-Liner company is based in Seattle, Washington (800) 458-6627. It was founded in 1989 by Jim Carlson, D.D.S., who, along with his son, Paul Carlson, now teaches clinicians across the United States about the latest advances in dental/cranial therapy. The Carlsons work closely with Runar Johnson, D.D.S., a Seattle-based clinical expert, (425) 455-1583, who helped develop the Accu-Liner.

For more information on cranial therapy contact: The Upledger Institute (561) 622-4334 or Kathleen Cliff, L.M.P., the originator of cranial sacral fulcrum therapy. Call (425) 885-6018 for information on workshops and other services.

Nontoxic Dentistry

Today there are thousands of dentists across the United States who practice a form of dentistry known as biological dentistry. This means that they use nontoxic dental restoration materials, and are "holistically oriented." In other words, they're aware of the very serious harmful effects that certain kinds of dental materials and dental procedures can have on the entire body.

European researchers estimate that up to half of all degenerative diseases may be directly or indirectly related to modern dental practices that involve the use of toxic, allergy-producing, or electrically charged metals, infections associated with root canals, problems with specific teeth in relation to acupuncture meridians, and TMJ. Sadly, vast numbers of people spend years searching for answers to chronic health problems, never realizing that the primary cause of their suffering may actually be in their mouths.

In recent years there has been lots of controversy surrounding the use of mercury amalgams (comprised of silver and mercury) to fill cavities. While all metals used in dental or orthodontic procedures can be toxic, many experts believe that mercury is the most dangerous. Mercury has been recognized as a poisonous substance for centuries, and the Environmental Protection Agency regards it as a hazardous waste that requires special handling. In Germany, the use of mercury amalgams has been banned since the early 1990s. Other European countries routinely issue public health advisories against the use of mercury fillings, especially for pregnant women.

The United States has been very slow to take action on this issue, chiefly because the dental establishment claims that mercury is safe when used in combination with other metals. Yet many clinicians insist that there is a wealth of evidence to show that mercury amalgams often cause allergies, chronic fatigue, immune dysfunction, thyroid deficiency, intestinal problems, headaches, depression, cardiovascular irregularities, memory loss, neuropathy, rheumatoid arthritis, dizziness, intestinal problems, and a host of other disorders.

Root canals are another potential health hazard. As early as the 1930s, Dr. Weston Price claimed that pockets of infection beneath root canals may cause cardiovascular disease, kidney disease, and disorders of the nervous and endocrine systems. Today, overwhelming numbers of biological dentists agree with this perspective. Since root canal seals are somewhat permeable, bacteria can easily penetrate and thrive in these oxygen-starved environments. This produces chronic infections and resulting toxins that escape into the body and have the potential to interfere with normal metabolic functions.

Although there is widespread agreement among biological dentists that root canals can create serious health problems, there are differences of opinion as to how to resolve the problem. Some dentists are convinced that the best solution is tooth extraction. Others believe that new procedures like laser treatment to kill bacteria, combined with the use of nontoxic root canal filler material (such as Bio Kalyx from France), offers a good alternative in many cases.

Yet another way in which modern dental practices can lead to chronic degenerative conditions is through the electrical conductivity of metal fillings or crowns. This is a phenomenon with which I have a great deal of personal experience. The mineral content of your saliva acts as a "conductant." This means it can combine with various kinds of metal alloys to create an actual electrical current.

If the electrical charge given off by a filling or crown is strong enough, it can irritate a remote organ or gland through the meridian system. As you may know, acupuncture is based on the concept of meridians—pathways of energy that run up and down your body and correspond to individual organs and organ systems. All your upper and lower teeth are also associated with specific internal organs through meridians.

About five years ago, I needed a crown for one of my lower right teeth. Since I prefer not to have any metal in my mouth, I requested a porcelain crown, and my dentist complied with my request. Shortly thereafter, however, I began to develop hypoglycemic problems quite unlike anything I had ever experienced before. Over the course of a year my condition deteriorated to an extraordinary degree, to the point where I was in very bad shape and literally had to eat every two hours, even in the middle of the night.

Then one day I happened to glance at a dental meridian chart and noticed that the pancreas is associated with the very same tooth that had the porcelain crown. Soon I consulted another dentist who had equipment to detect electrical currents in the mouth. Sure enough, there was an extremely powerful electrical charge coming off the tooth in question. To my surprise, I discovered that the crown I thought was made entirely of porcelain actually had a metal underjacket. I immediately had it removed and replaced with a crown made of nonmetal composite material. On that day, my very severe hypoglycemia disappeared and has never returned.

I later learned that the electrical charge from this particular tooth was causing a 24-hour-a-day irritation to the pancreas. This resulted in a loss of normal regulatory control over insulin secretion. My pancreas was being continuously overstimulated, and this had a disastrous effect on my blood sugar balance and overall health.

As you can see, dentistry can be a very challenging arena. It's easy for people to feel overwhelmed by some of the issues involved. But the good news is that awareness is the critical first step in resolving any problem, and there really are good options and alternatives available to those who take the time to do some research.

Remember that it's always best to investigate issues on your own and get a number of opinions on any given topic. Don't necessarily rely on what any dentist tells you, whether he or she is a biological dentist or a traditional dentist. Do your homework and rely on your own best judgment. Also, talk to friends who are knowledgeable in the area of biological dentistry and learn from their experiences. As in any area, it's best to consult with clinicians who come highly recommended by people whose judgment you trust.

Bear in mind that it's highly unlikely that any single clinician will have all the expertise you need. For instance, if your dentist is a top expert in the area of structural problems like TMJ, chances are he or she will not have the in-depth expertise you might need in other areas such as nontoxic dental restoration. You may need different types of dental specialists for different kinds of procedures. Here are some excellent information resources:

Information

Dr. Douglas L. Cook, D.D.S., 10971 Clinic Road, Surling, Wisconsin 54174, tel.: (920) 842-2083, fax: (920) 842-4203, E-mail: dlcook1@ez-net.com.

Dr. Cook is a leading expert in biological dentistry. He can provide information on many important topics, such as how to identify the safest possible composite materials for fillings and crowns (i.e., materials that are most "biocompatible").

Environmental Dental Association, 9974 Scripps Ranch Boulevard, Suite 36, San Diego, California, 92131, tel.: (800) 388-8124.

The Environmental Dental Association is an organization of alternative dentists that provides books and other information products to the public. For a free packet of literature, call their toll-free number.

DAMS (Dental Amalgam Mercury Syndrome) is an excellent nonprofit educational and advocacy group that provides free information packets to consumers on dental toxins and related health issues. For information, call (800) 311-6265 or visit: www.amalgam.org.

Books

The Key to Ultimate Health by Richard T. Hansen, D.M.D., FACAD, Advanced Health Research, Fullerton, California, tel.: (888) 792-1102. This book covers a broad range of important current topics in the field of biological dentistry.

Uninformed Consent: The Hidden Dangers in Dental Care by Hal Huggins, D.D.S., and Thomas Levy, M.D., Charlottesville, VA: Hampton Roads Publishing, 1999.

Whole Body Dentistry: Discover the Missing Piece to Better Health by Mark Breiher, D.D.S., Fairfield, CT: Quantum Health Press, 1999.

Newsletters

Dental & Health Facts, published by Sam Ziff, founder of the Foundation for Toxic-Free Dentistry, P.O. Box 608010, Orlando, Florida 32860-8010.

eHealthy News is a free online newsletter published by Dr. Joseph Mercola, a highly regarded alternative medical practitioner. The biweekly newsletter contains up-to-the-minute information on a wide range of health topics, including important dental issues. To subscribe, visit Dr. Mercola's Web site at: www.mercola.com.

Water: The Most Vital Nutrient

Did you know that your body is composed of approximately 87 percent water? That's why it's not an exaggeration to say that water is our most vital nutrient. You can live for many days without food, but the average length of survival without water is just three days. A loss of a mere 10 to 20 percent of the water in your body would be fatal. Water carries nutrients and oxygen to your cells, acts as a natural cooling system, provides a protective cushion for your tissues, and is essential to digestion and the removal of metabolic waste products through perspiration and urine. When you don't drink enough water, the fluid volume in your system decreases, your blood thickens, and it becomes very difficult for your body to detoxify or your cells to receive adequate nourishment.

Many people are unaware that dehydration is a very widespread problem that routinely causes breakdowns in fundamental physiological processes. Symptoms may include headache, fatigue, chronic pain, high blood pressure, and digestive disturbances. Interestingly, the point at which your mouth goes dry usually represents an advanced stage of dehydration. To avoid the problems associated with dehydration, be sure to drink at least three quarts of water each day (between meals), and increase that to a gallon when the weather is warm or you're perspiring a lot due to physical exertion. Note that juice, soda, tea, alcohol, and other beverages are not adequate substitutes for pure water, since they often contain substances that act as diuretics. For important information on the effects of dehydration, read *Your Body's Many Cries for Water* by F. Batmanghelidj, M.D., Global Health Solutions, 1992. Call (703) 848-2333 to obtain the book.

As important as the amount of water you consume is the quality of water you are drinking. As you know, many of our rivers, lakes, and underground water supplies (aquifers) have been heavily contaminated by herbicides, pesticides, fertilizers, acid rain, heavy metals such as arsenic and lead, radioactive wastes, and thousands of industrial chemicals. Yet many public water purification systems, now 30 to 40 years old, were designed to treat good-quality water for bacteria, not to eliminate the kinds of chemical toxins that now saturate the environment. Besides, expecting public health officials to effectively purify the millions of gallons of water used every day in local areas is neither feasible nor practical, especially when only about 1 percent of the water is used for human consumption. That's why the best solution is to have "end user" purification, i.e., a water purification system in your own home. Needless to say, it's not wise to drink tap water!

There are three basic types of water purification methods: filtration, distillation, and reverse osmosis. Filtration devices such as granular charcoal and solid block carbon remove particulate matter and metals such as lead and cadmium but generally lack the ability to remove organic chemicals (and suspected carcinogens) such as fluorine. Although distillation was a great option for many years, that was before the widespread introduction of chlorine. In the distillation process, particulate matter tends to bind with chlorine to form toxic compounds that are converted into a gaseous state but then recondense into freshly distilled water. Reverse osmosis systems use an advanced membrane technology that removes bacteria as well as chemical contaminants, so they're probably the best choice for most situations.

However, all purification methods have their limitations, so you'll want to shop around and do plenty of research before choosing a system for home use. You may also want to have your water supply (i.e., your tap) tested by an independent laboratory to determine the extent of contamination. This will help you choose the best system for your particular situation. There are many good labs and equipment suppliers nationwide, but here's one I like: Ozark Water Services & Air Quality, 114 Spring Street, Sulphur Springs, Arkansas 72768-0218. Tel.: (800) 835-8908.

If you do use bottled water, it's a good idea to buy it in glass bottles as opposed to plastic containers, which generally leach traces of chemicals into the water. The brands that come in glass bottles are more expensive, but many of them taste great and are of superior quality. Try Mountain Valley Water, available in most supermarkets.

Filter Toxins from Shower Water

Believe it or not, your exposure to toxic chemicals is even worse in the shower than it is through your tap! Studies by the Environmental Protection Agency have shown that people can obtain up to sixty percent more volatile chemicals from bathing and showering than they would absorb by drinking the same water. The reason for this is that hot water creates a steam vapor that gets inhaled and goes directly into the bloodstream. That's why it's a great idea to get a shower filter to reduce chlorine and other chemicals, and heavy metals. For shower filters and other products to enhance the quality of your home environment, check out the Healthy Home Center in Clearwater, Florida (www.healthyhome.com).

Simple Ways to Purify Your Air

Unfortunately, our atmosphere has been saturated with tens of thousands of man-made chemicals and toxins. For many people, this situation is made worse by spending hours each day in fresh-air-starved office buildings, and hours more in airtight, fuel-efficient houses loaded with indoor air pollutants from "outgassing" carpets, furniture, fabrics, and building construction materials. This "sick-building syndrome" is exacerbated during the winter months in colder climates, when outside air flow is at a minimum and indoor air quality drops through the use of wood stoves, gas furnaces, and so on.

Yet the oxygenation of all your body tissues is essential to good health. For example, cancer thrives in an anaerobic (without oxygen) environment. That's why it's important to get plenty of fresh air and exercise (and to do deep breathing) on a daily basis. You might also want to consider the use of an air purification device. Here again, there are many options to choose from, including HEPA (high-efficiency particulate attentuation) filters, electrostatic furnace filters, ozone machines, and negative-ion generators. Check out the Cutting Edge Catalog (www.cutcat.com) in Southampton, New York, for great up-to-date information on air purification.

Alternatively, here's a "low-tech" approach to purifying your air:

Consider the strategic use of houseplants! Researchers have found that many common houseplants thrive on the very chemicals that make humans ill and can neutralize many indoor air pollutants. Some experts believe that just fifteen to twenty houseplants such as English ivy, Chinese evergreens, corn plants, spider plants, weeping figs, and Boston ferns have the capacity to purify an 1800-square-foot home. Read *How to Grow Fresh Air: 50 Houseplants That Purify Your Home or Office* by B. C. Wolverton.

Another Vital Nutrient: Natural Light

Like food, water, and oxygen, sunlight is a vital nutrient necessary for all life-sustaining metabolic processes. Many experts believe that ongoing exposure to poor light poses a serious health risk. Poor light is defined as any kind that does not contain the full wavelength spectrum found in natural sunlight. Most artificial lighting, both incandescent and fluorescent, is not full spectrum. In addition, windows, windshields, eyeglasses, and air pollution all filter out parts of the light spectrum and contribute to this problem.

Studies show that deficient lighting interferes with the body's ability to absorb nutrients and contributes to problems such as fatigue, tooth decay, depression, hostility, immune suppression, hair loss, skin damage, strokes, alcoholism, seasonal affective disorder, Alzheimer's disease, and even cancer. Sunlight is also the primary source of vitamin D, which plays many important roles in human health. That's why it's important for everyone to try to be outdoors a minimum of 30 minutes each day, exposed to natural light and fresh air.

Throughout history, light has been highly valued for its healing properties, and today "light therapy" is an important emerging discipline. Various forms of light therapy—including natural sunlight, full-spectrum light, colored light, and ultraviolet light—are currently being investigated by major hospitals and research centers worldwide. Experts believe there are many ways in which light can be used to improve people's physical and psychological well-being. Many light therapy devices, including full-spectrum light bulbs, are now widely available for use at home or in the office.

Some clinicians predict that in the future people will regard exposure to natural light as a very basic component of a healthful lifestyle, in the same way they now regard diet and exercise as fundamental to health and well-being. For information on the effect of light on human health, read *Health & Light*, by John Nash Ott, Old Greenwich, CT: The Devin-Adair CO., 1988. For information on the use of light in the treatment of depression, visual problems, stress, learning disabilities, weakened immunity, PMS, and various kinds of cancer, read *Light: Medicine of the Future,* by Jacob Liberman.

Steer Clear of Electromagnetic Fields

Our environment is full of electromagnetic fields (EMFs) produced by electrical wiring and appliances in our homes and offices. Scores of scientists and researchers worldwide believe that these fields exert subtle but very damaging effects on human health. Many professionals remain skeptical of the dangers of EMF environmental pollution. However, even the United States Congress's Office of Technology Assessment recommends a policy of prudent avoidance of EMFs.

Stay at least five feet from microwave ovens and all kitchen and laundry appliances when they are in operation. Don't stand near copy machines or fax machines while operating. Always stay at least three feet from TV screens and the backs and sides of computers. Sit two to three feet away from your computer screen and use computer shields or low-radiation monitors. Use cell phones as little as possible. In your bedroom, keep appliances such as radios, alarm clocks, and lights at least three feet from your head and use battery-powered units when possible. Don't use hair dryers on children and minimize your own use of them. Use the lowest settings and keep them at least eight inches from your head. Don't use electric toothbrushes or razors or sleep under electric blankets or heating pads.

To measure the amount of electromagnetic radiation in your home or office, use a Gauss meter, a small and easy-to-use device available from many suppliers, including Safe Technologies, (800) 638-9121, and the Cutting Edge (800) 497-9516. These devices (which start at around $35) will show which spots in your home or office are safe from chronic EMF exposure and which spots you need to avoid. Before moving into a new house, apartment, or office, always test for high electromagnetic field levels. Also avoid living or working near power lines or generators. For more information read *Cross Currents: The Perils of Electropollution and the Promise of Electromedicine* by Robert O. Becker, M.D.

Avoid Toxic Household and Personal Products

What if you learned that a majority of the household products in your kitchen cupboard and the personal care items in your bathroom cabinet contain chemical ingredients that the Environmetal Protection Agency has designated as known or suspected carcinogens? The list of toxic chemicals contained in the products you buy and use every day—from hair spray and floor wax to cosmetics and weed killer—is endless.

Consider this: Most household cleaning agents are extremely hazardous (containing substances like ammonia, chlorine, phenol, ethanol, and formaldehyde) and can damage the liver, lungs, kidneys, and central nervous system. White paper products like towels, napkins, and tissues contain dioxin, a by-product that is formed when chlorine is used to bleach brown wood pulp white. Dioxin causes immune suppression, miscarriages, birth defects, and genetic damage and this is documented in animal studies. Deodorants contain aluminum, which has been linked to Alzheimer's disease. Many brands of lipstick and mascara contain PVP, a plastic resin that is a suspected carcinogen.

These are just a few examples of the toxic burden most of us confront on a daily basis. And, as Joseph D. Beasley, M.D., author of *The Betrayal of Health,* explains, the cumulative effect of these chemical "stressors" poses a major health hazard. So it makes good sense to avoid as many of them as you possibly can. Here are two books that provide hundreds of simple and practical alternatives to the unhealthy and ecologically unsafe products that currently clutter up and contaminate our lives: *Better Basics for the Home: Simple Solutions for Less Toxic Living,* by Annie Berthold-Bond, and *Home Safe Home: Protecting Yourself and Your Family from Everyday Toxics and Harmful Household Products,* by Debra Lynn Dadd, Putnam, 1997.

Uniquely Modern Health Hazards: Heavy Metals

Many people in modern societies are continuously exposed to high concentrations of heavy metals. Unfortunately, these toxic contaminants have become an integral part of our industrialized culture. Metals like aluminum, cadmium, lead, and mercury are commonly found in thousands of different food products, household products, personal products, and untold numbers of industrial products and chemicals.

Heavy metals accumulate in the body's vital organs and tissues (e.g., brain, liver, kidneys, spleen, and pancreas), thereby disrupting their ability to function normally. They also displace "good" minerals (e.g., calcium, magnesium, and zinc) that are necessary for vital enzyme reactions. In this way, heavy metals are often the primary cause of a very broad range of serious degenerative disorders.

The following chart summarizes the sources of each of nine heavy metals as well as their adverse effects on the body. If your job or living circumstances expose you to any of these toxic metals, I strongly urge you to minimize or eliminate your exposure as much as possible. Be aware that there are many ways these toxins can be absorbed into your body—through foods and beverages, skin exposure, and via the air you breathe. Whenever possible, wear gloves, use protective breathing apparatuses, and be sure there is adequate ventilation.

Although eliminating exposure entirely is almost impossible, the good news is that you can prevent heavy metals from collecting in your body. You can also get rid of them if they've already accumulated in your organs and tissues. The best way to do this is to balance your body chemistry by following the appropriate metabolic typing program. This will enable your body to pick up ("chelate") the heavy metals, mobilize them out of tissue storage sites, and eradicate them entirely from your system. Many health professionals use hair analyses to track the mobilization of heavy metals out of the body.

HOW HEAVY METALS HARM

HEAVY METAL	SOURCES	POSSIBLE EFFECTS
Aluminum	alum, aluminum foil, animal feed, antacids, aspirin, auto exhaust, baking powder, commercially-raised beef, bleached flour, cans, ceramics, commercial cheese, cigarette filters, color additives, construction materials, cookware, cosmetics, some dental amalgams, deodorants, drinking water, drying agents, dust, insulated wiring, medicinal compounds, milk products, nasal spray, pesticides, pollution, salt, tap water, tobacco smoke, some toothpaste, treated water, vanilla powder	ALS, Alzheimer's, anemia, appetite loss, behavioral problems, cavities, colds, colitis, confusion, constipation, dementia, dry mouth, dry skin, energy loss, excessive perspiration, flatuence, headaches, heartburn, hyperactivity, inhibition of enzyme systems, kidney dysfunction, lowered immune function, learning disabilities, leg twitching, liver dysfunction, memory loss, neuromuscular disorders, numbness, osteoporosis, paralysis, Parkinson's disease, peptic ulcer, psychosis, reduced intestinal activity, senility, skin problems, spleen pain, stomach pain, weak and aching muscles
Arsenic	burning of arsenate treated building materials, coal combustion, insect sprays, pesticides, soils (arsenic rich), seafood from coastal waters, especially muscles, oysters, and shrimp	abdominal pain, anorexia, brittle nails, diarrhea, nausea, vomiting, chronic anemia, burning in mouth/esophagus/stomach/bowel, confusion, convulsions, dermatitis, drowsiness, enzyme inhibition, garlicky odor to breath/stool, hair loss, headaches, hyper-pigmentation of nails and skin, increased risk of liver/lung/skin cancers, low-grade fever, mucus in nose and throat, muscle aches/spasms/weakness, nervousness, respiratory tract infection, swallowing difficulty, sweet metallic taste, throat corstriction
Beryllium	coal burning, manufacturing, household cleaners, industrial dust	disturbance of calcium and vitamin D metabolism, magnesium depletion, lung cancer, lung infection, rickets, vital organ dysfunction

HOW HEAVY METALS HARM

HEAVY METAL	SOURCES	POSSIBLE EFFECTS
Cadmium	airborne industrial contaminants, batteries, candy, ceramics, cigarette smoke, colas, congenital intoxication, copper refineries, copper alloys, dental alloys, tap water, electroplating fertilizers, food from contaminated soil, fungicides, incineration of tires/rubber/plastic, instant coffee, iron roots, kidney, liver, marijuana, processed meat, evaporated milk, motor oil, oysters, paint, pesticides, rubber, galvanized pipes, processed foods, refined grains/flour cereals, rubber, rubber carpet backing, seafoods (cod, haddock, oyster, tuna), sewage, silver polish, smelters, soft water, solders (including in food cans), tobacco, vending machine soft drinks, tools, vapor lamps, water (city, softened, well), welding material	alcoholism, alopecia, anemia, arthritis (osteo and rheumatoid), bone disease, bone pain in middle of bones, cancer, cardiovascular disease, cavities, cerebral hemorrhage, cirrhosis, diabetes, digestive disturbances, emphysema, enlarged heart, flulike symptoms, growth impairment, headaches, high cholesterol, hyperkinetic behavior, hypertension, hypoglycemia, impotence, inflammation, infertility, kidney disease, learning disorders, liver damage, lung disease, migraines, nerve cell damage, osteoporosis, prostate dysfunction, reproductive disorders, schizophrenia, stroke
Copper	congenital intoxication, copper cookware, copper IUDs, copper pipes, dental alloys, fungicides, ice makers, industrial emissions, insecticides, swimming pools, water (city/well), welding, avocado, beer, bluefish, bone metal, chocolate, corn oil, crabs, gelatin, grains, lamb, liver, lobster, margarine, milk, mushrooms, nuts, organ meats, oysters, perch, seeds, shellfish, soybeans, tofu, wheat germ, yeast, birth control pills (elevate copper levels in the body)	acne, adrenal insufficiency, allergies, alopecia, anemia, anorexia, anxiety, arthritis (osteo and rheumatoid), autism, cancer, cystic fibrosis, depression, diabetes, digestive disorders, dry mouth, dysinsulinism, estrogen dominance, fatigue, fears, fractures, fungus, heart attack, high blood pressure, high cholesterol, Hodgkin's disease, hyperactivity, hypertension, hyperthyroid, low hydrochloric acid, hypoglycemia, infections, inflammation, insomnia, iron loss, jaundice, kidney disorders, libido decreased, lymphoma, mental illness, migraines, mood swings, multiple sclerosis, myocardial infarction, nausea, nervousness, osteoporosis, pancreatic dysfunction, panic attacks, paranoia, phobias, PMS, schizophrenia, senility, sexual dysfunction, spacey feeling, stuttering, stroke, tooth decay, toxemia of pregnancy, urinary tract infection, yeast infection

HOW HEAVY METALS HARM

HEAVY METAL	SOURCES	POSSIBLE EFFECTS
Iron	drinking water, iron cookware, iron pipes, welding, foods: black-strap molasses, bone meal, bran, chives, clam, heart, kidney, leafy vegetables, legumes, liver, meat, molasses, nuts, organ meats, oysters, parsley, red wine, refined foods, shellfish, soybeans, wheat germ, whole grains	amenorrhea, anger, rheumatoid arthritis, birth defects, bleeding gums, cancer, constipation, diabetes, dizziness, emotional problems, fatigue, headache, heart damage, heart failure, hepatitis, high blood pressure, hostility, hyperactivity, infections, insomnia, irritability, joint pain, liver disease, loss of weight, mental problems, metallic taste in mouth, myasthenia gravis, nausea, pancreas damage, Parkinson's disease, premature aging, schizophrenia, scurvy, shortness of breath, stubbornness
Lead	ash, auto exhaust, battery manufacturing, bone meal, canned fruit and juice, cigarette smoke, coal combustion, colored inks, congenital intoxication, cosmetics, electroplating, household dust, glass production, hair dyes, industrial emissions, lead pipes, lead-glazed earthenware pottery, liver, mascara, metal polish, milk, newsprint, commercial organ meats, paint, pencils, pesticides, produce near roads, putty, rainwater, pvc containers, refineries, smelters, snow, tin cans with lead solder sealing (such as juices, vegetables), tobacco, toothpaste, tap water, wine	abdominal pain, adrenal insufficiency, allergies, anemia, anorexia, anxiety, arthritis (rheumatoid and osteo), attention deficit disorder, autism, back pain, behavioral disorders, blindness, cardiovascular disease, cartilage destruction, coordination loss, concentration loss, constipation, convulsions, deafness, depression, dyslexia, emotional instability, encephalitis, epilepsy, fatigue, gout, hallucinations, headaches, hostility, hyperactivity, hypertension, hypothyroid, impotence, immune suppression, decreased IQ, indigestion, infertility, insomnia, irritability, joint pain, kidney disorders, learning disability, liver dysfunction, loss of will, memory loss (long term), menstrual problems, mood swings, muscle aches, muscle weakness, muscular dystrophy, multiple sclerosis, myelopathy (spinal cord pathology), nausea, nephritis, nightmares, numbness, Parkinson's disease, peripheral neuropathies, psychosis, psychomotor dysfunction, pyorrhea, renal dysfunction, restlessness, retardation, schizophrenia, seizures, sterility, stillbirths, sudden infant death syndrome, tingling, tooth decay, vertigo, unintentional weight loss

HOW HEAVY METALS HARM

HEAVY METAL	SOURCES	POSSIBLE EFFECTS
Mercury	adhesives, air conditioner filters, algicides, antiseptics, battery manufacturing, body powders, broken thermometers, burning newspaper and building materials, calomel lotions, commercial cereals, congenital intoxication, cosmetics, dental amalgams, diuretics, fabric softeners, felt, floor waxes, fungicides, germicides, commercial grains, industrial waste, insecticides, laxatives, lumber, manufacture of paper and chlorine, medications, mercurochrome, paints, paper products, pesticides, photoengraving, polluted water, Preparation H, psoriasis ointment, seafoods (especially tuna and swordfish), sewage disposal, skin-lightening creams, some soft contact lens solutions, suppositories, tanning leather, tattooing, water (contaminated), wood preservatives	adrenal dysfunction, allergy, alopecia, anorexia, birth defects, blushing, brain damage, cataracts, cerebral palsy, poor coordination/jerky movements, deafness, depression, dermatitis, discouragement, dizziness, drowsiness, eczema, emotional disturbances, excess saliva, fatigue, gum bleeding and soreness, headaches (band type), hearing loss, hyperactivity, hypothyroidism, forgetfulness, immune dysfunction, insomnia, irritability, joint pain, kidney damage, loss of self-control, memory loss, mental retardation, metallic taste, migraines, nervousness, nerve fiber degeneration, numbness, pain in limbs, rashes, retinitis, schizophrenia, shyness, speech disorders, suicidal tendencies, tingling, tremors (eyelids, lips, tongue, fingers, extremities), vision loss, weakness
Nickel	butter, fertilizers, food processing, fuel oil combustion, hydrogenated fats and oils, imitation whipped cream, industrial waste, kelp, margarine, nuclear device testing, oysters, stainless steel cookware, tea, tobacco smoke, unrefined grains and cereals, vegetable shortening	anorexia, kidney dysfunction, apathy, disruption of hormone and lipid metabolism, fever, hemorrhages, headache, heart attack, intestinal cancer, low blood pressure, muscle tremors, nausea, oral cancer, skin problems, vomiting

Natural Solutions for
Women's Hormonal Imbalances

In recent decades, malnutrition has had an extremely negative impact on women's health. In previous generations, before the dawn of modern farming techniques, a wholesome food supply enabled women to maintain a healthy hormonal balance between estrogen and progesterone. This is because crops grown on nutrient-rich soils contained naturally occurring "phytoestrogens" and "phytoprogesterones." Unfortunately, these substances have all but disappeared today due to food processing and preservation techniques. The absence of these substances in commercially grown food has resulted in serious hormonal deficiencies and imbalances. This in turn has contributed to a situation peculiar to Western, industrialized societies—epidemic numbers of conditions like fibroid tumors, ovarian cysts, premenstrual syndrome, menstrual problems, menopausal problems, breast/ovarian/uterine cancers, and osteoporosis.

Since natural phytoestrogens and phytoprogesterones are no longer in our food supply, the need for natural hormone replacement therapy is now common. And, thanks to the pioneering research of John Lee, M.D., we now know that conditions like fibroids, PMS, and osteoporosis are often the result of a progesterone—not an estrogen—deficiency. Lee pointed out, for example, that even though estrogen can slow the rate of bone loss in osteoporosis, progesterone can actually reverse it.

As Lee and many other physicians point out, there are numerous hazards associated with the traditional use of synthetic hormone replacement therapy. This is apparent just by glancing through the list of side effects (see the *Physician's Desk Reference*) associated with drugs like Premarin and Provera. A much smarter course currently being adopted by progressive physicians is the use of readily available natural hormones.

An absolutely indispensable book for women is *What Your Doctor May NOT Tell You About Menopause,* by John Lee, M.D., Warner Books, 1996. It's a practical guide to natural hormone replacement therapy. However, it's actually a very valuable book for women of any age, because it covers an extensive range of female problems related to hormonal imbalances. Another good book on this topic is *Natural Hormone Replacement,* by Jonathan Wright, M.D., Smart Publications, 1997.

The natural hormone creams recommended by Dr. Lee and others are widely available in health food stores, or via mail order from places like Women's International Pharmacy, (800) 279-5708, or Professional Arts Pharmacy, (800) 832-9285.

The Unrecognized Epidemic: Parasitic Infections

Parasites are a very widespread but frequently undiagnosed source of illness in America today. A common misconception among health professionals and health consumers alike is that parasites are a problem only in third world countries, not in clean, modern, highly developed societies like our own.

Since many Western clinicians do not expect to encounter parasitic infections, they're simply not prepared either to recognize or to treat these conditions. Yet researchers estimate that up to twenty-five percent of the population in places like New York City are infected with one or more parasites. There are roughly three hundred varieties of parasites thriving in the United States today, including many different types of worms (e.g., tapeworms, roundworms, and hookworms), flukes (liver flukes and heart flukes), and amoebic organisms (e.g., Giardia lamblia), ranging in size from microscopic to twenty feet in length. Many of these unwanted invaders flourish in people's systems for years on end (primarily in the intestinal tract), without any awareness on the part of the host.

Parasites place a relentless burden on the immune system, rob the body of vital nutrients, poison the body with their toxic wastes, and disrupt normal metabolic functions. Common symptoms may include fever, asthma, coughing, abdominal pain, anemia, diarrhea, weakness, weight loss, nausea, chronic fatigue, arthritic pain, immune dysfunction, teeth grinding, irritable bowel syndrome, allergy, skin conditions, joint and muscle aches and pains, nervousness, sleep disturbances, and candida infections.

It's very easy to pick up parasites by eating undercooked food, by eating raw fruits and vegetables contaminated with parasite eggs, from contaminated drinking water, by exposure to household pets and other infected animals, in restaurants with inadequate sanitation practices, or from shaking hands with or other minimal exposure to infected individuals. Children are particularly susceptible to picking up parasites from contact with family pets or other children, and they in turn frequently spread parasites to other family members.

Sometimes doctors misdiagnose parasitic infections as bacterial infections and prescribe antibiotics, but of course antibiotics are of no use in these situations. Or, when physicians do recognize the problem, they often recommend synthetic drugs designed specifically to kill parasites. But drugs can't eradicate parasitic infections; the best they can do is suppress them temporarily. And when these infections recur after a course of drug therapy, they're often worse than they were originally.

One of the difficulties in dealing with parasites is that laboratory tests designed to detect them are unreliable; there is a very high incidence of false negative results. In other words, people often get negative test results even when they definitely have parasite infections. Another aspect to this problem is that most tests are designed to identify parasites in the GI tract, yet parasites (particularly the microscopic variety) can flourish in the respiratory tract and many other regions of the body.

Fortunately, there are a number of natural remedies that are very effective in eliminating parasite infections. For example, many cultures worldwide have used antiparasitic herbs successfully for centuries.

Currently, some of the best antiparasitic herbs I know of are available through *Healing Within Products*, P.O. Box 1013, Larkspur, California 94977-1013; tel.: (415) 454-6677. This company offers a wide selection of potent antiparasitic herbs imported from South America. They're expensive but superior products. The herbal formulations have been designed and made available in the United States by Hermann Bueno, M.D., a tropical disease expert who practices in New York City. For specific details on the use of these antiparasitic herbs, read the booklet *Parasites: An Epidemic in Disguise,* by Stanley Weinberger, available from *Healing Within Products.*

For more general information on parasitic infections, including their effects on the body and ways to avoid your exposure, read the booklet *Uninvited Guests,* by Hermann Bueno, M.D., Keats Publishing, 1996. Or the book *Guess What Came to Dinner: Parasites and Your Health,* by Ann Louise Gittleman, Avery Publishing, 1993. Ms. Gittleman's antiparasitic products (Para/Verma Systems) are also very effective. Call (800) 888-4353.

A particularly unique and valuable resource that covers parasitic infections and related topics is a newsletter called *Sharing Health from the Heart,* an inexpensive consumer publication available by subscription. Call (866) 777-4273 or write to Sharing Health Inc., P.O. Box 1817, Oroville, WA, 98844.

The *Sharing Health* newsletter contains a great deal of interesting and practical information on the use of electromagnetic devices (designed for consumer use) to neutralize infectious organisms of all kinds. For many years now, scientists worldwide have been actively researching the use of microcurrents of electricity to combat infections and to treat other kinds of health disorders. This appears to be a very promising emerging area in the realm of alternative medicine.

Another good resource is SOTA Instruments Incorporated, P.O. Box 1269, Revelstoke, BC, VOE 2S0 Canada; tel.: (800) 224-0242; Web site: www.sotainstruments.com. This company manufactures a range of innovative and relatively inexpensive electromagnetic consumer products designed by award-winning researcher/physicist Robert Beck and researcher Hulda Clark.

Hulda Clark is the author of *The Cure for All Diseases,* a widely available book that contains some interesting insights into the reasons parasites have achieved epidemic status in modern industrialized cultures and valuable tips on antiparasitic herbal regimes. Although Hulda Clark's herbal protocols are not as potent as Dr. Bueno's formulations, they've proven to be useful for some applications and far less expensive.

Remember though, whenever you're attempting to fight an infection of any kind, parasitic, yeast, bacterial, viral, the essential first step is to eat a metabolically appropriate diet! Without adequate nutrition you won't be able to mobilize your own natural immunity and you'll never manage to get the upper hand over the invading organisms. Eating right will immediately help to alleviate the symptoms of your infection and provide a foundation that will greatly enhance the efficacy of remedies such as herbs and other modalities used to zap the bugs.

Identifying Food Sensitivities

If you have food intolerances, you'll want to avoid eating the offending foods, at least for a while. This will enhance your ability to reestablish metabolic balance and efficiency, a necessary first step in eliminating the underlying cause of your allergy problems.

Until recently, the only available methods for identifying food allergies—elimination diets, skin tests, and certain blood tests—have been difficult, time-consuming, and subject to inaccuracy. However, within the last several years, a new kind of blood test has emerged, one that offers an efficient and precise way of identifying food sensitivities. The ALCAT test uses advanced electronic technology that detects highly specific changes in your blood cells when they're exposed to foods that you're allergic to. It eliminates the subjective nature of other types of blood tests and is less time-consuming than the trial-and-error approach of elimination diets. Most important, it picks up responses that may be mediated by both immune and nonimmunologic mechanisms.

It's important to correctly identify and eliminate the foods to which you are intolerant as a means of preserving the vital energy your body needs to repair and rebuild itself. The immune responses triggered by ingestion of offending foods needlessly divert energy from other, more important bodily processes.

You and your doctor can obtain more information about the ALCAT test by contacting American Medical Testing Laboratories (AMTL Corp.) at One Oakwook Boulevard, Suite 130, Hollywood, Florida, 33020; tel: (800) 881-2685 or (954) 923-2990. Web site: www.ALCAT.com.

Homeopathy: Healing for the Mind/Body/Spirit

For many of us living in the Western world, it's difficult to imagine that there might be more to human beings than what we can see or hear or touch. In the world's oldest and most advanced cultures, however, the physical or material realm is considered to be far less significant than the invisible, or "energetic," realm.

All the great ancient philosophies and medical traditions are based on the idea that a "life force" permeates and supports the health and well-being of every living thing. Although this sounds like a mystical notion, modern physics now endorses the concept that the world and everything in it is comprised entirely of vibrating energy fields—not solid objects, as Isaac Newton and his seventeenth-century colleagues once believed.

For centuries now, physicians, healers, and shamans from China, Japan, India, Tibet, Peru, Indonesia, Egypt, Greece, and Native American and Australian Aboriginal cultures have all shared the fundamental belief that human illness originates at an intangible, or metaphysical, level—a level well beyond ordinary physical reality.

In these systems, physical ailments have always been viewed as mere outward reflections of much deeper disturbances within the energy fields or emotional/spiritual dimensions of a human being. That's why healers through the ages have developed a rich and varied assortment of "vibrational" or "energetic" therapeutic modalities—acupuncture, shiatsu, qi gong, tai chi, and numerous other techniques involving the naturally occurring vibrations of light, color, sound, flowers, minerals, and herbs.

The idea is that we are all much more than "meat and bones" or "molecules and chemicals," and, therefore, healing approaches, in order to be effective, must somehow renew or enhance or facilitate the abundant invisible energy that gives us each life and breath.

Some people are intuitively aware of subtle energies, but if you're doubtful, here's a way to "tune in" to this invisible realm: Imagine yourself on a tropical island, soaking up sun while listening to the sounds of waves lapping against the shore. Or think about a mountain retreat full of wonderful vistas and the scent of pine trees and the peaceful sounds of birds or falling rain. These things are universally appealing to human beings. Why? Simply because we're all attuned to nature on an energetic level. Our own vibrational energy is profoundly affected by, connected to, and replenished by the vibrations of nature.

Many energetic healing approaches are well known for producing very tangible health benefits, but one of the most significant is homeopathy. It's actually one of the single largest and most successful medical disciplines in the world, now in use by an estimated five hundred million people around the globe.

Unlike drugs, herbs, and vitamins, homeopathic remedies have no chemical ingredients. Though they're made with naturally occurring substances from plants, minerals, and animals, they're so highly diluted (with water or alcohol) that no trace of the original chemical constituent remains in the remedies. Instead, they're believed to contain the "vibration," or "electromagnetic frequency," of the substances from which they're extracted.

The popularity of homeopathy is the result of its outstanding 200-year track record of safety and efficacy. Although it's based on therapeutic principles that date back thousands of years, homeopathy was first developed as a formal clinical discipline in the late 1700s by the legendary German physician Samuel Hahnemann.

Throughout the 1800s, vast numbers of physicians across the United States and Europe embraced Hahnemann's work. Unfortunately, because of the threat it posed to the pharmaceutical industry and its divergence from conventional medical beliefs, homeopathy was heavily maligned and effectively suppressed in the United States for well over a century. Nonetheless, it flourished in Europe and eventually became a dominant force within the worldwide health care community.

Today homeopathic hospitals and clinics are part of Britain's national health care system, and in France pharmacies are required to carry homeopathic remedies alongside conventional drugs. It's also widely practiced in North America, South America, and the Far East. The World Health Organization has even recommended that homeopathy be integrated with conventional medicine in order to upgrade global standards of health care.

Homeopathy is a highly individualized therapeutic approach that recognizes many different kinds of "constitutional types." The typing system helps practitioners select remedies that are tailored to the unique aspects of each patient's situation—including remedies to address the underlying psychological dimensions of illness, or disruptions in what Hahnemann referred to as the "vital force."

For example, let's say you have a chronic health disorder such as arthritis or colitis. Your symptoms could be the result of a negative emotion like anger or resentment or fear, or a difficult life experience like growing up in an abusive or alcoholic environment.

If that's the case, no amount of dietary or structural therapy will ever be sufficient to resolve your ailment. You may succeed in diminishing the symptoms to some extent, or they may even disappear for a while. But they'll inevitably reappear at some point, or you'll develop new symptoms to take the place of the old.

Karen Gorney, R.N., a leading homeopath in New York, who has taught at Cornell Medical College at New York University, focuses on the emotional basis of illness. She believes that emotional trauma affects everyone on a deep level, and is particularly devastating, on a physical level, to people with highly sensitive natures. Karen views the combination of emotional trauma and temperament as a major factor in the development of many forms of physical and psychological illness. As a result, she, like other homeopaths, uses the remedies to help dissolve conflicts that are lodged in the unconscious mind. Since the unconscious mind is inextricably linked to the body, homeopaths see it as the source of much pathology seen in the body.

Karen summarizes the value of homeopathy this way: "Emotional stress and conflict can ultimately manifest in virtually any kind of disease or physical disorder, from asthma to AIDS to chronic fatigue to cancer. Many forms of psychotherapy are also geared toward dealing with underlying emotional causes of illness, but they're limited to working with cognition as a way of reaching unconscious conflict. Traditional psychotherapy uses only the psychological clues without exploring the physical symptomology, and therefore misses half of the manifested information about the 'disease block.' Without all the cues, the cure is elusive."

Vinton McCabe, president of the Connecticut Homeopathic Association, and author of *Let Like Cure Like: The Definitive Guide to the Healing Power of Homeopathy* (St. Martin's Press, 1996), shares similar perspectives on the origins of illness. He writes: "All healing demands change—a change in our thinking, a change in our living. If some aspect or aspects of our lives didn't need to change, we wouldn't be sick to start with."

In the United States today there are approximately 3,000 physicians and other licensed health care professionals practicing homeopathy, but not all have equivalent levels of training and skill. Those with more limited experience tend to practice allopathically—in other words, they tend to "match remedies to symptoms"—whereas highly skilled homeopaths generally look beyond specific ailments and seek a more "holistic" understanding of the mind/body/spirit dimensions of each individual.

For further information on homeopathy, here are more excellent books:

1. *Beyond Flat Earth Medicine,* by Timothy Dooley, Timing Publications, 1995.
2. *A New Model for Health and Disease,* by George Vitoulkas, North Atlantic Books, 1992.
3. *The Science and Art of Healing,* by Ralph Twentyman, Floris Books, 1996.
4. *Poisons That Heal,* by Dr. Eileen Nauman, Light Technology Publications, 1997.

12

Chapter

INDISPENSABLE TIPS
FOR SAVVY CONSUMERS

Food Purity and Safety

As we all know, most of the food available in supermarkets today is radically different from what our grandparents were used to. Have you noticed how hard it can be to find commercial produce that even tastes good? So much of it is totally bland and unappealing. It's difficult to find tomatoes, berries, melons, corn, carrots, cucumbers, peaches, apples, or any other fruits and vegetables that are anywhere near as rich and flavorful as they're meant to be. The lack of flavor is due to the fact that most crops are grown in soil that's severely deficient in nutrients. Fruits and vegetables lose even more nutrient value and freshness because of all the time involved in shipping, warehousing, and product distribution. In addition, much of our commercial food has been sprayed, chemically treated, or otherwise processed in ways that can be damaging to our health.

Fortunately, there are lots of places where savvy consumers can still obtain fresh, natural, chemical- and toxin-free meats, produce, and dairy products—health food stores, farmer's markets, food co-ops, even mail-order suppliers. Roughly half of all supermarkets in the United States have small but growing selections of organic products. This is due to a sharp increase in consumer demand for organic food in recent years. According to the CROPP Cooperative, the largest organic farm cooperative in North America, the market for organic food is expanding by approximately 20 percent each year.

Even though organic food products are more expensive than regular commercial products, demand is surging because consumers everywhere are becoming keenly interested in food that is both safe and good tasting. They're tired of bland food, and they don't want to gamble with their health. People realize that organic food is a sound investment, i.e., a good form of health insurance.

It's a great idea to incorporate organic food into your diet if you haven't already done so. Of course, you don't need to be fanatical about trying to avoid food contaminants. That's impossible anyway, since even the best-quality organic food is sometimes exposed to a degree of contamination from polluted groundwater and other environmental influences. On the other hand, it's wise to be aware of the serious hazards of modern agricultural practices, and to increase your consumption of pure food as much as possible.

Where to Buy Organic Food

Check Out Health Food Stores

Many health food stores sell high-quality organic produce and have large and varied selections of organic fruits and vegetables and numerous other food products. In smaller stores, selections are sometimes limited.

Look for a Food Co-op in Your Area

Most cities have food cooperatives, member-owned food stores that sell organic produce from local farms and other natural food products by local manufacturers. Food co-ops are typically organized for the purpose of empowering consumers by making healthy foods available at reduced prices and encouraging the preservation of the environment. To find a food co-op in your area, visit this Web site: www.prairienet.org/co-op/directory.

Shop at Farmer's Markets

Many areas have farmer's markets, where local farmers gather, usually on a weekly basis, to sell fruits and vegetables and other food products directly to the public. The produce is usually much fresher than the produce you find at supermarkets. Often it was picked that day, and much of it is likely to be organic.

Buy Organic Produce by Mail

There are a number of companies that ship excellent organic produce to consumers nationwide. Overnight delivery is available, and foods are expertly packed and shipped. Here are well established mail-order companies you may want to check out:

1. Azure Standard: (541) 467-2230 or www.azurestandard.com
2. Diamond Organics: (888) ORGANIC;
   Web: www.diamondorganics.com

Obtain an Organic Food Directory

Try contacting your state agricultural department and asking for referrals to organic farmers in your region. Or purchase a copy of the 1999 National Organic Directory. It lists growers and other food producers throughout the United States, costs about $40, and can be ordered through the mail by calling (800) 852-3832.

Check the Supermarket

Don't forget that your local supermarket is likely to carry organic produce and other food products. Look for labels on fruits and vegetables that say "certified organic"; don't necessarily go by handwritten signs. Though most states have no government-regulated organic certification programs, there are about forty independent agencies throughout the country that provide credible certification.

Tips on Buying Nonorganic Produce

There will no doubt be times when you have to buy nonorganic fruits and vegetables. Check the labels on regular produce (including package labels on frozen vegetables) and try to avoid food grown in Mexico, Central America, or South America. Even though certain toxic pesticides have been banned in the U.S., we routinely export these chemicals to other countries, where they're used on fruits and vegetables that are then shipped right back to us!

When buying waxed produce such as apples, cucumbers, and eggplants, peel them, since pesticides are frequently sealed in with the wax. Also, talk to your local health food store manager and ask for recommendations on natural products that can be used to wash produce and remove pesticide residues.

Choose Dairy Products Carefully

Whenever possible, buy organic milk, cheese, yogurt, butter, and ice cream. These products are widely available in health food stores and many supermarkets. Look for package labels that indicate the product has been produced under organic conditions—in other words, derived from dairy cows that have not been given growth hormones, antibiotics, or anything other than organic (pesticide-free) feed or grain.

Two high-quality and widely available brands of organic dairy products are:

1. Organic Valley: www.organicvalley.com
2. Horizon Organic: www.horizonorganic.com

When buying dairy products, you might also want to try *raw* milk and cheese products—i.e., natural products that have not been *either* pasteurized *or* homogenized.

Pasteurization is a heating process designed to kill bacteria. But, along with bacteria, pasteurization destroys naturally occurring enzymes in milk. Though pasteurization is often necessary in this age of mass distribution and extended product shelf lives, it's not quite what nature intended. Homogenization is a mechanical process that involves whipping whole milk so rigorously that the healthy clumps of butterfat are transformed into microscopic spheres of fat, which are then permanently suspended in the waterlike portion of the milk.

Remember those popular old TV commercials that featured yogurt enthusiasts, leading healthy and vigorous lives in remote mountain villages in Europe? Elderly people in their nineties and beyond? You can be sure that, in the real world, people like this have never consumed factory-produced milk products. Their healthy native diets would naturally only incorporate dairy foods in a raw, unprocessed state.

Raw cheese is available in virtually every health food store nation-wide, though raw milk is harder to obtain. In California, state law permits raw milk to be sold in stores, but in most other states raw milk cannot be distributed through stores. As a result, many people throughout the country buy raw milk directly from small dairy farms.

In health food stores and even some supermarkets you can also find a few dairy products that have been *pasteurized but not homogenized*. For instance, if you see bottles of milk or containers of yogurt that have cream collected at the top, they most likely have not been homogenized.

Some researchers believe that excessive consumption of homogenized milk contributes to hardening of the arteries. Studies have shown that in countries where people use large amounts of homogenized milk, the death rate from heart attack is high, while in countries where the milk is nonhomogenized, the heart attack rate is much lower, even if the diet is high in cholesterol.

For more information on this topic, read *The XO Factor: Homogenized Milk May Cause Your Heart Attack,* by Kurt Oster, M.D.

Here are two sources of nonhomogenized yogurt:

1. Erivan Yogurt. For almost thirty years, the small and highly specialized Erivan Dairy in Pennsylvania has produced a tangy and delicious, traditional European yogurt that is one of the few *non-*

homogenized yogurt products on the market. Currently it's widely available in health food stores on the East Coast and in the Midwest. For more information, write to company founder Paul Fereshetian at: Erivan Dairy, 105 Allison Road, Oreland, PA 19075.

2. Brown Cow Yogurt. This popular brand of nonhomogenized yogurt is widely available in health food stores and supermarkets nationwide.

Be Finicky About Meat and Poultry

In a previous era, cattle used to graze on grass in natural, unspoiled environments. But today's commercially raised cattle are grain-fed, and the grain is most often laced with antibiotics, growth hormones, and tranquilizers. This situation applies to poultry as well, so most of the beef and poultry sold in supermarkets and meat markets today is contaminated with these substances. Organically raised beef and poultry are safer and have a far better taste than chemically raised varieties.

The use of antibiotics in livestock is emerging as a particularly controversial issue. Each year, farmers dump close to 20 million pounds of antibiotics into the food and water of farm animals, which amounts to roughly a third of all the antibiotics produced in the U.S. on an annual basis. The drugs are not intended to fight disease; they're primarily used as a cheap way to fatten livestock. This is helping to create new strains of bacterial organisms that are resistant to existing antibiotics.

Public health organizations worldwide are calling for cutbacks on the use of antibiotics on farms. The World Health Organization has even called for a ban on antibiotics as growth stimulants for livestock, and in 1998, the European Union announced a ban on four antibiotics used in animal feed. But very little is being done in the United States. Naturally the pharmaceutical industry and large agricultural interests are vehemently opposed to any restrictions on the use of drugs in food production.

Fortunately, organic beef and poultry are becoming increasingly available nationwide. Here are some sources you may want to investigate:

1. Daily Blessing Organic Farms, (888) 236-1424 or www.yc2.net/organics

2. D' Artagnan Organic Game & Poultry: www.dartagnan.com
3. Homestead Healthy Foods (organic beef and chicken):
   www.homesteadhealthyfoods.com
4. Petaluma Poultry: www.healthychickenchoices.com

Many stores also carry a few brands of *natural* beef and poultry. This generally means that the livestock have not been given antibiotic and growth hormones, but may have been raised on regular commercial feed, i.e., feed that is not necessarily free of pesticides. Check out Coleman Natural Beef at: www.colemannatural.com

Avoiding Irradiated and Genetically Engineered Food

Here's another reason why it's a great idea to support local farmers, co-ops, and organic food producers of all kinds: you can avoid food that's been irradiated and fruits and vegetables that have had their genetic composition altered.

Food irradiation involves zapping foods with cobalt gamma rays for the purpose of killing bacteria and extending product shelf life. It's been used to a limited extent for many years for spices and several other food products. However, the FDA recently approved the use of irradiation to treat beef, and food industry coalitions are currently pressuring government regulators to expand the use of the technology to other food categories.

The meat industry and other food producers contend that irradiation is an excellent means of improving food safety and reducing problems such as product recalls. Yet there is not uniform agreement within the meat industry on these issues. Some companies and industry experts believe that irradiation is not an effective solution to meat contamination, and in some instances may even exacerbate bacterial problems. In general, many knowledgeable observers believe that irradiation is no substitute for proper sanitation, packaging, storage, and preparation.

Radiation kills vitamins, friendly bacteria, and enzymes, effectively rendering the food "dead," and therefore useless to the body. Many researchers report that it also breaks up the molecular structure of food and creates chemical by-products like benzene, formaldehyde, and a number of known mutagens and carcinogens.

The genetic manipulation of crops is an even more complex and controversial issue. In the last five years, over 45 million acres of American farmland have been planted with "transgenic" crops, such as corn, soybeans, and potatoes. The gene-altered seeds used to grow these crops are patent-protected by large chemical and biotech companies, and therefore a source of huge potential profits.

New breeds of crops are being "engineered" in the hope that they'll have the ability to produce toxins to repel insects and to resist the toxic effects of herbicides (weed killers). The corporations that manufacture transgenic seeds claim that this will facilitate a sweeping new agricultural revolution—one that will make farming more sustainable, feed the world, and improve health and nutrition.

However, organic farmers and health-conscious consumers are strongly opposed to the biotech industry's tampering with the food supply. Researchers simply don't know what the eventual consequences might be to the ecosphere or to human health from tampering with the DNA of crops.

For more information on this topic, read *Farmageddon: Food and the Culture of Biotechnology*, by Brewster Kneen, or *Against the Grain: Biotechnology and the Corporate Takeover of Your Food*, by Marc Lappe and Britt Bailey.

For information on a broad range of topics pertaining to the safety and purity of food, including news, background information, and practical advice related to consumerism and citizen activism, visit these web sites:

1. The Organic Consumers Association: www.organicconsumers.org
2. The Campaign for Food Safety: www.campaignforfoodsafety.org

Oceanic Marvel: Pure Sea Salt from France

To be healthy, you need a sufficient amount of salt for many different kinds of metabolic activities. For example, salt (in the form of sodium chloride) plays a key role in your ability to digest and absorb nutrients. When you chew your food, salt is what activates the critical first enzyme in your mouth, salivary amylase. In the parietal cells of the stomach wall, sodium chloride is used to make hydrochloric acid, an enzyme that is essential for digestion.

What's important to realize is that not all salt is created equal. Even though all salts come from the sea, there are big differences in the way various salts are harvested and processed. In its naturally occurring state, salt contains a rich assortment of other minerals, such as magnesium, calcium, and potassium. However, most table salts and sea salts are treated with chemicals and stripped of their accompanying nutrients. This disruption of the natural mineral complex interferes with the salt's ability to function normally in the body.

Fortunately, the French government has preserved thousands of acres of pristine wild marsh in northern France, for the purpose of enabling farmers' cooperatives to harvest extraordinary, mineral-rich sea salt, known as Celtic Sea Salt. People all over Europe treasure this salt, which is never treated with chemicals and is harvested by hand in order to protect fragile trace elements. It's called Celtic Salt because it's harvested using a 2,000-year-old method of gathering salt with wooden tools (as opposed to metal tools) that do not disturb the salt's delicate ionic balance.

In addition to being much healthier than factory-processed varieties, pure organic Celtic Sea Salt has a sensational taste. For information contact: The Grain & Salt Society, 273 Fairway Drive, Asheville, NC; tel: (800) 867-7258; Web: www.celtic-seasalt.com.

Stevia, the Natural Herbal Sweetener

Stevia is an herb with extraordinary sweetening power. It has a mild, licoricelike taste and is actually many times sweeter than white sugar. Unlike other sweetening agents, stevia is completely calorie-free, never initiates a rise in blood sugar, contains no chemicals or artificial ingredients, is completely nontoxic, can be used in baking, and actually inhibits the formation of cavities and tooth plaque. Although it's a plant indigenous to South America, stevia has been used by cultures all over the world for hundreds of years. It's especially popular in countries like Korea and Japan, where people are very cautious about the use of artificial sweeteners.

In the United States, however, stevia remains quite obscure, while artificial sweeteners like aspartame, saccharin, and sorbitol dominate the marketplace. For years, health experts in the U.S. have warned consumers of potential health risks associated with these kinds of chemicals. In his book *Natural Health Natural Medicine*, Andrew Weil, M.D., advises people to avoid the use of artificial sweeteners, which he regards as more hazardous than food preservatives. Anne Louise Gittleman shares a similar perspective in *Super Nutrition for Women*. Both books describe numerous health problems that many researchers believe are associated with artificial sweeteners, including headaches, dizziness, seizures, allergies, and even cancer.

Ironically, stevia, a natural substance that has proved to be perfectly safe, has been kept off the market in the United States for years, due to very tight restrictions by the Food & Drug Administration (FDA). In the meantime, the market here is glutted with chemical sweeteners that are known to pose health risks. Fortunately, however, government restrictions on stevia have eased recently, and it's now possible to purchase it in health food stores as a supplement.

The history of stevia's availability and use in the United States is an example of how patents, politics, and profits dictate what types of products consumers ultimately have access to. Unfortunately, healthy natural substances are frequently suppressed, while questionable or obviously unhealthy products are often vigorously promoted and made widely available. For details on this interesting topic, read *The Stevia Story: A Tale of Incredible Sweetness and Intrigue*, by Linda Bonvie, Bill Bonvie, and Donna Gates.

Food Preparation Dos and Don'ts

1. Don't overcook your food, as it will result in a loss of vital enzymes and nutrients. Vegetables should be cooked until slightly tender, yet still retain their bright color. Steaming vegetables in purified water is

the best option. Salt your food after cooking, not during cooking, since salt helps leach nutrients into the water. To retain nutrients, use the water in which you steam vegetables to make soup. Note that the dark color of the water is from minerals leached in the steaming process.

2. To guard against parasites and harmful bacteria, don't undercook meat. At the same time, meat that is slightly on the "rare" side retains more enzymes than "well done" meat, and it's certainly never a good idea to eat blackened or charred meat. The best way to ensure that meat retains its enzymes, juices, flavors, and nutrients best is to cook it at lower temperatures for longer periods of time. Preferable means of cooking include roasting and baking.

3. Eggs are best when they're cooked lightly, as in soft boiling or poaching. A good way to cook eggs is to place them in water and let them come to a boil for only a few seconds; then remove the pan from the heat, and let the eggs stand for a few minutes until the desired consistency is reached. Look for fertile eggs from hens raised in free-ranging circumstances and given unmedicated feed.

4. To preserve the nutrient content of whole grains or legumes, simmer them slowly at a low temperature. Buy whole or uncut grains in health food stores, as opposed to processed commercial brands.

5. To maximize your ability to digest whole grains, beans, or legumes, soak them overnight in purified water, and then cook them in the same water.

6. Limit or refrain from eating microwaved foods. Microwaving actually changes the molecular structure of food in a way that nature did not intend.

7. Always strive to obtain whole, fresh foods. Fragmented foods (e.g., whole wheat flour as compared to the whole wheat berry itself) impart significantly less energy than whole foods. The same holds true for food that is not fresh. For instance, if you spent a week eating

nothing but leftover, stale, frozen, canned, or microwaved food, you would feel very poorly—physically, emotionally, and mentally.

8. The ions and molecules in both raw and cooked foods react with metallic and synthetic ions in cookware. Whenever possible, choose nonreactive cookware such as porcelain enamel, glass, or earthenware. Even though stainless or surgical steel is the least reactive metal, and far superior to aluminum or popular synthetic cookware products that feature nonstick surfaces, remove cooked food from metal as soon as it is cooked to minimize its metallic taste. Don't use porcelain cookware that's chipped or severely scratched.

Easy Ways to Organize and Implement Your Diet

Getting Started

1. Here's a simple way to get familiar with the foods that are right for you: Photocopy your Allowable Foods chart in Chapter 7. Then cross off any food you may dislike or to which you are allergic.

2. Next, make four copies of the list. Post one on your refrigerator, keep one in your office, and one at your desk at home. For shopping convenience, carry a copy in your wallet or purse.

3. Glance through your list often, and before long you'll know it by heart.

4. When shopping, opt for fresh foods as much as possible, with frozen vegetables and meats as a second choice. Some canned foods, such as tuna, salmon, and sardines, are okay if they're on your list, but look for these items in nonleaded cans in health food stores.

5. Review the twelve steps in Chapter 7 to learn how to combine your proteins, carbohydrates, and fats in the ratio that's right for you.

Planning Ahead

1. Always plan your meals a day ahead. Think about where you'll be the following day and how you can obtain your metabolically appropriate foods.

2. If you cook at home, prepare double to triple the amount called for in each recipe. This will help keep your refrigerator adequately stocked.

3. Buy a small soft lunch box and get in the habit of carrying food with you.

4. After a while these steps will become a habit and you will have mastered the most important aspect of successful meal planning—*preparation*.

If You Don't Cook

1. Find a good deli that prepares simple foods such as tuna salad, chicken salad, and wholesome entrees. Many health food stores have excellent deli counters.

2. When eating out, select restaurants with simple, high-quality foods that are appropriate for your metabolic type. A diner is better for the Protein Type, a vegetarian restaurant for the carbohydrate type.

3. Many cities and towns have excellent health food restaurants that serve great tasting organic foods appropriate for all metabolic types. Look for one near you.

4. Stock your kitchen with plenty of good snack foods—wholesome breads, nut butters, fruits, cheeses, yogurt—whatever's appropriate for your metabolism.

5. Learn to do just a couple of things well, like making an omelet or a great-tasting salad or sandwich. Or consider taking a basic cooking course at a local adult education center.

For the Traveling Person

1. When traveling, avoid getting stuck without decent food. Pack a sandwich and some snacks or, if you're driving, pack a cooler with at least a couple of meals.

2. Bring foods that won't go bad, like nuts, seeds, crackers, fruits, cheese, and nut butter.

3. When selecting a hotel, make food a high priority. Consider the availability of restaurants or room service where you can get simple but high-quality food.

4. Always carry pure water with you and avoid getting dehydrated.

5. Ask the hotel to pack a dinner or lunch for you to eat on the way home.

APPENDIX A

Troubleshooting Test

If you're still not sure of your metabolic type for some reason, or you tried the diet recommended for your type and the fine-tuning guidelines but still did poorly, you can use this troubleshooting test either to confirm or to determine your metabolic type. But before you proceed, make sure that you have followed your diet to the letter, eating only your recommended foods, and that you have exhausted the fine-tuning methods.

This troubleshooting test will take four days to complete. Here's a brief synopsis of what you need to do:

OVERVIEW OF TROUBLESHOOTING TEST	
DAYS 1 & 2	**DAYS 3 & 4**
Follow Diet Plan #1	*Follow Diet Plan #2*
• Fill out a dietary intake record	• Fill out a dietary intake record
• Record before and after meal symptoms	• Record before and after meal symptoms
• Indicate if your symptoms were made better or worse	• Indicate if your symptoms were made better or worse

During the four days of the test, you should:

• Eat only the recommended foods specified on the Daily Record Sheets

• Record the way you feel *both* before each meal and after each meal

The following provides a real-world example to illustrate how to use your Daily Record Sheet for Days 1 to 4:

EXAMPLE OF HOW TO COMPLETE A DIETARY RECORD SHEET

FOOD INTAKE			REACTIONS			
consume only the listed foods			record any reactions you may have to your food and beverage intake			
		Before	Two Hours After	Better	Worse	Overall
BREAKFAST 1 cup coffee, toast and jam, orange juice	Appetite	strong	already hungry	not hungry	(still hungry)	
	Cravings	sweets	still want sweets	less craving/none	(still cravings)	☐ Better
	Physical	tired	jittery	better, improved	(same or worse)	☑ Worse
	Energy	low	hyper but exhausted	better, improved	(same or worse)	
	Mind	slow, spacy	nervous	better/improved	(same or worse)	
	Emotions	ok	anxious	better/improved	(same or worse)	

Clearly, the effect of this meal on this person was not very good. Within two hours after eating, hunger was present once again. The desire for sweets did not go away. Tiredness was replaced with jitteriness. Low energy changed into a hyper sensation, with exhaustion underneath. Mentally, the slow, spacey quality had transformed into a nervous quality. And emotional stability prior to breakfast turned into anxiety after breakfast. As a result of these reactions, the overall effect of the meal was negative, so "Worse" was checked in the far right column.

Days 1 and 2

On Days 1 and 2, you'll follow a very precise diet of allowable foods, listed for you on your Day 1 and Day 2 charts. You can eat as much as you'd like to of those foods. But it's critical that you eat those foods and those foods only. No cheating. If you do cheat, you won't get reliable results and you may not be able to determine your metabolic type.

You will also complete daily symptom records, just like the one described in the example above. If you should feel poorly on the diet recommended, then you're "lucky" because you won't have to follow it for the whole two days. If it really makes you feel much worse, stop it at that point. Skip this test diet for the rest of the day and eat the way you want to eat. The next day, start the Days 3 and 4 diet.

Days 3 and 4

On Days 3 and 4, you'll follow a very precise diet of allowable foods, but one very different from the one on Days 1 and 2. You can eat as much as you'd like to of the allowable foods. But it's critical that you eat those foods, and *those foods only*. No cheating on this diet. If you do cheat, you won't get reliable results and you may not be able to properly determine your metabolic type.

If you should feel poorly on this diet, then you're "lucky" because you won't have to follow it for the rest of the test time. If it really makes you feel much worse, stop it at that point. Eat as usual for the rest of the day. The end of Day 4 marks the end of the Troubleshooting Test. You're now ready for final scoring.

Final Scoring

Here's how to score your results:

• If you felt poorly on Days 1 and 2 and well on Days 3 and 4, then consider yourself a *Protein Type.*

• If you felt poorly on Days 3 & 4 and well on Days 1 & 2, then consider yourself a *Carbo Type.*

• If you felt *either* good *or* bad on *both* diets, then consider yourself a *Mixed Type.*

After you determine the *right foods,* don't forget to fine-tune your macronutrient ratio to your individual needs.

Keep in mind that some people have sensitive (quick-to-react) metabolisms. For others, changes take a lot longer to manifest. Give your metabolic type diet adequate time to make changes in your metabolism before you judge its effectiveness. I suggest you monitor effects over a 3 to 4 week period.

Ultimately, if this section is not helpful to you, there is no need to give up. Your next step may be to work with a professional who is trained in helping people implement the metabolic typing program. (See Metabolic Typing Education Center in Appendix E.)

On the following pages are the complete charts for Days 1 to 4. Good luck. And have fun as a metabolic detective!

DIETARY RECORD SHEET FOR DAYS 1 & 2

FOOD INTAKE	REACTIONS				
consume only the listed foods	record any reactions you may have to your food and beverage intake				
		Before	Two Hours After	Better	Worse	Overall

FOOD INTAKE		Before	Two Hours After	Better	Worse	Overall
BREAKFAST 1 cup coffee, toast and jam, orange juice	Appetite			not hungry	still hungry	
	Cravings			less craving/none	still cravings	☐ Better
	Physical			better/improved	same or worse	☐ Worse
	Energy			better/improved	same or worse	
	Mind			better/improved	same or worse	
	Emotions			better/improved	same or worse	
LUNCH 1 cup coffee (optional), chicken breast, rice, salad: lettuce, tomato, onion, steamed broccoli, half tablespoon olive oil, lemon juice to taste	Appetite			not hungry	still hungry	
	Cravings			less craving/none	still cravings	☐ Better
	Physical			better/improved	same or worse	☐ Worse
	Energy			better/improved	same or worse	
	Mind			better/improved	same or worse	
	Emotions			better/improved	same or worse	
SNACK fruit, low-fat yogurt (optional)	Appetite			not hungry	still hungry	
	Cravings			less craving/none	still cravings	☐ Better
	Physical			better/improved	same or worse	☐ Worse
	Energy			better/improved	same or worse	
	Mind			better/improved	same or worse	
	Emotions			better/improved	same or worse	

DIETARY RECORD SHEET FOR DAYS 1 & 2 (cont.)

FOOD INTAKE		REACTIONS			
consume only the listed foods		record any reactions you may have to your food and beverage intake			
		Before	Two Hours After		Overall
			Better	Worse	
DINNER turkey breast or Cornish game hen or chicken breast or ham or cod or halibut, millet or rice, steamed zucchini, salad: lettuce, cabbage, cucumber, tomato, half tablespoon olive oil, lemon juice to taste	Appetite		not hungry	still hungry	
	Cravings		less craving/none	still cravings	❑ Better
	Physical		better/improved	same or worse	❑ Worse
	Energy		better/improved	same or worse	
	Mind		better/improved	same or worse	
	Emotions		better/improved	same or worse	
SNACK fruit, low-fat yogurt (optional)	Appetite		not hungry	still hungry	
	Cravings		less craving/none	still cravings	❑ Better
	Physical		better/improved	same or worse	❑ Worse
	Energy		better/improved	same or worse	
	Mind		better/improved	same or worse	
	Emotions		better/improved	same or worse	

DIETARY RECORD SHEET FOR DAYS 3 & 4

REACTIONS

record any reactions you may have to your food and beverage intake

FOOD INTAKE (consume only the listed foods)		Before (Two Hours After)	Better	Worse	Overall
BREAKFAST bacon, eggs (2–3), sausage(s), half slice toast, butter	Appetite		not hungry	still hungry	
	Cravings		less craving/none	still cravings	☐ Better
	Physical		better/improved	same or worse	☐ Worse
	Energy		better/improved	same or worse	
	Mind		better/improved	same or worse	
	Emotions		better/improved	same or worse	
LUNCH steak, steamed cauliflower, butter, half cup rice	Appetite		not hungry	still hungry	
	Cravings		less craving/none	still cravings	☐ Better
	Physical		better/improved	same or worse	☐ Worse
	Energy		better/improved	same or worse	
	Mind		better/improved	same or worse	
	Emotions		better/improved	same or worse	
SNACK hard boiled egg or nut butter and half slice bread or nuts	Appetite		not hungry	still hungry	
	Cravings		less craving/none	still cravings	☐ Better
	Physical		better/improved	same or worse	☐ Worse
	Energy		better/improved	same or worse	
	Mind		better/improved	same or worse	
	Emotions		better/improved	same or worse	

DIETARY RECORD SHEET FOR DAYS 3 & 4 (cont.)

FOOD INTAKE		REACTIONS				
consume only the listed foods		record any reactions you may have to your food and beverage intake				
		Before	Two Hours After	Better	Worse	Overall
DINNER lamb or salmon, steamed spinach, butter, half cup rice	Appetite			not hungry	still hungry	
	Cravings			less craving/none	still cravings	
	Physical			better/improved	same or worse	❑ Better
	Energy			better/improved	same or worse	❑ Worse
	Mind			better/improved	same or worse	
	Emotions			better/improved	same or worse	
SNACK hard-boiled egg or nut butter and half slice bread or nuts	Appetite			not hungry	still hungry	
	Cravings			less craving/none	still cravings	
	Physical			better/improved	same or worse	❑ Better
	Energy			better/improved	same or worse	❑ Worse
	Mind			better/improved	same or worse	
	Emotions			better/improved	same or worse	

Appendix B

The Nine Fundamental Homeostatic Controls

This book is based on a technology I developed known as The Healthexcel System of Metabolic Typing. Since 1987, the technology has been used by health professionals for the purpose of evaluating patient's nutritional requirements and developing customized nutritional protocols.

There are many thousands of biochemical reactions that take place on a daily basis as part of the innumerable life-supporting processes of metabolism. But they occur neither independently nor without the direction of *fundamental homeostatic controls*.

The potential for sufficient adaptation, continual homeostatic balance, metabolic efficiency, and thereby good health, is a measure of the body's ability to manage stressors, which can be mental, emotional, structural, biochemical (quantity and quality of nutrients), or environmental (chemical, electromagnetic, thermal). This is made possible by the body's capacity for the creation, maintenance, and control of energy via the Fundamental Homeostatic Control Mechanisms.

The Healthexcel System of Metabolic Typing incorporates and utilizes nine separate Fundamental Homeostatic Control Mechanisms. They are:

Autonomic Nervous System
• master regulator of metabolism, neuro-endocrine/hormonal balance
AUTONOMIC TYPE
Sympathetic vs. Parasympathetic

Carbo-Oxidative System
• conversion of nutrients to energy via intermediary metabolism, involving glycolysis, citric acid (Krebs) cycle, beta oxidation
OXIDATIVE TYPE
Fast Oxidation vs. Slow Oxidation

Lipo-Oxidative Processes
• involving fatty acid/sterol balance, selective membrane permeability, aerobic/anaerobic metabolism
CATABOLIC/ANABOLIC BALANCE
Catabolic vs. Anabolic

Electrolyte/Fluid Balance
ELECTROLYTE/FLUID BALANCE
Electrolyte Excess vs. Electrolyte Deficiency

Acid/Alkaline Balance
• six potential acid/alkaline imbalances:
metabolic acidosis, metabolic alkalosis, respiratory acidosis, respiratory alkalosis, potassium excess acidosis, potassium depletion alkalosis
ACID/ALKALINE BALANCE
Acid vs. Alkaline

Prostaglandin Balance
PROSTAGLANDIN BALANCE
Series 1 + Series 3 Prostaglandins vs. Series 2 Prostaglandins

Endocrine System
• Endocrine Type as per dominant energy gland
ENDOCRINE TYPE
Pituitary vs. Thyroid vs. Adrenal vs. Gonad

ABO Blood Type
BLOOD TYPE
Type O vs. Type A vs. Type B vs. Type AB

Constitutional Elements
• constitutional qualities of foods interacting with constitutional qualities of the body
CONSTITUTIONAL TYPE
Vata vs. Pitta vs. Kapha

The Fundamental Homeostatic Controls are involved in the regulation of all metabolic processes. Adverse symptoms and disease processes involve imbalances in one or more of these control mechanisms. Every nutrient and every food has specific stimulatory or inhibitory effects on one or more of the Fundamental Homeostatic Control Mechanisms listed above. Genetic inheritance, along with the impact of environmental and lifestyle factors, define one's Metabolic Type as expressed through the Fundamental Homeostatic Controls, thus forming the basis for the determination of individual nutritional requirements.

Following is a brief overview of the Fundamental Homeostatic Controls.

Autonomic Type

The clinical model for the Autonomic Type originated from the work of Francis M. Pottenger, M.D., on the autonomic nervous system (ANS) in 1919. The Autonomic Type is more accurately termed the Neuro-Endocrine Type, since it concerns the interrelationship of the autonomic nervous system and the endocrine system.

The human nervous system may be considered from the standpoint of two grand divisions: the voluntary or cerebrospinal (CNS), and the involuntary or autonomic nervous system (ANS). The ANS is the master regulator of metabolism and, along with the endocrine system, controls most all metabolic processes. Through the five senses, the sensory-motor system perceives the condition of the external environment and after processing this information in the CNS, mobilizes the musculoskeletal system to adapt appropriately. The ANS has the task of perceiving the internal environment, and after processing the information in the CNS, regulating the functions of the internal environment in response to both internal and external environmental pressures. In other words, the autonomic nervous system has the job of maintaining life. The ANS is divided into two parts or divisions on the basis of anatomical and physiological grounds: the sympathetic and the parasympathetic divisions. Nerves from both divisions connect the brain (the hypothalamus) to the various organs and glands in the body. In a sense, the ANS acts as an information transport system. If the brain is thought of as the central switchboard, the ANS is like the telephone lines leading to all the branches.

The sympathetic and parasympathetic systems work together in the regulation of all the involuntary activities of the body: control of the heart rate, blood pressure, digestion, repair and rebuilding, rate of cellular activity, secretion of sweat, contraction of the pupils in the eyes, activities of the immune system, and so forth. Each division is in charge of "turning on," or innervating, various functions of the body. In turn, the other system has the task of "turning off" the activity or inhibiting the function.

The organs, glands and systems thought to be "dominated" (turned on) by, or associated with the sympathetic system are: posterior hypothalamus, anterior pituitary, thyroid, heart, adrenal medulla, kidneys, bladder, uterus, prostate, testes, ovaries, skeletal system, cardiovascular system, neuromuscular system, urinary system, reproductive system, and calcium metabolism.

The organs, glands, and systems thought to be associated with the parasympathetic system are: anterior medial hypothalamus, posterior pituitary, parathyroid, thymus, tonsils, parotid, lungs, adrenal cortex, pancreas, liver, gallbladder, spleen, stomach, intestines, appendix, bone marrow, digestive system, immune system, lymphatic system, respiratory system, excretory system, protein metabolism, carbohydrate metabolism, and fat metabolism.

Most people are neurologically influenced more strongly by either the sympathetic or parasympathetic system, but everyone is different in the degree to which their bodies are influenced. The result of these genetically inherited differences in the degrees of sympathetic and parasympathetic dominance, coupled with varying levels of efficiency of function, is what determines the individual differences in metabolism from the standpoint of the influence of the autonomic nervous system. For example, parasympathetics typically have strong digestion and elimination, while sympathetics display weaknesses in this area. On the other hand, sympathetics tend to have strong adrenal and thyroid function, and are often lean, energetic, and highly motivated.

Different nutrients and foods have varying effects on the different divisions of the autonomic nervous system. Some stimulate, strengthen, or support the sympathetic system, thereby producing an acidic shift in metabolism, while having an opposite effect on the parasympathetic system. Others have the opposite effects, i.e., stimulating the parasympathetic system and causing an alkaline shift in metabolism. For example, potassium is a powerful stimulant to the parasympathetic system, and magnesium has an inhibiting influence on the sympathetic system. Thus, these nutrients tend to increase the parasympathetic activity and decrease the sympathetic activity. On the other hand, phosphorus and calcium powerfully activate the sympathetic system, thereby increasing sympathetic qualities and decreasing parasympathetic qualities.

Significantly, it should be noted that those foods and nutrients (in general) that produce an acidic shift through sympathetic stimulation have the opposite pH effect on the oxidative system, producing an alkaline shift. And those foods and nutrients that have an alkaline influence through acceleration of the parasympathetic system will actually produce an acidic response via the oxidative system. I observed this phenomenon in 1983 and named it "The Dominance Factor." This explains why what works for one person can fail or even worsen the same condition in another person and exemplifies the necessity of first determining the metabolic type before making dietary or nutritional recommendations.

Catabolic/Anabolic Balance

The extraordinary and far-reaching impact of the dualistic, diphasic catabolic/anabolic balance was discovered and evolved over some sixty years by the great Emanual Revici, M.D., and expounded in his epic work, *Research in Physiopathology as a Basis of Guided Chemotherapy*. It concerns fundamental processes involving both membrane permeability and oxidative energy metabolism. Revici found that in

OXIDATIVE TYPE

GLYCOLYSIS

Metabolism of carbohydrates is a step-by-step process, each of which requires specific nutrients. Responsible for about 20% of potential energy.

Group 1 Nutrients
potassium, magnesium, chromium, copper, iron, manganese, vitamins B_1, B_2, B_3, B_6, C, D, PABA, biotin, folic acid, etc., low-fat, low-purine proteins, high carbohydrate

BETA OXIDATION

Metabolism of fats.

Group 2 Nutrients
calcium, iodine, phosphorus, zinc, choline, inositol, bioflavonoids, vitamins A, B_5, B_{12}, E, etc., high-fat, high-purine proteins, low carbohydrate

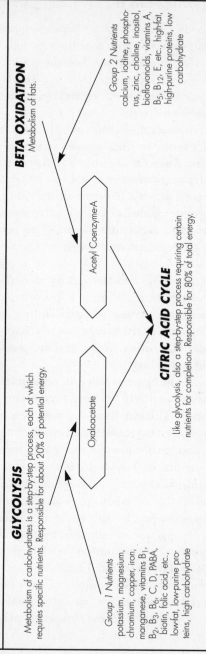

Oxaloacetate → Acetyl Coenzyme-A

CITRIC ACID CYCLE

Like glycolysis, also a step-by-step process requiring certain nutrients for completion. Responsible for 80% of total energy.

First researched by George Watson, Ph.D., the oxidative types relate to intermediary metabolism, the metabolic processes that relate to the conversion of nutrients to energy, specifically glycolysis, beta oxidation and CAC (Citric Acid Cycle or Krebs Cycle). Approximately 20% of total energy comes from Glycolysis and the other 80% from the CAC. The successful completion of these processes is dependent on the availability of proper amounts of oxaloacetate (primarily from carbohydrate) and Acetyl CoA (primarily from fat). The availability of proper amounts of each initiate the Citric Acid Cycle. Watson's clinical, objective research found that certain foods and nutrients (here referred to as Group 1) increased the rate of glycolysis and thereby the production of oxaloacetate. He also found that certain people were overly reliant on glycolysis for energy and deficient in beta oxidation. These individuals he classified as fast oxidizers through a number of objective indicators, including venous plasma pH. Other foods and nutrients (Group 2 nutrients) he determined increased beta oxidation activity and thereby Acetyl CoA production. Those who were overly reliant on beta oxidation for energy production and "slower" at glycolysis, he classified as slow oxidizers. *Both fast and slow oxidizers suffer from deficient energy production but for totally opposite biochemical reasons.* Whereas fast oxidizers burn carbohydrate excessively and overproduce oxaloacetate while remaining deficient in Acetyl CoA, slow oxidizers metabolize carbohydrates too slowly in glycolysis while overproducing Acetyl CoA in beta oxidation. Correction of these imbalances requires that fast oxidizers increase protein and fat relative to carbohydrate in their diet in order to slow down glycolysis and provide raw materials necessary for the production of Acetyl CoA, as well as increase the levels of nutrients required to activate and increase the rate of beta oxidation. Conversely, slow oxidizers need to decrease fat and protein in order to decrease Acetyl CoA production, while increasing carbohydrates and those nutrients required to activate and increase the rate of glycolysis and the production of oxaloacetate.

a state of good health, the body naturally cycles between catabolic and anabolic influences throughout a twenty-four-hour period. But when chronic imbalance sets in, the body can become "stuck" in either a catabolic or anabolic mode. More often than not, this is the result of a defense mode that, when unable to resolve a stressor, becomes a basis for degenerative processes.

This fundamental control involves the balance of fatty acids (negative polar groups) and sterols (positive polar groups) as well as specific biochemical constituents. Anabolic imbalance is characterized by an excess of sterols to fatty acids, resulting in a loss of selective membrane permeability toward a decrease in permeability. Additionally, there is a shift into anaerobic (without oxygen) metabolism. As a result, instead of energy production through the use of oxygen, an anabolic imbalance produces a reliance on the less efficient fermentation metabolism.

Conversely, catabolic imbalance is characterized by an excess of fatty acids and a deficiency of sterols, resulting in a loss of selective membrane permeability toward an increase in permeability. Additionally, there is a shift into aerobic (with oxygen) metabolism. The result is oxidation out of control, causing free radical and peroxide formation, which are harmful to the body.

The loss of selective membrane permeability is undesirable in both cases: When membranes are too tight, nutrients and other good factors can't get into the cells, and toxins can't get out. When too porous, the loss of membrane regulation allows for an outflow of good factors from within the cell, and "free" inflow of toxins into the cell.

An anabolic imbalance results in a systemic alkalinity as the body's defense against abnormal tissue acidity (caused by the build-up of lactic acid from the anaerobic metabolism). Catabolic imbalance produces the reverse (a systemic acidic defense against abnormal tissue alkalinity (caused by the fixation of chlorides by fatty acids, which allows sodium to remain free to combine with carbonate, forming alkaline compounds in the interstitial fluids).

Revici found a number of clinical indications of an anabolic imbalance, including: high cellular potassium, low cellular calcium, high urinary surface tension, low specific gravity, low urine pH, low sedimentation rate, low indican, high eosinophils. These indicators are reversed in a catabolic imbalance.

Clinical indications commonly seen in catabolic/anabolic imbalances include:

ANABOLIC	IMBALANCE	CATABOLIC
osteo	ARTHRITIS	rheumatoid
hypertension	BLOOD PRESSURE	hypotension
constipation	BOWEL	diarrhea
tachycardia	HEART RATE	bradycardia
increased	OXYGEN CAPACITY OF BLOOD	decreased
somnolence	SLEEP	insomnia
polyuria	URINATION	oliguria
Common to both: dyspnea, hearing loss, itching, manic/depressive, pain		

Electrolyte/Fluid Balance

The Electrolyte / Fluid Balance fundamental control is based on the work of Guy Schenker, D.C., who adapted it from the original research of John Riddick. It concerns the balance between electrolytes and body fluids. Imbalances in this fundamental control system can produce electrolyte excess or electrolyte deficiency. Either of these conditions can result in significant metabolic disturbances.

It is vital for the effective transport of nutrients and other vital factors throughout the body that nutrients in suspension remain discrete. In normal fluids, this is accomplished by the fact that particles remain negatively charged, creating dispersion and preventing clumping or flocculation. As long as this is the case, all vital substances (nutrients, enzymes, toxins, hormones, and so forth) are effectively transported to where they need to go.

When this particle separation is lost, serious problems can result, producing an imbalance known as electrolyte excess. Thickened fluids can no longer reach their destinations in an effective or timely manner. It becomes increasingly difficult for fluids to circulate through arterioles, and in some capillaries circulation is virtually cut off, since blood cells move through capillaries one cell at a time. Additionally, transport across cell membranes is disrupted. This can result in insufficient oxygen and nutrient delivery, inefficient detoxification, increased load on the heart, causing increased blood pressure and pulse, poor circulation, diminished efficiency of vital organs, particularly the kidneys, arterial depositions, embolism formation, as well as other problems.

Electrolyte deficiency can occur due to insufficient electrolyte intake or the loss of the body's ability to retain electrolytes. Insufficient electrolytes produce disruption to the endocrine and cardiovascular systems and can result in chronic fatigue, low blood pressure, and poor circulation.

In comparison to some of the other fundamental controls such as the autonomic nervous system, the oxidation rate, and the catabolic/anabolic balance, all of which are actively involved in metabolic processes, this fundamental control is more passive in that it is concerned not with metabolic processes but with the balance of electrolytes and fluids. However, because it involves the electrolyte balances throughout all of the body's fluid compartments and determines to a great degree the capacity for circulation, it works at a primary level and it's impact is significant and far-reaching.

Acid/Alkaline Balance

One of the indicators commonly used by alternative practitioners to determine nutritional protocols in clinical evaluations is pH, yet it is the least understood. Typically, pH is thought to be related to the acid or alkaline ash of a food after it is metabolized, and is commonly gauged through urine pH. In actuality, the ash pH can have an effect, but it is both the least common precipitator of pH imbalance and has the weakest influence. Other Fundamental Homeostatic Controls are far more significant in determining pH.

There are at least seven factors known to influence pH:

1. Autonomic [sympathetic (acid)/parasympathetic (alkaline)]
2. Oxidative [fast oxidation (acid)/slow oxidation (alkaline)]

3. Catabolic (alkaline tissues/acid system)/anabolic (acid tissues/ alkaline system)
4. Electrolyte/fluid balance
5. Endocrine (pituitary, thyroid, parathyroid, adrenal, gonads and their regulation of acid/alkaline minerals)
6. Respiration
7. Acid/alkaline ash of foods (only when the above influences are not present) due to chronic dietary imbalances

Thus, changes in pH are more often due to the effect of foods on the fundamental homeostatic controls, than on the pH of the foods' ash. For example, even though fruit typically has an alkaline ash, it will shift an oxidative dominant metabolizer acid, due to its stimulation of fast oxidation (and the production, thereby, of increased CO_2 and carbonic acid).

There are, however, also six kinds of "pure" acid/alkaline imbalances that have been identified that are not due to influences of the other Fundamental Control Mechanisms. They have been adapted from the work of Guy Schenker, D.C., and his Nutri-Spec System. Each of these imbalances manifest through differing clinical markers and require different protocols to resolve.

The six imbalances are metabolic acidosis, metabolic alkalosis, respiratory acidosis, respiratory alkalosis, potassium excess acidosis, and potassium depletion alkalosis.

These six acid/alkaline imbalances always involve respiratory and renal function. Respiration will be involved as either the source of the problem or part of the defense. Kidney function is always part of compensatory activity. So although urine pH can be used to identify the type of acid/alkaline imbalance, by itself it is not sufficient to determine the presence of an acid/alkaline imbalance. Since respiration is always involved as either the problem or the compensation, all six acid/alkaline imbalances will involve respiratory-related aberration. This fact, coupled with the understanding of the pH of the ash of foods expressed above, debunks the utilization of urine pH along with "acid" and "alkaline" foods to "treat" pH imbalance.

Properly addressing pH imbalance requires evaluation of all of the fundamental homeostatic controls, including the six acid/alkaline imbalances before an objective course of action can be chosen.

Prostaglandin Balance

Prostaglandins are derived from fatty acids and are believed to play a role in virtually every metabolic activity, controlling body responses involving inflammation, neurotransmission, hormones, immune efficiency, circulation, cholesterol production, fluid balance, and platelet aggregation. There are a number of prostaglandins, but the most important for our purposes are the Series 1 (PG1), Series 2 (PG2), and Series 3 (PG3) prostaglandins.

Disruptions to the prostaglandin balance involve excess PG2 relative to both PG1 and PG3. Arachidonic acid found in butter, meat, mollusks, and shellfish is the precursor to PG2 production. However, the impact from the diet is limited as compared to other dietary factors that block production of PG1, as well as the lack of dietary factors that typically would inhibit PG2 production. For example, EPA, an Omega-3 fatty acid found in fish oils, blocks arachidonic acid production, but fish is generally deficient in the American diet. Additionally, alcohol and trans fatty acids (found in all commercial oils and fats) block the body's own production of EPA.

Beyond the factors that increase PG2, others can contribute to a deficiency of PG1. The precursor to PG1 is the Omega-6 fatty acid, GLA, which is found in primrose, black currant and borage oils. The body can also produce GLA from the Omega-6 linoleic acid (LN), which is found in almonds, avocados, and pecans, as well as corn, cottonseed, olive, peanut, primrose, safflower, and sunflower oils. But production can be inhibited by aspirin, anti-inflammatory drugs, steroids, trans fats and alcohol, as well as a deficiency in vitamins B_3, B_6, C, E, and the minerals magnesium and zinc.

Finally, a deficiency of PG3 relative to PG2 can also cause problems. EPA (from fish) is the precursor to PG3 and the body's production of EPA is from the Omega-3 alpha linolenic acid (LNA). A deficiency of LNA (found in beans, chestnuts, flax, soy, walnut, and wheat germ) can result in a deficiency of PG3 and thereby an elevation of PG2. As with GLA, EPA production can be inhibited by aspirin, anti-inflammatory drugs, steroids, trans fats and alcohol, as well as a deficiency in vitmins B_3, B_6, C, E, and the minerals magnesium and zinc.

It is believed that Americans consume anywhere from an 11:1 up to a 30:1 ratio of Omega-6 (vegetable oils) to Omega-3 (fish, flax oil) fatty acids. But a more ideal ratio, based on evolutionary and anthropological data, would be in the range of 1:1 to 4:1.

In cases where a prostaglandin imbalance exists, it is necessary to prevent the elevation of arachidonic acid and PG2 and prevent the suppression of PG1 and PG3. To do so one should avoid trans fats, alcohol, aspirin, and anti-inflammatory drugs, and minimize intake of butter, meat, mollusks, and shellfish. And to increase PG1, one should get the proper amounts and quality of Omega-3 and Omega-6 in the daily diet. For Omega-3, people can eat fish or take fish oil capsules.

The best supplement I have found to restore the proper Omega-3 and Omega-6 levels in the body is Balanced EFA. It has a 1:1 ratio of Omega-3:Omega-6 and is available from Ultra Life, (800) 323-3842.

Endocrine Type

Researchers such as Henry Bieler, M.D., and Elliot Abravanel, M.D., discovered that certain foods stimulate particular endocrine glands. They also learned that, in every individual, one of the four primary endocrine glands (pituitary, thyroid, adrenals, and gonads) tends to be responsible for how excess weight accumulates on the body. When excess weight does accumulate, it may be due in part to an over-stimulation and subsequent exhaustion of the "dominant gland." Consequently, eating foods that naturally stimulate the dominant gland, if done to excess, may result in a weakening or exhaustion of the gland and in turn, a lowering of metabolic rate. This can contribute to the accumulation of excess weight. However, our experience has suggested that other fundamental controls, such as the autonomic and oxidative systems, play the primary role in weight management, but that the endocrine type influence can be a significant consideration in some cases.

Blood Type

Our understanding of the effect of blood type on metabolism and diet is derived from the combined research of James D'Adamo, N.D., and Peter D'Adamo, N.D. In my experience, the influence of blood type on dietary requirements is secondary to the primary regulatory influences of other fundamental homeostatic controls (e.g., autonomic, oxidative, electrolyte, catabolic/anabolic). However, blood type does have an important role to play and can make a significant difference in those to whom it applies. In our experience, the blood type actually has far more to do with what foods you *should avoid* than what foods you *should eat*.

For a discussion of blood types, see page 277.

Constitutional Type

The significance of the constitutional elements of foods relative to the constitutional elements of individual metabolism is drawn from Ayurvedic and Chinese medicine. This aspect of metabolic individuality does not concern the application of specific vitamins and minerals. Rather, it pertains to the proper application of herbs and foods.

For example, nature always provides more than one herb for any given condition. If the nature and the constitution of an herb or food runs contrary to the nature of the human metabolism on whom it is employed, it will have an aggravating influence on the constitution. This will override the symptom-specific nature of the herb or food, contributing to existing imbalances or creating new ones. For example, valerian, hops, and skullcap are commonly employed for insomnia. But, people frequently complain that they "don't work." It so happens that two of these herbs actually have a stimulatory influence on certain constitutional qualities in certain types. Used in these types, the calming aspects of the herb are offset by their constitutionally stimulatory action, effectively neutralizing the desired result.

APPENDIX C

Nutritional Supplememts for Your Metabolic Type

Your Vitamin/Mineral Requirements Are Unique

Today we know with great certainty that different people have distinctly different requirements for macronutrients—proteins, carbohydrates, and fats—in their daily diets. The same holds true for micronutrients—vitamins and minerals. Your body has its own unique need for certain amounts and ratios of micronutrients in order to function efficiently.

While each of us needs a complete spectrum of vitamins and minerals in our daily diet, the need for specific quantities of each nutrient can vary dramatically from person to person. For instance, your daily requirement for a given nutrient such as calcium might be anywhere from two to ten times greater than for someone else with a different metabolism.

The right supplements for your metabolic type can greatly enhance the results of a metabolically correct diet. Similarly, the wrong supplements for your type will not only neutralize the health benefits of a metabolically appropriate diet—they can also worsen existing ailments, or create entirely new health problems where none existed.

Why Nutritional Supplements Are Essential

Today, supplements are critically important because our food supply has lost much of its nutritional value—due to modern methods of growing, storing, transporting, processing, and preserving food. Unfortunately, what looks like an ear of corn or a tomato is in many cases very different in composition (and taste!) from the corn or tomato of a hundred or even fifty years ago. In addition to compensating for a deteriorated food supply, nutritional supplements are essential for your health because they:

1. stimulate and support weak areas in your body
2. supply concentrated raw materials that your body needs to repair and rebuild itself
3. substitute for functions in the body that are deficient (for example, enzymes are essential for people with insufficient digestion)

Over time, if you fail to give just what your body needs, physical breakdown and degenerative disease are almost assured. But if you consistently meet your body's unique need for specific nutrients, you'll greatly increase your chances of staying healthy and fit for a lifetime.

Obtaining Supplements for Your Metabolic Type

To obtain supplements for your metabolic type, contact Ultra Life, an excellent company in Carlyle, Illinois. For over twenty-five years, Ultra Life has been a leader in the manufacture of high quality metabolic type nutritional products.

As a basic daily regimen, you'll want to take: 1) a multiple vitamin/mineral formula specific to your metabolic type; 2) a digestive enzyme formulation specific to your metabolic type; and 3) a balanced essential fatty acid supplement. Depending on your metabolic type, select from the following products:

- Protein Type Formula (multiple vitamin/mineral formula)
- Carbo Type Formula (multiple vitamin/mineral formula)

- Mixed Type Formula (multiple vitamin/mineral formula)
- Protein Type Enzymes
- Carbo Type Enzymes
- Mixed Type Enzymes
- Balanced EFA (essential fatty acid for all metabolic types)

For product information, call Ultra Life at (800) 323-3842; or visit: www.CustomizeYourDiet.com.

APPENDIX D

Free Reports for Health Consumers

"Quick Start Guide"

The "Quick Start Guide" is a free report—a perfect companion to the Metabolic Typing Diet. If you're a busy person with little or no time to devote to customizing your meals or fine-tuning your diet, you'll definitely want to obtain a copy of the "Quick Start Guide."

The guide is a brief report that you can obtain online. It provides highlights of the techniques provided in the Metabolic Typing Diet. By using the guide, you'll learn how to focus on a few easy steps that will enable you to master the essentials of metabolic typing in a matter of hours.

In no time you'll discover just how easy it can be to identify your metabolic type and fine-tune your diet. You'll learn how to get the most out of the Metabolic Typing Diet and how to rapidly achieve the many incredible health benefits that come from eating a diet that's right for you.

To obtain your free copy of the "Quick Start Guide," send an e-mail to: QuickStart@CustomizeYourDiet.com. You'll receive a document that you can download to your computer.

"Computer-Based Metabolic Profiling"

This report provides information about advanced forms of metabolic typing, made possible with computerized evaluations known as "metabolic profiles." It's ideal for health consumers who are already using the dietary customization techniques provided in the Metabolic Typing Diet, but would like more information about high-precision approaches to metabolic type testing.

A computer-based metabolic profile is a test that provides an in-depth look at what makes you unique on a biochemical level, and reveals a great deal of information about imbalances in your regulatory systems. It is these imbalances that define your metabolic type and determine what type of nutritional support you need to balance your body chemistry and in turn optimize your health and fitness.

A metabolic profile is a computer-based inventory and subsequent analysis of many of your unique characteristics. It's an especially useful tool for people who are seeking precise guidance in the area of nutritional supplementation.

To obtain a free report on the health benefits of Computer-Based Metabolic Profiling, send an e-mail request to: profiles@ CustomizeYourDiet.com. You'll receive a document that you can download to your computer.

"Quick and Delicious Recipes for Your Metabolic Type"

This report contains a series of great tasting and easy-to-prepare recipes for people of all metabolic types. It's great information you can use to prepare meals and snacks for you or other members of your family (who may have dietary needs that are different from yours!). For a free report, send an e-mail request to: recipes@CustomizeYourDiet.com.

"Maximize Your Child's Potential with Customized Nutrition"

This report contains a series of excellent tips that make it easy for you to provide your kids with the benefits of customized nutrition. You'll be amazed at the many dramatic improvements in your children's health and well-being when they eat according to their metabolic type. The report covers the special dietary needs of growing children and the profound influence that nutrition has on every area of a child's life—including his or her scholastic performance, behavior, energy, weight, and future health. For a free report, send an e-mail request to: kids@CustomizeYourDiet.com.

Free Reports for Health Professionals

"The Coming Revolution in Patient-Specific Health Care"

This report addresses important emerging trends in the field of health care. Of central significance is the ongoing, rapidly accelerating revolution in alternative medicine. Health consumers are increasingly interested in natural therapies, and studies show that Americans now spend more out-of-pocket money (i.e., discretionary, noninsurance dollars) on alternative medical modalities than they do on orthodox medical procedures.

An important related trend is the growing significance of clinical nutrition. However, a major problem that currently confronts clinicians who offer nutritional counseling is their inability to achieve consistent, predictable results. In other words, standardized nutritional regimens that produce positive results in some patients often produce limited or no success with other patients. This is deeply frustrating for clinicians as well as patients, since it is now widely understood that nutritional science holds enormous potential for preventing and reversing many kinds of chronic health disorders.

In every area of medicine there is now increasing recognition of the importance of shifting away from standardized, "one-size-fits-all" therapeutic protocols toward "patient specific" modalities. Nowhere is this trend more significant than within the realm of clinical nutrition.

Fortunately, new technologies now enable clinicians to address patients' individualized nutritional needs with an unprecedented degree of specificity and precision. These technologies promise to unleash the real power inherent in clinical nutrition—and in turn revolutionize many aspects of health care delivery.

For a free report, send an e-mail request to: trends@Metabolic Typing.com. You'll receive a document that can be downloaded to your computer.

"Build Your Practice with Customized Nutrition"

This report contains information on leading-edge approaches to nutritional counseling. It's ideal for health professionals seeking to integrate new and innovative nutritional modalities into their clinical practices. The focal point of the report is metabolic typing, an advanced nutritional discipline that enables clinicians to evaluate the unique nutritional status of patients, and to offer customized nutritional programs that address each patient's highly individualized needs. Included in the report is commentary by clinicians who have used metabolic typing technology very successfully.

For a free report, send an e-mail request to: YourPractice@ MetabolicTyping.com. You'll receive a document that can be downloaded to your computer.

"Metabolic Typing: A Scientific Overview"

This report contains information on the science and historical evolution of metabolic typing, including technical details of how it works and why it's so effective. Included is a discussion of the effects of nutrition on key regulatory control systems such as the autonomic nervous system and the cellular oxidative system. These control systems are akin to "executive command centers" that manage the millions of biochemical reactions which are continually taking place within the body. By keeping these "executive" systems in balance, metabolic typing can be used to "balance total body chemistry" and, in turn, address a wide range of physiological and psychological imbalances.

For a free report, send an e-mail request to: science@Metabolic Typing.com. You'll receive a document that can be downloaded to your computer.

Appendix F

Metabolic Typing Resources

www.MetabolicTyping.com

This is a key Web portal on customized nutrition for health consumers as well as health professionals. Here you'll find links to a wide range of metabolic typing information resources, products, and services.

www.CustomizeYourDiet.com

A great Web site for health consumers, bringing you a wealth of information, including news, features, success stories, and important tips to help you manage your diet and achieve a whole new level of health and fitness.

www.MetabolicTypingPro.com

A key Web site for health professionals interested in the rapidly emerging realm of customized nutrition. Important news and information related to current scientific developments and breakthroughs, educational opportunities, and clinical success stories.

Healthexcel

Healthexcel is the world's leading metabolic typing analytical laboratory. The company provides computer-based evaluations and technical support services to health professionals engaged in nutritional counseling and ecological lifestyle management. Healthexcel's innovative metabolic typing technology enables clinicians to assess the highly individualized nutritional status of patients, and to provide them with high precision, customized health protocols. For information, visit: www.healthexcel.com.

Metabolic Typing Education Center

The Metabolic Typing Education Center (MTEC) provides education, training, and metabolic typing evaluation services to health professionals and health consumers throughout the United States. MTEC offers a range of programs in the form of seminars, workshops, and educational counseling services. Educational programs are based on leading-edge developments in the field of customized nutrition. For information, call (650) 325-1840; or visit: www.Metabolic Ed.com.

Customized Nutrition Systems

Customized Nutrition Systems (CNS) is a business-to-business consulting organization that assists corporations, health care provider organizations, and clinical professionals with the implementation of customized dietary programs. Programs are based upon breakthrough developments in metabolic typing and related areas of lifestyle enhancement. CNS services are designed to optimize the business and financial opportunities of its clients. Services include business strategy, program management, and marketing communications. For information, call (212) 688-6853; or visit: www.Custom NutritionSystems.com.

Ultra Life

For over twenty-five years, Ultra Life has been the leading provider of customized nutritional formulations for clinicians and consumers who utilize advanced metabolic typing programs. Ultra Life's products are based on the scientific discoveries of Healthexcel, the world's leading metabolic typing testing and research center. These unique metabolic type formulations are highly regarded by consumers around the world for their exceptional level of quality and effectiveness. For product information, call (800) 323-3842; or visit: www.CustomizeYourDiet.com.

Metabolic Typing Resources Outside the U.S.

For information on metabolic typing services and resources in Canada, Europe, Asia, South America, Australia, and New Zealand, please visit: www.healthexcel.com.

Price-Pottenger Foundation

The Price-Pottenger Foundation is a nonprofit educational organization that was organized in 1965 for the purpose of preserving the archives and research of Weston Price, an American dentist widely regarded as the "Charles Darwin of Nutrition." The foundation publishes a quarterly journal and distributes books and tapes related to the prevention and reversal of degenerative disease resulting from modern dietary habits. For information, call (619) 574-7763; or visit: www.price-pottenger.org.

SELECTED REFERENCES

Chapter 1: One Man's Food Is Another's Poison

Abrams, Leon H., Jr. "Anthropological Research Reveals Human Dietary Requirements for Optimal Health." *Journal of Applied Nutrition* 34 (1) (1982).

Archives of the Price Pottenger Nutrition Foundation, Curator, Marion Patricia Connolly, P.O. Box 2614, La Mesa, CA 91943-2614, (619) 574-1314, 1-800-366-3748. Web site: www.price-pottenger.org.

Atkins, Robert. *Dr. Atkins' Super Energy Diet.* New York: Crown Publishers. 1976.

Barnard, Neal, M.D., *Food for Life: How the New Four-Food Groups Can Save Your Life.* Pittsburgh, PA: Three Rivers Press, 1993.

CBS Evening News. A 3-part series on long-lived cultures in remote regions of the world: Richard Threlkeld reporting from Azerbaijan, Barry Petersen reporting from Okinawa, Japan, Mark Philips reporting from Crete. May 11–13, 1998.

Cheraskin, E., M.D., et al. *Diet and Disease.* Emmaus, PA: Rodale Books, 1975.

Eaton, S. B., and M. Konner. "Paleolithic nutrition: A consideration of its nature and current implications." *New England Journal of Medicine*, 312:283–89, Jan. 31, 1983.

Eisenberg, D. M., et al. "Unconventional Medicine In the United States: Prevalence, Cost, and Patterns of Use." *New England Journal of Medicine* 328 (Jan, 1993): 246–252.

Fallon, Sally. *Ancient Wisdom for Tomorrow's Children.* La Mesa, CA: Price-Pottenger Foundation, 1985.

Fallon, Sally, Connolly, Pat and Enig, Mary, Ph.D. *Nourishing Traditions.* La Mesa, CA: Price Pottenger Foundation, 1995.

Gittleman, Ann Louise. *Your Body Knows Best.* New York: Pocket Books, 1996, 1997.

Griffin, Edward G. *World Without Cancer.* Westlake, CA: American Media, 1974.

Hall, Ross Hume. *Food for Thought: The Decline in Nutrition.* New York: Vintage Books, 1976.

Kushi, Michio. *Healing Through Macrobiotics.* Tokyo and New York: Japan Publications, 1978.

Martin, Katahn, Ph.D. *The T-Factor Diet.* New York: Bantam Books, 1994.

McCamy, James, M.D., and James Presley. *Human Life Styling: Keeping Whole in the 20th Century.* New York: Harper Colophon Books, 1975.

McDougall, John A. *The McDougall Program for Maximum Weight Loss.* New York: Plume, 1995.

Moore Lappe, Frances. *Diet for a Small Planet.* New York: Ballantine, 1971.

Null, Gary, et al. *Body Pollution.* New York: Arco, 1973.

Ornish, Dean. *Dr. Dean Ornish's Program for Reversing Heart Disease.* New York: Random House, 1990.

Pottenger, Francis M., Jr., M.D. *Fragmentation and Scarring of Bones.* La Mesa, CA: Price Pottenger Foundation, 1975.

Price, Weston. *Nutrition and Physical Degeneration: A Comparison of Primitive and Modern Diets and their Effects.* La Mesa, CA: Price Pottenger Foundation, 1945.

Pritikin, Nathan. *Live Longer Now.* New York: Bantam Books, 1974.

Robbins, John. *Diet for a New America.* Tiburon, CA: H. J. Kramer, 1998.

Schaefer, Otto. "When the Eskimo Comes to Town," *Nutrition Today*, November 10, 1971, 8–16.

Schmid, Ronald F., N.D. *Native Nutrition: Eating According to Ancestral Wisdom.* Rochester, VT: Healing Arts Press, 1987.

Sears, Barry. *The Zone.* New York: Regan Books, 1995.

Steward, H. Leighton, et al. *Sugar Busters: Cut Sugar to Trim Fat.* New York: Ballantine Books, 1998.

Chapter 2: A Brief History of Metabolic Typing

Bannister, R. *Autonomic Failure.* Oxford University Press, 1992.

Hockmann, C. *Essentials of Autonomic Function.* C. Thomas, 1987.

Kelley, William D. *One Answer to Cancer.* Kelley Foundation, 1969.

————. *The Metabolic Types.* Kelley Foundation, 1976.

Lee, Royal, DDS. *Protomorphology: The Principles of Cell Auto-Regulation.* Lee Foundation, 1947.

Low, P. *Clinical Autonomic Disorders.* Little, Brown and Co., 1993.

Pottenger, Francis M., M.D. *Symptoms of Visceral Disease.* C. V. Mosby Co., 1919.

Valentine, Tom and Carole. *Medicine's Missing Link: Metabolic Typing and Your Personal Food Plan.* Rochester, VT: Thorson's Publishers, 1987.

Watson, George, Ph.D. *Nutrition and Your Mind.* Harper and Row, 1972.

Wiley, Rudolph. *BioBalance.* Life Sciences Press, 1989.

Williams, Roger. *Biochemical Individuality.* New York: Wiley and Sons, 1956, New Canaan, Connecticut: Keats Publishing, 1998.

————. *Nutrition Against Disease.* Pitman Publishing, 1971.

————. *Nutrition In A Nutshell.* Doubleday, 1962.

————. *Physician's Handbook of Nutritional Science.* Thomas, 1977.

————. *Physician's Handbook of Orthomolecular Medicine.* New Canaan, Connecticut: Keats Publishing, 1979. For information on all Williams's books, see the Web site at http://www.cm.utexas.edu/williams

Wolcott, W. L. "A Theoretical Model for Clinical Application of the Relationship Between the Autonomic Nervous System and the Oxidation Rate in the Determination of Metabolic Types and the Requirements of Nutritional Individuality." *Metabolic Technology I.* International Health Institute, 1983.

————. *Therapeutic Food Manual.*

Chapter 3: Paradigm Shift

Armstrong, David, and Elizabeth Metzger Armstrong. *The Great American Medicine Show*. Prentice-Hall, 1991.

Harrower, Henry. *Practical Endocrinology*. Pioneer Printing Co., 1932.

Jennings, Isabel. *Vitamins in Endocrine Metabolism*. William Heinemann Medical Books, 1970.

Page, Melvin E. *Body Chemistry in Health and Disease*. Biochemcial Research Foundation, 1949.

―――. *Degeneration-Regeneration*. Biochemcial Research Foundation, 1949.

Page, Melvin E., and H. Leon Abrams, Jr. *Your Body Is Your Best Doctor*. New Canaan, CT: Keats Publishing, 1972.

Pizzorno, J.E., and Murray Susser, M.T., eds. *A Textbook of Natural Medicine*. Seattle, WA: John Bastyr College Publications, 1988–89.

Pottenger, Francis M., M.D., *Symptoms of Visceral Disease*. C. V. Mosby Co., 1919.

Radetsky, Peter. *Allergic to the Twentieth Century*. Little, Brown & Company, 1997.

Rea, William J. *Chemical Sensitivity*, 4 vols. Lewis Publishers, 1992–1996.

Rosenbaum, M., M.D., and M. Susser, M.D. *Solving the Puzzle of Chronic Fatigue Syndrome*. Tacoma, WA: Life Sciences Press, 1992.

Starr, Paul. *The Social Transformation of American Medicine*. Basic Books, 1982.

Strauss, S., M.D. "Chronic Fatigue Syndrome." U.S. Department of Health and Human Services, Public Health Service, NIH Publication no. 90-3059 (June 1990): 5.

Walker, Lynne Paige, and Ellen Hodgson Brown. *The Alternative Pharmacy*. Prentice-Hall, 1998.

Watson, George. *Nutrition and Your Mind*. Harper and Row, 1972.

Weil, Andrew, M.D. *Health and Healing*. Houghton Mifflin Company, 1988.

Wolcott, W. L. "The Death of Allopathic Nutrition." Winthrop, WA: Healthexcel Publications, 1998.

Chapter 4: A Revolution in Patient-Specific Nutrition

Hattersly, J. G. "Acquired Atherosclerosis: Theories of Causation, Novel Therapies." *Journal of Orthomolecular Medicine* 6:2 (1991), 83–98.

Hausman, Patricia. *The Right Dose*. New York: Ballantine, 1989.

Kowalski, Robert E., *The 8 Week Cholesterol Cure*. Harper & Row, 1987.

Lieberman, Shari, Ph.D. *The Real Vitamin and Mineral Book: Using Supplements for Optimum Health*. Garden City, NY: Avery, 1997.

Mindell, Earl. *Earl Mindell's Vitamin Bible*. Warner Books, 1991

Muller, R.O. *Autonomics in Chiropractic*. Chiro Publishing Co., 1954.

Pizzorno, Joseph, N.D. and Michael Murray, N.D. *The Encyclopedia of Natural Medicine*. CA: Prima, 1998.

Pizzorno, J. E., and M. T. Murray, eds. *Hypertension: A Textbook of Natural Medicine*. Seattle, WA: John Bastyr Publications, 1988.

Robbins, S. L., R. S. Cotran, and V. Kumar, eds. *Pathological Basis of Disease* (New York: W.B. Saunders, 1984).

Schenker, Guy. *An Analytical System of Clinical Nutrition*. Mifflintown, PA: Nutri-Spec, 1989.

Smith, R. L., "Dietary lipids and heart disease: The contriving of a relationship." *American Clinical Laboratory*, November 1989, 26–33.

Revici, Emanuel. *Research in Physiopathology as a Basis of Guided Chemotherapy*. New York, 1961.

Tenney, Lousie. *Today's Herbal Health*. Woodland Books, 1992.

Tolstoi, L. G., and Levin, R. M. "Osteoporosis—the Treatment Controversy," *Nutrition Today* (July/Aug 1992), 6–12.

Walker, Lynne Paige; and Ellen Hodgson Brown. *The Alternative Pharmacy*. Prentice-Hall, 1998.

Watson, George, Ph.D., *Nutrition and Your Mind*. Harper & Row, 1972.

Wilson, George. *The Second Factor in Chiropractic*. 1959.

Wolcott, W. L. "Core Premises: The Healthexcel System of Metabolic Typing." Winthrop, WA: Healthexcel Publications, 1986.

———. "The Death of Allopathic Nutrition." Winthrop, WA: Healthexcel Publications, 1998.

Chapter 5: The One and Only You

Abravanel, Elliot. *Body Type Diet*. Bantam, 1983.

Aihara, Herman. *Acid & Alkaline*. Macrobiotic Foundation, 1971.

Bieler, Henry. *Food Is Your Best Medicine*. Random House, 1966.

Cohen, Jordan J., and Jerome P. Kassirer. *Acid/Base*. Little, Brown and Co., 1982.

Foster, George M. *Hippocrates' Latin American Legacy: Humoral Medicine in the New World (Theory and Practice in Medical Anthropology and International Health, Vol. 1)*. Gordon and Breach Science Publications, 1994.

Frawley, David. *Ayurvedic Healing*. Passage Press, 1989.

———. *The Yoga of Herbs*. Lotus Press, 1986.

Hawkins, Harold. *Applied Nutrition*. Second Edition. International College of Applied Nutrition, La Habra, CA, 1977.

Hills, A. Gorman. *Acid-Base Balance*. Williams and Wilkins Co., 1973.

Kaptchuk, Ted. *The Web That Has No Weaver*. Congdon & Weed, 1983.

Lad, Vasant. *Ayurveda*. Lotus Press, 1985.

Lesser, Michael. *Nutrition and Vitamin Therapy*. Grove Press, Inc. 1980.

Lu, Henry. *Chinese System of Food Cures*. Sterling Publishing Co., 1986.

McMurray, W. C. *Essentials of Human Metabolism*. Harper & Row, 1977.

Revici, Emanuel. *Research in Physiopathology as a Basis of Guided Chemotherapy*. New York, 1961.

Sheldon, W. H. *The Varieties of Human Physique*. C. V. Mosby, 1944.

Shils, Maurice. *Modern Nutrition In Health And Disease*. Lea & Febiger, 1994.

Vithoulkas, George, and William A. Tiller. *The Science of Homeopathy*. Grove Press, 1980.

Watts, David. *Clinical Application of Tissue Mineral Analysis*. T.E.I., 1995.

Chapter 9: Fine-Tuning Your Diet

Ahlgren, Andrew, and Halbero, Franz. *Cycles of Nature: An Introduction to Biological Rhythms.* National Science Teachers Association, 1990.

Brand, Jennie, et al. *The Glucose Revolution: The Authoritative Guide to the Glycemic Index, the Groundbreaking Medical Discovery.* Marlowe & Co., 1999.

D'Adamo, James. *One Man's Food.* Richard Marek Publishers, 1980.

————. *The D'Adamo Diet.* McGraw-Hill, 1989.

D'Adamo, Peter. *Eat Right 4 Your Type.* G. P. Putnam's Sons, 1996.

Dries, Jan. *The Complete Book of Food Combining: A New Approach to Healthy Eating.* Element, 1998.

Doris Grant, Jean Joice, and John Mills. *Food Combining for Health: Get Fit with Foods That Don't Fight.* Inner Traditions Intl. Ltd., 1990.

Freed, David L. J., M.D. "Lectins in Food: Their Importance in Health and Disease." *Journal of Nutritional Medicine* (1991) 2, 45–64.

Orlock, Carol. *Inner Time: The Science of Body Clocks and What Makes Us Tick.* Birch Lane Press, 1993.

Podell, Richard N. and Proctor, William. *The G-Index Diet: The Missing Link That Makes Permanent Weight Loss Possible.* Warner Books, 1994.

Power, Laura, Ph.D. "Dietary Lectins: Food Allergies and Blood-Type Specificity," *The Townsend Letter for Doctors*, June 1991, 474–478.

Refinetti, Roberto. *Circadian Physiology.* CRC Pr., 1999.

Wolcott, W. L. "Core Premises: The Healthexcel System of Metabolic Typing." Winthrop, WA: Healthexcel Publications, 1986.

Chapter 10: Customized Weight Loss

Allred, J. B., "Too much of a good thing? An overemphasis on eating low-fat foods may be contributing to the alarming increase in overweight among us adults," *Journal of the American Dietetic Association*, April 1995; 95(4): 417–18.

Cappon, J. P., et al, "Acute effects of high fat and high glucose meals on the growth hormone response to exercise," *J Clin Endocrinol*, 1992; 76(6):1418–22.

Corpas, E., et al. "Human growth hormone and human aging," *Endocrin Rev*, 1993; 14(1):20–39.

Editorial Staff. "Alterations on Metabolic Rate after Weight Loss in Obese Humans," *Nutrition Reviews* 43, no. 2 (Feb. 1985): 41–42.

Farquhar, J. W., et al. "Glucose, insulin, and triglyceride responses to high and low carbohydrate diets in man," *J Clin Invest*, 1966; 45(10):1648–56.

Galbo, H. "Endocrinology and Metabolism in Exercise." *International Journal of Sports Medicine* 2 (1981):125–30.

Piatti, P. M., et al. "Hypocaloric high-protein diet improves glucose oxidation and spares lean body mass: Comparison to hypocaloric high-carbohydrate diet," *Metabolism*, December 1994; 43 (12):1481–87.

Porte, D., Jr., and Woods, S. C. "Regulation of Food Intake and Body Weight by Insulin." *Diabetologia* 20 suppl. (Mar. 1981): 274–280.

Sears, Barry. *The Zone*. Regan Books, 1995.

Van Dale, D., and Saris, W. H. "Repetitive Weight Loss and Weight Regain: Effects on Weight Reduction, Resting Metabolic Rate, and Lipolytic Activity Before and After Exercise and/or Diet Treatment." *American Journal of Clinical Nutrition* 49, no. 3 (Mar. 1989): 409–416.

Watson, George, Ph.D. *Nutrition and Your Mind*. Harper & Row, 1972.

Westphal, S. A., et al. "Metabolic response to glucose ingested with various amounts of protein," *American Journal of Clinical Nutrition*, 1990; 52:267–72.

Widmaier, Eric P., Ph.D. *Why Geese Don't Get Obese and We Do*, W. H. Freeman & Company, 1998.

Wiley, Rudolph. *BioBalance*. Life Sciences Press, 1989.

Williams, Roger. *Biochemical Individuality*. Wiley and Sons, 1956; Keats Publishing, New Canaan, Connecticut, May 1998.

Wolcott, W. L. "Core Premises: The Healthexcel System of Metabolic Typing." Winthrop, WA: Healthexcel Publications, 1986.

Chapter 11: Key Considerations Beyond Diet

Abramovitz, Janet N., and Peterson, Jane A. *Imperiled Waters, Impoverished Future: The Decline of Freshwater Ecosystems.* Worldwatch Institute, 1996.

Cone, James E., and Hodgson, Michael J. *Occupational Medicine: Problem Buildings: Building-Associated Illness and the Sick Building Syndrome.* Hanley and Belfus, 1989.

Coulter, H. L. *Divided Legacy: A History of the Schism in Medical Thought.* Vol 2. Washington, D.C.: Wehawken Book Co., 1973–1977.

Duesberg, Peter H. *Infectious AIDS: Have We Been Misled?* Berkeley, CA: North Atlantic Books, 1995.

———. *Inventing the AIDS Crisis.* Washington, D.C.: Regnery Publishing, Inc., 1996.

Fryman, V. M. "A Study of the Rhythmic Motions of the Living Cranium." *Journal of the American Osteopathic Association* 70 (May 1971): 928–945.

Golub, Edward S. *The Limits of Medicine: How Science Shapes Our Hope for the Cure.* New York: Random House, 1994.

Gutfeld, G. "The New Science of Rays and Rhythms, Cutting Edge Light Therapies That Can Brighten Your Health," *Prevention* 45 no. 2 (Feb. 1993):67–71; 116–123.

Hyman, J. W. *The Light Book.* New York: Ballantine Books, 1991.

Melillo, W. "How Safe is Mercury in Denistry?" *The Washington Post Weekly Journal* of *Medicine, Science and Society.* (Sept. 1991):4.

Price, Weston A., DDS. *Dental Infections* Volume 1: *Oral and Systemic.* Cleveland, OH: Benton Publishing, 1973.

Rhodes, Philip. *An Outline History of Medicine.* London: Butterworths, 1985.

Rogers, Sherry, M.D. *Wellness Against All Odds.* Prestige Publishers, 1994.

Root-Bernstein, Robert. *Rethinking AIDS.* New York: The Free Press, 1993.

Samuels, Mike, M.D., and Hal Zina Bennett. *Well Body, Well Earth: The Sierra Club Environmental Health Sourcebook.* San Francisco: Sierra Club Books, 1983.

Tate, Nicholas. *The Sick Building Syndrome: How Indoor Pollution Is Poisoning Your Life and What You Can Do.* New Horizon Press, 1994.

Upledger, J. E. *Your Inner Physician and You: Cranial Sacral Therapy.* Berkeley, CA: North Atlantic Books, 1992.

Weil, A., M.D. *Natural Health, Natural Medicine: A Comprehensive Guide to Wellness and Self-Care.* Boston, MA: Houghton Mifflin, 1990.

Wertheimer, N., and Leeper, E. "Electrical Wiring Configurations and Childhood Cancer." *American Journal of Epidemiology* 109 (1979):273-284.

"Winter Blues? Try a Little Morning Light." *Bioenergy Health Newsletter* (Dec. 1987): 7.

World Health Organization. *Environmental Health Criteria for Inorganic Mercury* 118. Geneva: World Health Organization, 1991.

Ziff, S. "Consolidated Symptom Analysis of 1569 Patents." *Bio-Probe Newsletter* 9, no. 2 (Mar. 1993): 7–8.

Chapter 12: Indispensable Tips for Savvy Consumers

Anderson, Mark, and Jensen, Bernard. *Empty Harvest: Understanding the Link Between Our Food, Our Immunity And Our Planet*, Avery Publishing Group, 1993.

Douglass, William Campbell, M.D. *The Milk Book: How Science Is Destroying Nature's Nearly Perfect Food.* La Mesa, CA: Price-Pottenger Foundation, 1983.

"EU Scientific Committee Warns of Human Health & Cancer Hazards of Monsanto's recombinant Bovine Growth Hormone (rBGH)." *Scientific Committee of European Union on Veterinary Measures relating to Public Health Outcome.* March 15–16, 1999.

"Frankenstein Foods?" *Newsweek,* Sept. 13, 1999.

Gibbs, Gary, Dr. *The Food That Would Last Forever.* Avery Publishing Group, 1993.

Howell, Edward. *Enzyme Nutrition.* Wayne, NJ: Avery Publishing Group, 1985.

Jacobs, Paul. "Biotech in the USA Under Attack from All Sides." *Los Angeles Times,* October 7, 1999.

Kilman, Scott. "Wall Street Predicts a Major Upheaval Over Genetically Engineered Foods in the USA." *Wall Street Journal*, October 7, 1999.

Krebs, Al. "What's that glowing in the kitchen?" *Agribusiness Examiner* #26 (March 22, 1999). On-line newsletter. avkrebs@earthlink.net

Levy, Stuart B. *The Antibiotic Paradox: How Miracle Drugs Are Destroying the Miracle*. Plenum, 1992.

"Monsanto's Genetically Modified Milk Ruled Unsafe by the United Nations." *PR Newswire,* Aug. 18, 1999.

"Playing God in the Garden: New York Times Magazine on Genetically Engineered Crops." *The New York Times Sunday Magazine*, Oct. 25, 1998.

Pottenger, Francis M., Jr., M.D. *Pottenger's Cats*. La Mesa, CA: Price Pottenger Foundation, 1983.

Repetto, Robert, and Sanjay S. Baliga. *Pesticides and the Immune System: The Public Health Risks*. World Resources Inst., 1996.

"U.S. Factory Farm Antibiotic Use Threatens Public Health." *US News & World Report*, May 31, 1999.

Webb, Tony, Tim Langan, and Kathleen Tucker. *Food Irradiation: Who Wants It?* Rochester, VT: Thorson Publishers, 1987.

INDEX

Note: Page numbers in *italics* indicate charts or graphics.